TREATING TRAUMA
IN DIALECTICAL BEHAVIOR THERAPY

TREATING TRAUMA IN DIALECTICAL BEHAVIOR THERAPY

The DBT Prolonged Exposure Protocol (DBT PE)

Melanie S. Harned

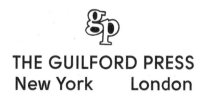

THE GUILFORD PRESS
New York   London

The author has checked with sources believed to be reliable in her efforts to provide information
that is complete and generally in accord with the standards of practice that are accepted at the
time of publication. However, in view of the possibility of human error or changes in behavioral,
mental health, or medical sciences, neither the author, nor the editors and publisher, nor any
other party who has been involved in the preparation or publication of this work warrants that the
information contained herein is in every respect accurate or complete, and they are not responsible
for any errors or omissions or the results obtained from the use of such information. Readers are
encouraged to confirm the information contained in this book with other sources.

Library of Congress Cataloging-in-Publication Data

Names: Harned, Melanie S., author.
Title: Treating trauma in dialectical behavior therapy : the DBT prolonged
    exposure protocol (DBT PE) / Melanie S. Harned.
Description: New York : The Guilford Press, [2022] | Includes
    bibliographical references and index.
Identifiers: LCCN 2021031113 | ISBN 9781462549122 (paperback) |
    ISBN 9781462549139 (cloth)
Subjects: LCSH: Post-traumatic stress disorder—Treatment. | Dialectical
    behavior therapy.
Classification: LCC RC552.P67 H373 2022 | DDC 616.85/21—dc23
LC record available at *https://lccn.loc.gov/2021031113*

To my children

May you be happy, fulfilled, and free from suffering

About the Author

Melanie S. Harned, PhD, ABPP, is Coordinator of the DBT Program at the VA Puget Sound Health Care System and Associate Professor in the Department of Psychiatry and Behavioral Science and Adjunct Associate Professor in the Department of Psychology at the University of Washington. She previously served as Research Director of the Behavioral Research and Therapy Clinics at the University of Washington, Director of Research and Development for Behavioral Tech, and Director of Behavioral Tech Research. Dr. Harned's research focuses on the development and evaluation of the DBT Prolonged Exposure protocol (DBT PE), as well as methods of disseminating and implementing this and other evidence-based treatments in clinical practice. She regularly provides training and consultation nationally and internationally in DBT and DBT PE, and has published numerous articles and book chapters.

Acknowledgments

Development of the DBT Prolonged Exposure protocol would not have been possible without the groundbreaking work of Marsha Linehan and Edna Foa who have spent their careers developing and disseminating the two highly effective treatments on which DBT PE is based. I am truly privileged to be able to stand on the shoulders of such giants and to have had their support as I worked to create DBT PE. I am also particularly indebted to my original DBT PE treatment development team—Katie Korslund, Annie McCall, Bob Goettle, and Julia Hitch—for agreeing to enter this uncharted territory with me before I really had any idea what I was doing. It is an unusual breed of therapist who says "yes" to treating posttraumatic stress disorder in highly suicidal clients when there is no evidence base to support this. I am also grateful to the many other therapists and consultants who have worked with me on my research over the years and helped to develop DBT PE's evidence base: Sara Schmidt, Samantha Yard, Trevor Schraufnagel, Dan Finnegan, Andrea Neal, Elizabeth Hembree, Tony DuBose, and the teams at Project Transition, COMHAR, Carson Valley Children's Aid, and Community Treatment Teams. Perhaps most importantly, I want to thank the clients who participated in this research, as well as those I have had the good fortune to work with in other contexts. Your courage and resilience inspire me to do this work, and the lessons you have taught me have helped to make this treatment better and more available to other people who need it.

The Behavioral Research and Therapy Clinics at the University of Washington was my professional home in the years that I was developing and starting to research DBT PE, and I am grateful to the many colleagues, students, and postdoctoral fellows who enriched my thinking and my life while I was there. Katie Korslund was especially helpful in keeping me going over those years with her combination of validation, wisdom, and quirky humor. To my current colleagues at the Seattle VA, thank you for welcoming me so warmly and for providing me with such a validating environment in which to move DBT PE forward.

Many expert trainers have helped me to disseminate DBT PE to therapists around the world and I greatly appreciate their contributions to this mission (and to making me a better teacher). Thanks are also due to the courageous therapists who have attended these trainings and are using DBT PE with some of the most challenging clients in the world. Without them, my work to develop DBT PE would be pointless.

Writing this book has been quite an undertaking that I sometimes thought would never end. I want to thank Kitty Moore at The Guilford Press for believing in me and for being such a steady guide and comforting presence throughout the process. Annie McCall read every word of this book more than once and her thoughts are reflected in many of them. She made sure the human element of this treatment didn't get lost in translation, allowed me to steal all her metaphors, and helped me to find my wise mind more times than I can count. I am especially grateful that she pushed me to become my own voice while writing this book even (and especially) when I was scared to do this. Lorie Ritschel also volunteered her time to read this entire book and it is undoubtedly better as a result. She helped me sharpen my thinking and tighten up my writing and provided support in numerous other ways (even when it required her to do exposure). I am also appreciative of the many other people who read portions of this book and gave valuable feedback: Sara Schmidt, Jill Rathus, Emily Cooney, Samantha Yard, Laura Meyers, Katie Smith, Vibh Forsythe Cox, Trevor Coyle, Natalia Garcia, Charlotte Brill, Colleen Sloan, David Pantalone, and Aaron Brinen.

Finally, thank you to my family and friends for supporting me through the many years I have been doing this work and the many challenges I encountered along the way. I could not have done it without you.

Author's Note

All of the case material in this book is fictional, disguised, or a composite of many cases. I have made every effort to use gender-neutral pronouns (*they/their/them*) throughout the book. The exceptions are examples that refer to specific individuals.

Contents

PART IV. **Troubleshooting and Tailoring Treatment**

PART V. **Next Steps**

PART I

BACKGROUND

CHAPTER 1

The Development
and Foundations of DBT PE

A history of trauma is the norm rather than the exception among individuals receiving dialectical behavior therapy (DBT). Many clients in DBT have experienced multiple traumas that often started in childhood, occurred repeatedly over a prolonged period of time, and were perpetrated by caregivers and other important people in their lives. Posttraumatic stress disorder (PTSD) is a common outcome of these traumatic experiences that causes tremendous suffering and often contributes to the primary problems targeted in DBT. People with PTSD are haunted by intrusive trauma memories, experience intense distress when reminded of their trauma, and feel as if they are constantly under threat. To cope with PTSD, clients in DBT often engage in high-risk and self-destructive behaviors—like suicide attempts, self-injury, substance use, and binge eating—that provide short-term relief but lead to long-term suffering. Over time, clients' lives typically become very restricted and disconnected due to efforts to avoid people and situations that elicit trauma-related distress and prompt dysregulated behavior. This difficulty functioning in daily life often strengthens the messages they internalized from past trauma—that they are bad, unlovable, and worthless people—and contributes to pervasive shame and self-hatred. Trapped in a life of trauma-related suffering that they feel unable to either change or tolerate, many clients come to view suicide as the only solution. As one of my clients aptly remarked, "It's all in the trauma."

Given the pervasiveness of trauma among individuals receiving DBT, it is critical that DBT therapists have the ability to effectively treat PTSD. Indeed, many DBT clients will not be able to fully reach their life-worth-living goals until PTSD has been resolved. The treatment described in this book is designed to provide a structured method of integrating PTSD treatment into DBT for the many clients who need such treatment. The treatment combines an adapted version of prolonged exposure (PE) therapy for PTSD (Foa, Hembree, Rothbaum, & Rauch, 2019), called the DBT Prolonged Exposure protocol (DBT PE), with standard DBT (Linehan, 1993, 2015). In this chapter, I begin by providing an overview of the treatment, including the history of its development, as well as its theoretical and empirical foundations.

The Origins of DBT PE

My primary goal in developing the DBT PE protocol was to make effective PTSD treatment available to high-risk, complex, and severely impaired clients who are typically unable to access these treatments. I first became aware of this treatment gap as a psychology intern at McLean Hospital in Belmont, Massachusetts, where I worked in a partial hospital program that provided intensive treatment for adults. In this setting, I encountered clients for the first time who were actively suicidal and self-injuring and had multiple severe conditions, such as mood, anxiety, personality, eating, and substance use disorders. Given my research background in interpersonal trauma, I was highly attuned to the presence and impact of trauma in many of these clients' lives, and PTSD often appeared to contribute greatly to their suffering. Armed with a healthy dose of naiveté and a limited therapeutic skill set, early in my training year I suggested to one of my supervisors that perhaps I could use the exposure procedures I had learned in graduate school to treat PTSD with one of my clients. While I don't remember my supervisor's exact response, the message was clear: No way! I was advised that these types of clients were too high risk and unstable for trauma-focused treatments. Instead, a skills-based treatment was needed to help them achieve safety and stability and learn to cope effectively with current life stressors. In this context, I was first exposed to DBT as a way to help clients achieve these important goals.

I then immersed myself in learning DBT and sought out a postdoctoral fellowship at Two Brattle Center in Cambridge, Massachusetts, that specialized in providing DBT in intensive outpatient programs. As I became more adept at delivering DBT, I was thrilled to see that many of my clients were clearly benefiting. Clients who began DBT with severe and often life-threatening behavioral dysregulation were able to gain control over these behaviors by using DBT skills to better tolerate and regulate the painful emotions that typically prompted them. I was convinced—these skills were truly lifesaving! At the same time, for some clients, achieving behavioral control was not enough to enable them to reach their life-worth-living goals. Although they were no longer trying to kill or harm themselves and generally had reasonable control over their behavior, they remained in a state of extreme emotional pain that was often driven by past unresolved traumas.

After searching the DBT manual for an answer, I became convinced that DBT's second stage of treatment, which was supposed to focus on targeting posttraumatic stress, was what was needed for these clients. I again approached my supervisors to ask about moving on to Stage 2 with some of my clients so that we could treat their PTSD. The answer this time: Not yet. It soon became clear that nobody was quite sure what this elusive Stage 2 was or when exactly it was supposed to occur. The DBT manual provided little guidance about how and when to approach the treatment of PTSD in Stage 2, while also clearly warning therapists about the potential of causing serious harm to their clients if they focused on trauma too soon. Given this, it was completely understandable that I was advised to remain focused on helping clients solve current life problems and to avoid trauma-focused treatment. At the same time, this felt both unsatisfying and insufficient.

I decided to go directly to the source to try to find a solution to this problem. In 2004, I began a postdoctoral fellowship with Marsha Linehan, the developer of DBT, at the University of Washington in Seattle. In my first meeting with her, she asked about my goals for my fellowship and I told her rather boldly that I wanted to help figure out how to do Stage 2 of DBT. I shared my prior clinical experiences with her and said that it seemed as if PTSD was often not treated during DBT because therapists, myself included, were unsure of when and how to do this. Marsha agreed that Stage 2 was not as well developed as Stage 1 of DBT, but was unconvinced that therapists were not already treating PTSD when it was needed. Always a scientist at heart, she told me that first I would have to prove to her that something more was needed and invited me to analyze data from her clinical trials of DBT to see what I could discover. I eagerly agreed to this plan and set off to evaluate my clinically driven hypothesis.

Several months later I returned with results showing that PTSD was both highly prevalent and unlikely to remit during DBT. Specifically, in a recent randomized controlled trial (RCT) with suicidal and self-injuring women with borderline personality disorder (BPD), 50% met criteria for PTSD at the beginning of treatment, and of these, 87% still had PTSD after 1 year of DBT (Harned et al., 2008). This 13% remission rate was considerably lower than what was typically found in active PTSD treatments in which about half of clients who start treatment and two-thirds of those who complete treatment achieve remission from PTSD (Bradley, Greene, Russ, Dutra, & Westen, 2005). In a second set of analyses, I also learned that by the end of 1 year of DBT a majority of the clients with PTSD had successfully eliminated behaviors, such as suicidal and nonsuicidal self-injury, that are commonly used as exclusion criteria for PTSD treatments (Harned, Jackson, Comtois, & Linehan, 2010). Marsha and I agreed that the data were clear: DBT was effective in stabilizing clients so that they would be suitable candidates for PTSD treatment, but needed to be better at treating PTSD itself. Marsha encouraged me to take on this project and, just as she had done when developing DBT, suggested that I start by trying to treat PTSD with some of my own clients. Thus, with equal parts fear and determination, I began my journey to develop what is now known as the DBT PE protocol or "DBT PE" for short.

The Foundations of DBT PE

Fortunately for me, I had an incredibly strong base of existing treatments from which to start. DBT is an evidence-based, principle-driven treatment that was originally developed to treat chronically suicidal individuals with complex clinical presentations and has become best known as a treatment for BPD. In its standard format, DBT is delivered across four treatment modes. DBT individual therapy focuses on helping clients to reduce, in hierarchical order, life-threatening behaviors (e.g., suicidal and nonsuicidal self-injury), therapy-interfering behaviors (e.g., nonattendance, noncompliance, noncollaboration), and serious quality-of-life-interfering behaviors (e.g., severe mental disorders, relationship problems, functional impairment), while increasing their use of behavioral skills. These skills are taught in DBT group skills training and include mindfulness, emotion regulation, distress tolerance, and interpersonal effectiveness. Brief telephone contact between sessions is used for problem solving and in-the-moment skills coaching. Finally, therapists attend a structured weekly consultation team meeting to assist one another in the implementation of the treatment.

Given the multiproblem nature of the client population, DBT is intended to be a comprehensive treatment that can address the full spectrum of problems that clients have. To that end, DBT has a variety of protocols that are used on an as-needed basis to flexibly target many different problems. However, DBT did not have a formal protocol for treating PTSD, and this, Marsha and I believed, was what was needed. Although other treatments were being developed that blended elements of DBT with trauma-focused treatments (Bohus et al., 2013; Cloitre, Koenen, Cohen, & Han, 2002), these treatments differed considerably from standard DBT. In contrast, my goal was not to change DBT, but rather to develop a new protocol that could be added to it for those clients who needed PTSD treatment. As she had written in the DBT manual, Marsha recommended the use of formal exposure procedures to treat PTSD and suggested that this could be done by either inserting or concurrently delivering a well-developed exposure-based PTSD treatment into DBT. My first task, therefore, was to identify an existing PTSD treatment on which to base this new protocol. After only a short deliberation, I selected PE (Foa et al., 2019).

PE was originally developed for women with sexual assault–related PTSD and is now used in a wide variety of trauma populations. PE is a structured protocol that is typically delivered in 9–15 weekly or biweekly 90-minute individual therapy sessions and includes three primary components: *in vivo* exposure to avoided but safe situations, imaginal exposure to trauma memories, and processing of the emotions and beliefs elicited by imaginal exposure. My primary reason for selecting PE was that it was the most well-studied manualized, exposure-based PTSD treatment available and had been shown to be highly effective in treating PTSD in multiple RCTs at the time (e.g., Foa, Dancu, et al., 1999; Foa, Rothbaum, Riggs, & Murdock, 1991). In addition, there was preliminary evidence suggesting that PE was effective in reducing PTSD in clients with borderline personality characteristics (Feeny, Zoellner, & Foa, 2002), which gave me hope that it would also work for clients with more severe BPD. Although I had some concerns about our clients' ability to tolerate PE, I was reassured by several studies that had shown that PE was unlikely to result in symptom exacerbation or treatment dropout (Foa, Zoellner, Feeny, Hembree, & Alvarez-Conrad, 2002; Hembree et al., 2003). Another notable benefit of PE was that it had recently been found to be readily transportable to therapists in community practice settings who were able to achieve outcomes comparable to PE experts (Foa et al., 2005). For these reasons, I believed that PE would make the ideal foundation of DBT's protocol for treating PTSD.

Theoretical Influences

While developing the DBT PE protocol, I was completely immersed in the theory and practice of DBT. As described in detail elsewhere (e.g., Linehan, 1993; Swenson, 2016), DBT is rooted in the theories of cognitive-behavioral therapy (CBT), incorporates acceptance strategies derived from Zen, and balances these two opposing approaches with dialectical theory. The three paradigms of DBT—change, acceptance, and dialectics—were my theoretical home base and influenced all aspects of my thinking about how to treat PTSD among high-risk, complex, and emotionally dysregulated clients. From CBT, I believed that effective treatment would require precision, technical skill, and a scientific approach to generating, testing, and evaluating theory-driven hypotheses about the factors maintaining PTSD. I also viewed the principles of acceptance as critical to reducing trauma-related suffering, including mindful awareness, radical acceptance of reality as it is, and compassion toward oneself and others. Consistent with a dialectical worldview, I believed in the importance of helping clients to let go of extreme trauma-related emotions, beliefs, and behaviors by actively searching for what was being left out, working to find a synthesis between opposing sides, and embracing change. As in DBT, I expected that therapists would need to skillfully and flexibly shift back and forth between change, acceptance, and dialectical strategies while treating PTSD to help clients keep moving toward their goal of a life without trauma-related suffering.

In addition to the three-paradigm framework of DBT, I was particularly influenced by the biosocial theory of the development of BPD that Marsha first articulated in the DBT manual (Linehan, 1993). According to this theory, BPD is primarily a disorder of pervasive emotion dysregulation that develops as a result of transactions between biological emotional vulnerability (increased emotional sensitivity and reactivity combined with a slow return to emotional baseline) and an invalidating environment. An invalidating environment is one that chronically and pervasively communicates to the individual that they are bad, wrong, and unacceptable, and, at its most extreme, may include abuse and trauma. This type of environment is a particularly poor fit for an emotionally sensitive child as it is likely to regularly prompt painful emotions and then respond to these emotions by minimizing, judging, and/or punishing their expression. In addition, the child is typically expected to maintain constant control over their emotions but is not taught how to do so effectively. As a result, the individual does not learn how to understand, regulate, or tolerate their emotional responses and instead learns to invalidate and inhibit them. To achieve this, they often rely on maladaptive strategies, such as self-injury, substance use, and dissociation, that provide short-term emotional relief but worsen emotion dysregulation in the long run by contributing to a pattern of oscillating between emotional inhibition and extreme emotional states. Other common consequences of the invalidating environment include learning to set unrealistic standards for one's behavior, distrust one's perceptions of reality, hold extremely negative views about oneself, and expect rejection from others.

The biosocial theory provided a unifying framework for understanding the many trauma-related problems I was observing in my clients as either having an emotion regulation function or as being the natural consequence of pervasive emotion dysregulation. In the case of clients with PTSD, the core problem that seemed to be fueling their suffering was extreme emotional avoidance. My clients were terrified to experience their emotions because they were sure, based on their history, that doing so would result in the loss of behavioral control, intolerable pain, and rejection by others. Indeed, the experience of emotion was so excruciating that they were willing to do just about anything to avoid it—even if it increased their misery, including PTSD, in the long run. Based on this conceptualization, I believed that successful treatment would therefore need to address this core deficit by building clients' capacity to experience and tolerate their emotions so that PTSD and many other problems that were being driven by emotional avoidance would improve.

The biosocial theory also made me aware of the profound effects of pervasive invalidation on my clients' lives, including their experiences of and responses to trauma. Nearly every client I treated blamed themselves for the traumas they had experienced, judged their reactions during and after these events, and believed these experiences meant they were bad and unacceptable people. These self-invalidating beliefs could almost always be traced back to the negative messages they had absorbed from the invalidating environments in which they had lived. Although the biosocial theory focuses primarily on invalidation in the family of origin, it became clear to me that many clients had experienced severe invalidation from other important people (e.g., intimate partners), groups (e.g., peers in school), institutions (e.g., the mental health system), and the broader culture (e.g., due to systemic sexism, racism, and heterosexism). Accordingly, I thought that successful treatment of PTSD would need to help clients contextualize their traumatic experiences within both the micro- and macro-level invalidating environments in which they had occurred and replace the negative messages they had internalized from these environments with self-validation and compassion.

Although I was a DBT therapist at my core, I was also heavily influenced by the theories underlying PE that explain why PTSD develops, how it is maintained over time, and what needs to be done to change it. PE is based on emotional processing theory (EPT; Foa & Kozak, 1986), which proposes that PTSD develops when pathological fear structures form after trauma. Fear structures include stimuli that elicit physiological and behavioral responses, as well as thoughts about the meaning of the stimulus and response. These fear structures become pathological when someone who has experienced a trauma (e.g., sexual abuse) encounters a stimulus that is objectively safe (e.g., a memory of the abuse or a person who resembles the perpetrator); responds with intense distress (e.g., racing heart, sweating, urges to run away); and assumes negative meaning about themselves, others, or the world (e.g., "I am incompetent" or "People are likely to harm me"). Pathological fear structures are maintained by avoidance of trauma-related stimuli, which provides short-term relief from distress but maintains PTSD in the long run by preventing inaccurate meanings from being disconfirmed. PE works to modify these fear structures through exposure to feared but safe trauma-related stimuli (e.g., talking to a person resembling the perpetrator or thinking about the abuse) so that the person can learn that their beliefs about the stimuli and their responses to it are inaccurate (e.g., they do not get attacked or become unable to function). With repeated exposure to feared stimuli in the absence of negative consequences, fear will eventually decrease through a process of extinction (commonly referred to as "habituation") and PTSD will improve.

While EPT provides a compelling and science-based conceptualization of problematic fear and how to change it, fear was not the primary trauma-related emotion many of my clients were experiencing. Instead, they were plagued by intense levels of shame, guilt, and disgust at themselves that stemmed from the invalidating environments in which they had lived and the extreme negative self-construct they had developed as a result. I felt sure that these negative self-directed emotions would also need to be directly targeted during PTSD treatment and that exposure alone may not be sufficient to do so. To that end, I relied on DBT's model of emotions and its full-system approach to emotion regulation to identify additional strategies that could be used to change emotions when needed.

Another point of divergence was PE's emphasis on the role of problematic trauma-related beliefs as the primary factor that fuels the avoidance that maintains PTSD. This conflicted with DBT's emotion-focused approach that formulates problems as related to emotions, including deficits in emotion regulation skills, intense emotions that interfere with skillful responses, and/or inhibited emotional experiencing. Indeed, it is considered anti-DBT to formulate problems solely in terms of cognition. Given this, I believed it was important to emphasize the role of intense trauma-related emotions and efforts to avoid them as core problems that also maintain PTSD over time. I soon came to realize that *in vivo* and imaginal exposure provided a powerful method not only of treating PTSD but also of teaching clients how to experience and tolerate intense emotions without engaging in maladaptive escape behaviors. To that end, I incorporated ideas from inhibitory learning theory (Craske et al., 2008), such as emphasizing emotional tolerance rather than habituation during exposure and viewing exposure as an opportunity to violate clients' expectancies (e.g., about the negative outcomes of experiencing and expressing emotions).

In sum, I believed we needed to help clients develop the capacity for normative emotional experiencing in the process of using exposure to treat their PTSD while also correcting the damaging messages of invalidating environments, all of which I viewed as necessary to enable clients to achieve freedom from trauma-related suffering.

The Development of DBT PE

When I first began to develop the DBT PE protocol, I was bolstered by the theory and research supporting both DBT and PE as independent treatments, as well as a strong sense of conviction that PTSD was an important problem that needed to be solved for many of our DBT clients. What I did not have were any data or experience to draw upon about exactly how to treat PTSD in this particular client population. As far as I knew, other than a few clients Marsha had treated earlier in her career, nobody had tried to treat PTSD—let alone with exposure!—with the types of high-risk and complex clients I was trying to reach. Given this, I proceeded with an abundance of caution due to concern that one misstep might literally result in the death of a client.

The first client I decided to try this with was a woman who had been brutally gang raped by a boyfriend and his friends 5 years before she began treatment with me. Prior to this trauma, she had also experienced intimate partner violence in two relationships, as well as physical and verbal abuse by her mother since early childhood. She had a long history of nonsuicidal self-injury (NSSI) beginning in adolescence; two prior suicide attempts, including one that occurred several months before treatment; and chronic problems with binge eating and impulsive spending. She met criteria for PTSD, BPD, and bipolar II disorder. The first stage of DBT primarily focused on helping her to obtain control over her self-injurious behaviors. She cut herself three times in the first 2 months of treatment and had one serious suicide attempt via overdose in the fourth month of DBT. Chain analyses reliably indicated that these behaviors were related to trauma-related problems, including intense guilt and shame, thoughts that she was "bad," and exposure to trauma reminders. Her PTSD was also negatively impacting her quality of life as evidenced by frequent nightmares and flashbacks, chronic irritability with her children and boyfriend, avoidance of many anxiety-provoking situations (e.g., leaving the house alone), and excessive time spent engaging in safety behaviors (e.g., checking the locks on her doors). Based on her learning of DBT skills and abstinence from suicidal and self-injurious behavior, at the end of her sixth month of DBT we agreed that she was ready to begin PTSD treatment.

Before I began PE with this client, I had already decided to make several changes to its standard format. In the preexposure sessions (Sessions 1 and 2), I thought it would be important to use DBT strategies to obtain, strengthen, and troubleshoot commitments to actively participate in completing exposure and to not engage in suicidal or self-injurious behaviors during the treatment. I also wanted clients to create a DBT skills plan that they could use during and between sessions to manage urges to self-injure or kill themselves that may arise. Due to my worry about clients' ability to tolerate trauma-focused exposure, I made several modifications designed to create a more titrated approach to exposure, including having clients complete their first *in vivo* exposure with the therapist rather than on their own, and then conducting several weeks of in-session *in vivo* exposure before starting imaginal exposure. To monitor risk and increase the focus on emotions and acceptance, I also created the Exposure Recording Form for clients to complete before and after every exposure task that tracked their urges to kill and harm themselves, obtained ratings of specific emotions (e.g., fear, shame, guilt, sadness, anger) in addition to the usual Subjective Units of Distress Scale (SUDS) rating, and assessed the degree to which they radically accepted that the trauma had occurred.

With these initial modifications in place, I began to deliver PE with my client in weekly sessions that occurred concurrently with her ongoing weekly DBT individual and group therapy. Although she regularly reported increases in urges to self-injure and, to a lesser extent, kill herself after exposure tasks, she did not engage in either behavior during PE. Since her PTSD was primarily related to the gang rape she had experienced, we used *in vivo* exposure to target situations related to this event, as well as imaginal exposure to the trauma memory itself. After 11 sessions, she reported that no trauma-related stimuli elicited a SUDS rating greater than a 5 (out of 100) and she no longer met criteria for PTSD. I remember beaming with happiness and pride as I shared these results with Marsha and my DBT team. At this point, another postdoctoral fellow, Lizz Dexter-Mazza, agreed to try out this new protocol with one of her clients, a woman with chronic rape-related PTSD, BPD, and alcohol dependence who had presented to DBT with a pattern of regular NSSI; more than 40 suicide attempts in the past 2 years; and repeated psychiatric hospitalizations. When Lizz succeeded in obtaining comparably positive results with her client, I began to think we might be on to something. The results of these first two case studies were eventually published (Harned & Linehan, 2008), and I began to try to obtain a grant to formally develop and test this fledgling protocol. Little did I realize what a struggle this would be.

In 2005, I submitted my first grant to the National Institute of Mental Health (NIMH). It did not even receive a score. On the positive side, reviewers described my proposal to develop Stage 2 of DBT as "being as innovative as a proposal can be, with tremendous potential benefit to the field." Nonetheless, they viewed my plans as "overly ambitious" and questioned whether "a recently minted PhD with minimal experience with this population is the right person to develop what will surely be one of the most important treatments to be developed over the next decade." One reviewer flat-out said, "It does not seem appropriate to delegate this to someone who is relatively new to the BPD and DBT field." I might have quit then if it were not for Marsha who, having weathered more than her fair share of criticism in the process of developing DBT, stood firmly by my side and told me I had to keep trying. I then began what felt like an unending process of revising and resubmitting this grant, each time attempting to address the critiques that were raised by modifying the research design, collecting more pilot data, and refining the proposed treatment approach. Along the way, I was also fortunate to have Edna Foa, the developer of PE, agree to join the research team as a consultant. By the sixth submission, the main critique I was up against was that some reviewers believed that adding PE to DBT "might make some patients worse." I gathered as much data as I could to support my stance that worsening was unlikely to occur, while also acknowledging that this remained a largely unanswered empirical question; indeed, this was why this research needed to be done. If not now, then when? If not this team of researchers, which included the developers of both DBT and PE, then who? This argument finally worked and, 4.5 years and two children later, I received my first grant.

In 2009, I began this 4-year treatment development grant by assembling a team of DBT therapists who agreed to work on this project with me, including Katie Korslund, Annie McCall, Bob Goettle, and Julia Hitch. Those of us who would be delivering individual therapy then set off to attend a 4-day intensive workshop in PE led by Edna Foa and her colleagues at the University of Pennsylvania in Philadelphia. It was both an eye-opening and sobering experience for us as the reality of what we were about to do set in: Nobody before us had tried to use PE with the kinds of high-risk and complex clients we were planning to treat. While we were there, I met with Edna to discuss the proposed treatment protocol in more detail, including describing the modifications to PE that I had made with our early pilot cases. She agreed with most of the changes I had made but expressed concern about the cautious approach I had taken to exposure. Instead, Edna encouraged me to adhere to PE's standard format without titrating it, including asking clients to begin *in vivo* exposure on their own following Session 2 and starting immediately with imaginal exposure in Session 3. Despite my urge to fragilize our clients, I agreed to try this. (Not surprisingly, Edna was right: Our clients were able to tolerate this less titrated approach.) We then returned to our clinic at the University of Washington and began the first phase of the project involving an open trial with 13 suicidal and self-injuring women with BPD and PTSD who came to call themselves—with good humor—"the guinea pigs."

I am forever grateful to my team of therapists as well as the clients who agreed to participate in this first study for trusting that we would figure out how to do this even if I was not yet entirely clear on the specifics. Our weekly DBT consultation team meetings became focused on identifying problems, generating solutions, trying out new strategies, and constantly refining what we were doing with precision and rigor. Just as important, we kept one another motivated and willing to "plunge in where angels fear to tread" even when we were terrified that it might all blow up in our faces (and when it sometimes did). Our clients taught us how to be better at what we were doing, suggested changes we could make, and inspired us to keep going with their courage and commitment. I met with Marsha and Edna regularly to discuss our progress, obtain their feedback, and learn from their enormous clinical wisdom. Our team also benefited greatly from the consultation provided by PE experts in Edna's clinic who watched many of our sessions and helped us to hone our skills and gain clarity about the similarities and differences between our DBT-infused approach and standard PE.

With the support of this impressive team, by the end of the open trial I had developed the key elements of the integrated DBT and DBT PE protocol treatment that are described in this book. In this process, I tried to stick as closely as possible to standard PE and make adaptations only when I believed it was necessary to either better address the needs of our clients or increase compatibility with DBT. We were also thrilled to discover that this new synthesis of DBT and PE seemed to be working: By the end of treatment, 60% of the clients who had started treatment and 71% of those who completed it had remitted from PTSD and nobody got worse (Harned, Korslund, Foa, & Linehan, 2012).

I then proceeded to the second phase of the project: an RCT that compared DBT with and without the DBT PE protocol in a sample of 26 suicidal and self-injuring women with BPD and PTSD. This time I had a larger team of therapists, including several graduate students and postdoctoral fellows, and an even higher-risk sample of clients who had twice the rate of suicide attempts in the year prior to treatment as our original group. We lost our first client to suicide in this study, a woman who was in the standard DBT condition and therefore did not receive DBT PE. This incredibly sad event both reminded us of the reality of the risk we were facing and made us even more determined to keep going. At the end of this study, we found that most clients who completed DBT PE remitted from PTSD (80%), whereas those who received DBT alone did not (40%). Yet again, nobody who received DBT PE got worse. Indeed, adding DBT PE to DBT appeared to be making clients less rather than more likely to attempt suicide and self-injure (Harned, Korslund, & Linehan, 2014).

As these positive results were emerging, there was an increasing demand for me to start providing training to DBT therapists in this newly developed approach. After completing the initial open trial in 2012, I had somewhat tentatively begun to provide an introductory 2-day workshop in DBT PE while being clear about the preliminary nature of the evidence. In 2015, bolstered by the findings of the RCT, I expanded this to a 4-day intensive DBT PE workshop and began to train DBT therapists around the United States and internationally. Determined to make sure that what I was doing was helpful rather than harmful, I collected data from over 260 therapists who attended these workshops to evaluate whether they seemed to be effective in promoting the use of DBT PE in ways that were beneficial to clients. The results indicated that most therapists who attended these workshops used DBT PE in the 6 months after training, and those who did reported that it was safe and typically resulted in improvements in PTSD for their clients (Harned, Ritschel, & Schmidt, 2021).

In 2015, I received a second grant from NIMH to evaluate the effectiveness of the integrated DBT and DBT PE treatment in community practice settings. For this project, I partnered with four public mental health agencies in Philadelphia that were providing DBT to adolescents and adults across multiple levels of care. Together with Katie Korslund and Sara Schmidt, we provided training and consultation to these teams to help them implement DBT PE in their existing DBT programs. Over the next 4 years, I became intimately familiar with the challenges of delivering treatment in these underresourced settings, which are characterized by high rates of clinician turnover and an incredibly disadvantaged client population. Despite these challenges, we found that DBT PE could be transported effectively to these settings and that it continued to improve PTSD and other outcomes beyond the effects of DBT alone (see Harned, Schmidt, Korslund, & Gallop, 2021).

> ## A Note on the Name
>
> I am often asked why this treatment is called the DBT PE protocol (or DBT PE for short) as opposed to one or the other of its component treatments. The main answer is that this treatment is a true synthesis of both DBT and PE. Calling the treatment DBT would fail to acknowledge the reality that it is based on PE. At the same time, calling it PE would leave out the ways in which DBT has been infused into all aspects of its delivery. Therefore, the inclusion of both DBT and PE in the name of the protocol is intended to reflect a dialectical "both–and" approach that honors the importance of both treatments while also acknowledging that their synthesis has yielded something new and distinct.

After 14 years of working as the director of research in Marsha's clinic at the University of Washington, in 2018, I accepted a position at the Seattle division of the VA Puget Sound Health Care System. As part of my new position, I was tasked with establishing a comprehensive DBT program and training staff in both DBT and DBT PE. Building on the work of Laura Meyers and her team at the Minneapolis Veterans Administration (VA) who had shown that DBT PE was effective in a veteran population (see Meyers et al., 2017), my team and I began using the treatment with high-risk and behaviorally dysregulated veterans with BPD. Nearly every veteran we treat in our VA DBT program has PTSD, and DBT PE has become a standard, and typically successful, part of the treatment they receive. In this process, I have learned a lot about how to make DBT PE fit the needs of a new population of clients: in this case, veterans of all genders who often have a complex history of both military and nonmilitary traumas. These lessons on how to tailor DBT PE to different client populations are reflected throughout this book, and I expect the treatment will continue to evolve as we learn more about how to make it work as effectively as possible for the diverse clients who need it.

Evidence Base

A significant benefit of basing the DBT PE protocol on two gold standard evidence-based treatments is that there was already a large body of research supporting the effectiveness of its component parts. At this point, more than 35 RCTs have demonstrated the efficacy and effectiveness of DBT in reducing suicidal and self-injurious behavior (DeCou, Comtois, & Landes, 2018), symptoms of BPD (Storebø et al., 2020), and a wide range of other problems in both adults and adolescents (Miga, Neacsiu, Lungu, Heard, & Dimeff, 2019). Similarly, more than 35 RCTs of PE have been conducted that support its efficacy and effectiveness in reducing PTSD among adults (Powers, Halpern, Ferenschak, Gillihan, & Foa, 2010) and adolescents (Foa, McLean, Capaldi, & Rosenfield, 2013; Gilboa-Schechtman et al., 2010) with a wide range of traumas. Given the large evidence base for DBT and PE, research on the integrated DBT + DBT PE treatment has focused on confirming that they remain effective when adapted and combined and that doing so is feasible, acceptable, and safe for high-risk and multidiagnostic clients.

Efficacy Studies

As described above, the two original studies of DBT + DBT PE were conducted in an outpatient research clinic at the University of Washington and included an open trial ($n = 13$; Harned et al., 2012) and an RCT that compared DBT with and without the DBT PE protocol ($n = 26$;

Harned et al., 2014). Both studies involved 1 year of treatment and included adult women with recent (past 2–3 months) and recurrent suicide attempts and/or NSSI, PTSD, and BPD. On average, clients had attempted suicide between two and three times and engaged in NSSI more than 60 times in the year prior to treatment. Participants were 33–39 years old on average, primarily White (69–80%), low income (75–91% earned <$20,000 per year), and 13–54% identified as a sexual minority. Additional information about the clinical characteristics of these samples is provided in Chapter 2, and the specific racial/ethnic and sexual minority subgroups are described in Chapter 17.

Acceptability and Feasibility

Across both studies, 74% of clients reported a preference for DBT + DBT PE at intake compared to DBT alone (26%) or PE alone (0%), and this was predicted by more severe PTSD reexperiencing symptoms and an index trauma that occurred in childhood (Harned, Tkachuck, & Youngberg, 2013). Over the course of DBT, 46–77% of clients initiated the DBT PE protocol and this occurred after an average of 20 weeks of DBT; of these, 70–75% completed it in an average of 13 sessions (range = 6–19) during which two to three trauma memories were typically targeted. The primary barrier to initiating the DBT PE protocol was treatment dropout during Stage 1 of DBT, which occurred for 23–41% of clients and, in the RCT, was related to lower therapist adherence to DBT. Overall, the treatment was highly acceptable to clients and therapists in terms of positive treatment expectancies and satisfaction.

Safety

The DBT PE protocol was found to be safe to deliver. During the year of treatment, few clients in the open trial attempted suicide (9%) or self-injured (27%). In the RCT, clients who completed the DBT PE protocol were 2.4 times less likely to attempt suicide (17% vs. 40%) and 1.5 times less likely to self-injure (67% vs. 100%) than those completing DBT alone. These findings suggest that adding the DBT PE protocol to DBT is likely to decrease rather than increase the risk of suicidal and self-injurious behaviors. In addition, completing *in vivo* and imaginal exposure tasks was not associated with an increased risk of engaging in self-injurious behaviors. During the DBT PE protocol, urges to attempt suicide and self-injure rarely increased immediately following exposure tasks (6–11% of tasks) and, in the RCT, average pre- and postsession urges to engage in these behaviors were higher in DBT than in DBT + DBT PE. Overall, 20–25% of clients engaged in suicidal and/or self-injurious behavior during the DBT PE protocol portion of the treatment, which is no higher than what is found during DBT.

Clinical Outcomes

At posttreatment, DBT + DBT PE clients in the intent-to-treat samples (i.e., those who had the option to receive the DBT PE protocol) showed large and significant improvements in PTSD severity (Hedges's g effect sizes = 1.6–1.8), as well as high rates of reliable improvement (70–83%) and diagnostic remission of PTSD (58–60%). Clients who completed the DBT PE protocol showed even larger improvements in PTSD severity (gs = 1.9–2.9), as well as higher rates of reliable improvement (86–100%) and diagnostic remission of PTSD (71–80%). In the RCT, clients who completed the DBT PE protocol were two times more likely than those who completed DBT alone to achieve diagnostic remission from PTSD (80% vs. 40%). In both studies, clients in DBT + DBT PE also showed large improvements in dissociation, depression, anxiety, guilt, shame, and social and global functioning and, in the RCT, these improvements were larger in DBT + DBT PE than in DBT.

Mechanisms and Processes of Change

Using data from these efficacy trials, several studies have evaluated factors associated with improvement in PTSD during DBT + DBT PE. The first study examined the pattern of change in emotions during imaginal exposure and found that only global distress (SUDS) and fear significantly decreased during imaginal exposure trials (within-session habituation), whereas global distress, fear, guilt, shame, and disgust each showed significant reductions across imaginal exposure trials (between-session habituation; Harned, Ruork, Liu, & Tkachuck, 2015). This study also found that achieving remission from PTSD was predicted by greater between-session habituation, but not within-session habituation or emotional activation. Another study found that clients with higher levels of shame, guilt, experiential avoidance, and posttraumatic cognitions exhibited a slower rate of improvement in PTSD during treatment, suggesting the need to specifically target these maintaining factors to accelerate treatment gains (Harned, Fitzpatrick, & Schmidt, 2020).

Two studies have examined the timing of change in PTSD and other outcomes over the course of DBT + DBT PE. Across the three stages of the treatment, PTSD severity does not change in Stage 1 but does significantly improve in Stages 2 and 3, whereas BPD severity and state dissociation significantly improve only in Stage 3 (Harned, Gallop, & Valenstein-Mah, 2018). In addition, improvements in PTSD severity and posttraumatic cognitions both predict subsequent improvements in functional outcomes, such as social adjustment, global functioning, and health-related quality of life (Harned, Wilks, Schmidt, & Coyle, 2018).

Taken together, these findings indicate that (1) PTSD is unlikely to significantly improve in DBT until it is directly targeted in Stage 2 via the DBT PE protocol; (2) reducing trauma-related emotions, experiential avoidance, and posttraumatic cognitions are critical to achieving improvement in PTSD; and (3) improvements in many comorbid problems are likely to occur after, and as a result of, successful treatment of PTSD.

Effectiveness Studies

Since these original efficacy trials, two effectiveness studies have examined DBT + DBT PE in community practice settings. Meyers and colleagues (2017) evaluated the treatment in a 12-week intensive outpatient program at a VA medical center. This open trial included 33 veterans (mean age = 43, 52% male, 76% White) with PTSD and BPD traits that had interfered with prior attempts to receive standard PTSD treatments, including PE, in the VA. To accommodate the intensive outpatient model, the treatment was shortened to 12 weeks of standard DBT (three DBT skills groups and one DBT individual session per week) with the DBT PE protocol integrated into treatment beginning in Week 2. On average, clients received 12 DBT PE sessions. Overall, 67% of clients successfully completed the program, no clients dropped out during DBT PE, and there were no adverse events. Among treatment completers, there were large and significant reductions from pre- to posttreatment in PTSD severity, suicidal ideation, and dysfunctional coping. At posttreatment, 91% had experienced a reliable improvement in PTSD and 64% were below the clinical cutoff for a PTSD diagnosis.

As mentioned previously, my second NIMH grant involved a nonrandomized controlled trial that compared DBT with and without DBT PE in four public mental health agencies in Philadelphia (Harned, Schmidt, et al., 2021). These agencies included an adult outpatient DBT program, two residential DBT programs (one for adults, one for adolescents), and one DBT program embedded within an Assertive Community Treatment program for adults with severe mental illness. Clients were required to meet criteria for PTSD and to be enrolled in DBT in one of these programs; no exclusionary criteria were applied. The sample included 35 clients ranging in age from 12 to 56 years old (average = 30) of whom 80% were female, 65% were racial/ethnic minorities (primarily African American [41%] and Latinx [27%]), and 44% identified as sexual minorities. Most clients (85%) earned less than $5,000 per year and were receiving state or federal financial assistance or benefits. In the past year, 60% had engaged in NSSI, 46% had attempted suicide, and 49% had been psychiatrically hospitalized. Per clinician report, the most common co-occurring diagnoses were BPD (54%), bipolar disorder (34%), major depression (31%), substance use disorder (20%), and psychotic disorder (17%).

In this demographically and clinically diverse sample, 46% of clients initiated the DBT PE protocol during the course of DBT. The primary barrier to initiating DBT PE was therapist turnover: 58% of clients who did not receive DBT PE lost their therapist due to turnover during the course of their treatment. The rate of client-initiated dropout from treatment was 29% and did not differ between those who did or did not receive DBT PE. Clients who initiated and/or completed DBT PE had very large pre–post improvements in PTSD severity (gs = 1.1–1.4), high rates of reliable improvement of PTSD (54–71%), and 40–44% no longer met criteria for PTSD by posttreatment. In contrast, clients who did not initiate DBT PE exhibited moderate improvements in PTSD severity (g = 0.5) and had relatively low rates of reliable improvement (31%) or remission (23%) of PTSD. Similarly, clients who initiated DBT PE showed significant improvements in posttraumatic cognitions, emotion dysregulation, general psychological distress, and functional impairment, whereas clients who received DBT only either did not significantly change or improved less on these outcomes. The rate of suicide attempts and/or NSSI during treatment was significantly lower among clients who initiated DBT PE (27%) than those who received DBT alone (65%), and there was no evidence of increases in these behaviors or use of crisis services among clients who received DBT PE. Client age, gender, race/ethnicity, and sexual orientation did not significantly predict DBT PE initiation or impact the rate of improvement in PTSD and other outcomes, suggesting that the effects of DBT PE may generalize to clients from diverse sociodemographic groups.

Benchmarking analyses compared these results to those obtained in the two original efficacy studies (Harned et al., 2012, 2014) and found that the degree of improvement in PTSD severity in this sample, although very large, was significantly smaller than in the efficacy trials. This was likely due to differences in how the treatment was implemented in these settings—for example, clients received both shorter and less adherent DBT as well as fewer DBT PE sessions on average than in the efficacy trials. In addition, differences in the client samples may have contributed to these reduced treatment gains, as the effectiveness trial included a higher rate of racial/ethnic minorities, clients living in extreme poverty, clients with and without BPD, and individuals with psychotic and bipolar disorders.

Dissemination and Implementation Studies

Two studies have examined methods of training therapists to deliver the DBT PE protocol. The first study surveyed 266 therapists who self-selected to attend 2- or 4-day DBT PE workshops (Harned, Ritschel, et al., 2021). These therapists were delivering DBT in a wide variety of practice settings and, prior to the workshop, 78% reported feeling "very" comfortable using DBT. The workshops were effective in increasing therapists' confidence in DBT PE and their ability to deliver it, while also decreasing their concerns about potential client worsening. In the 6 months after training, therapists who attended the 4-day workshop were significantly more likely to use DBT PE in their practice than those who attended the 2-day workshop (66% vs.

39%) and use of DBT PE was predicted by greater self-efficacy and perceived treatment credibility at posttraining. The primary reason therapists reported for not using DBT PE in the 6 months after training was a lack of appropriate clients.

Among therapists who used DBT PE, 81% reported that on average their clients' PTSD had improved and 67% reported that PTSD was much to very much improved on average. In addition, most therapists reported that their clients' comorbid problems did not get worse during DBT PE. If worsening occurred, it typically involved temporary increases in internal distress (e.g., emotion dysregulation, dissociation, depression) and not loss of behavioral control. Few therapists reported having clients who exhibited temporary increases in suicide attempts (5%) or NSSI (17%), and sustained worsening of these behaviors was rare (NSSI = 3%) to nonexistent (suicide attempts = 0%). Taken together, these findings suggest that workshops, particularly the standard 4-day DBT PE workshop, appear to be an effective method of training therapists to deliver DBT PE in a manner they experience as being safe and effective for their clients. This workshop-only training model may be most effective for therapists who are motivated to learn and use DBT PE and have a high degree of confidence in their ability to deliver DBT.

The second therapist training study was embedded in the grant that evaluated DBT PE in public mental health agencies in Philadelphia. In this project, we used a more intensive implementation model that included the 4-day DBT PE workshop followed by 16 months of bimonthly team-based consultation with an expert who also regularly reviewed DBT and DBT PE sessions and provided adherence feedback (Harned, Schmidt, et al., 2021). Therapists in this study (n = 28) did not self-select to attend the training (they were asked to participate by their team leaders) and were primarily master's-level counselors and social workers who had been providing DBT at their agency for an average of 15 months. Half of these therapists (50%) reported feeling "very" comfortable using DBT prior to the workshop. From the beginning to the end of the workshop, there were significant increases in therapists' confidence in DBT PE and their ability to deliver it, as well as a decrease in negative beliefs about exposure therapy. Overall, 62% of eligible therapists used DBT PE after training and did so with high levels of adherence (96% of rated DBT PE sessions were deemed adherent). These findings support the potential effectiveness of a multicomponent implementation model for providing training and ongoing support to therapists learning to deliver DBT PE, perhaps particularly those who are less confident in their ability to deliver DBT.

Concluding Comments

The integrated DBT and DBT PE protocol treatment described in this book was born out of my determination to find a way for even the most high-risk and complex clients to receive effective treatment for PTSD. Starting from the tremendously strong foundations of DBT and PE, the DBT PE protocol was developed using an iterative trial-and-error approach that was guided by the theories underlying these treatments and the needs of the clients we were treating. Along the way, many therapists, clients, the DBT and PE treatment developers, and other experts have helped to shape it into its current form and make it better than it otherwise would have been. The research to date supports the feasibility, acceptability, safety, and effectiveness of this treatment approach in a variety of client populations and treatment settings, and when delivered by DBT therapists with diverse training backgrounds. After many years of treatment development and research, I am excited to share this manual with you and hope that it helps you to provide effective treatment for PTSD and change the lives of clients who have been trapped in a seemingly endless cycle of trauma-related suffering.

CHAPTER 2

The Target Population

The integrated DBT and DBT PE treatment is designed for individuals with PTSD who are too high risk and unstable to receive trauma-focused treatments as a first-line intervention. Prototypical clients receiving this treatment have suffered from PTSD for as long as they can remember, have spent many years engaged in mental health services, and have never received effective treatment for PTSD. In most cases, the nature and severity of these clients' problems has kept therapists from even attempting to provide a trauma-focused treatment. Indeed, many clients have been told that their problems are too complex to allow them to receive treatment for PTSD or that they should not talk about their traumas because it would be unsafe or destabilizing. Often clients have spent years stuck in this catch-22 situation in which trauma and PTSD are the cause of behaviors that contraindicate trauma-focused treatment. One of my clients described this dilemma by saying, "I haven't had a chance to tell my story and am derailed by it. I feel like a hamster running in circles because I haven't been able to talk about it." While the goal is clear—to reach people who both need PTSD treatment and are not yet stable enough to receive it—it is often less clear who exactly these people are. In this chapter, I provide a framework for determining who is appropriate for DBT + DBT PE and describe the common characteristics of clients who receive this treatment.

Stages of Disorder and Approaches to Treating PTSD

Decades of research have not provided a clear answer to the question of which approach to treating PTSD is best for whom, and there is a lack of consensus among trauma experts on this topic. One of the most debated issues is how to decide which types of clients are appropriate for trauma-focused treatments alone versus stage-based treatments that include a stabilization phase prior to trauma-focused treatment. Efforts to resolve this issue have typically focused on identifying specific comorbid conditions that do or do not contraindicate trauma-focused treatments. For example, research has shown that individuals with nonacute suicidal ideation, borderline personality characteristics, dissociation, major depression, and substance abuse can benefit from PE alone (van Minnen, Harned, Zoellner, & Mills, 2012).

But what happens if a person has all five of these problems plus five more that are potentially crisis level, such as panic attacks that interfere with working, restrictive eating, a verbally abusive partner, frequent occurrences of drunk driving, and an unstable housing situation? And what if the person attends therapy inconsistently and is often disengaged during sessions? While any one of these problems in isolation may not contraindicate trauma-focused treatment, the whole is likely to be more complex than the sum of its parts. In addition, there are certain types of problems that are widely viewed as requiring stabilization prior to trauma-focused treatment, such as those that create an imminent danger to self or others. Therefore, decisions about which treatments are appropriate for whom must take into account not only the types of problems that clients have but also the overall level of disorder these problems create. Accordingly, I use DBT's stages of disorder model (Linehan, 1993, 1999) as a framework for identifying the types of clients who are appropriate for DBT + DBT PE.

Stages of Disorder Model

In DBT, a client's level of disorder is defined according to five dimensions: (1) *imminent threat*: behaviors that create a high risk of imminent death, (2) *disability*: the inability to fulfill critical societal and/or social roles, (3) *severity*: the frequency and intensity of psychological and functional problems, (4) *pervasiveness*: the degree to which psychological and functional problems are limited to a specific context and/or are widespread, and (5) *complexity*: the number of co-occurring problems. As shown in Table 2.1, there are four levels of disorder that map onto four stages of treatment, with each stage associated with distinct treatment goals and approaches to addressing PTSD.

Stage 1

In Stage 1, clients have the most severe level of disorder, which is characterized by life-threatening behavioral dyscontrol, multiple mental disorders and out-of-control behaviors, pervasive emotion dysregulation, and severe disability. The treatment goals for the Stage 1 client include acquiring the behavioral skills needed to eliminate suicidal and self-injurious behaviors, achieve control over other impulsive and damaging behaviors, and participate effectively in treatment. Trauma-focused treatment is proscribed for clients with a Stage 1 level of disorder, as these individuals lack the ability to safely and effectively engage in these treatments. For example, I once worked with a client with severe PTSD who began treatment with a recent history of multiple suicide attempts and psychiatric hospitalizations. In the first several weeks of treatment she attempted suicide two times, first by overdose and then by trying to provoke the police to kill her. After the second attempt, she was taken to the emergency room where she then assaulted a nurse, was charged with a felony, and transferred to jail. Upon being released from jail a few days later, she returned home to discover that she was being evicted, which precipitated the next suicidal crisis and psychiatric hospitalization. Although her PTSD clearly needed to be treated and was contributing to this cycle of unrelenting crisis, it was simply not possible (let alone advisable) to attempt to deliver a trauma-focused treatment to a client with this level of disorder. Instead, a present-focused approach must be used in which clients are taught skills to cope effectively with PTSD without directly targeting the underlying disorder. Overall, treatment for the Stage 1 client with PTSD is viewed as the necessary preparation for subsequent trauma-focused treatment.

TABLE 2.1. Stages of Disorder and Approaches to Addressing PTSD

Stage of treatment	Level of disorder	Treatment goals	Approach to addressing PTSD
Stage 1: Behavioral dyscontrol	• Behaviors posing imminent threat to life • Pervasive behavioral and emotion dysregulation • Multiple mental disorders • Severe disability	• Increase commitment to living • Achieve behavioral control • Decrease behaviors that interfere with therapy • Acquire behavioral skills	Focus is on achieving safety and stability by increasing behavioral skills. PTSD is addressed using a present-focused approach that focuses on coping effectively with PTSD symptoms. Trauma processing is proscribed due to safety concerns.
Stage 2: Quiet desperation	• No imminent threat to life • Reasonable control of behavior • Intense emotional pain • One or more mental disorders • Significant and potentially disabling psychosocial problems	• Reduce posttraumatic stress • Increase nonanguished emotional experiencing • Decrease isolation and disconnection from others • Enhance sense of personal validity	Trauma-focused treatment is provided. For clients with other severe disorders or a recent history of behavioral dyscontrol, another treatment may be provided concurrently to target co-occurring disorders and reduce the risk of relapse to a Stage 1 level of disorder.
Stage 3: Problems in living	• Mild or no mental disorders • Able to function in normative social roles • Ordinary problems in living	• Reduce any residual disorders • Increase self-validation, self-respect, and mastery • Expand connections and increase engagement in the world	Focus is on building a life without PTSD, including addressing remaining barriers to achieving functional goals.
Stage 4: Incompleteness	• No mental disorders • Sense of incompleteness	• Build capacity for sustained joy • Increase peak experiences • Find spiritual fulfillment	No trauma intervention needed.

Stage 2

In contrast, individuals with a Stage 2 level of disorder are sufficiently stable to engage in treatments that focus directly on treating PTSD. These individuals may have multiple problems in addition to PTSD, but they are not severe enough to pose a clear barrier to engaging in trauma-focused treatment. For example, these individuals may have suicidal thoughts and urges to harm themselves, but they are in control of these behaviors and there is no immediate threat to life. Although Stage 2 clients experience intense emotional pain, they are typically able to cope with these emotions without consistently relying on maladaptive behaviors to alleviate immediate suffering. When problem behaviors occur, they are sufficiently controlled so as to not cause crises or routinely interfere with treatment. As an example, I recently began DBT PE with a client who was thinking about killing herself multiple times every day, using cannabis daily, and having regular anger outbursts toward staff and residents in the transitional housing facility where she lived. However, she consistently used skills to manage her suicide urges without acting on them, limit her substance use so that it did not cause serious problems, and reduce the frequency and intensity of her anger outbursts. This behavioral control had been achieved even though she continued to experience extreme emotional misery that began as soon as she woke up in the morning and was flooded with memories of past traumas. This state of pervasive emotional pain in the context of reasonable behavioral control is referred to in DBT as "quiet desperation."

For Stage 2 clients, the primary treatment goals are to reduce PTSD, increase nonanguished emotional experiencing (i.e., the ability to experience and regulate a range of emotions, including those related to past trauma), decrease isolation and disconnection from others, and enhance the person's sense of personal validity. For clients with a history of Stage 1 disorder, PTSD treatment should be provided as soon as possible to reduce the risk of relapsing back to Stage 1 behaviors. For clients without such a history, treating PTSD is likely to prevent them from ever reaching Stage 1 levels of dysfunction.

Stage 3

At Stage 3, clients may have one or more mental disorders, but they are not severe or disabling. For example, a client may have periodic major depression that does not seriously interfere with the ability to function in expected social roles. Overall, clients have what is referred to in DBT as "ordinary problems in living," which may include normative life stressors (e.g., conflict with family members, dissatisfaction with school or work) and ordinary unhappiness. Treatment goals in this stage focus on improving quality of life by increasing meaningful connections and participating in productive and value-driven activities. When needed, residual mental disorders may be treated and issues related to one's self-concept may be addressed. For clients who completed PTSD treatment in Stage 2, PTSD is typically gone or greatly reduced and the focus of treatment shifts to building a life that is no longer restricted by trauma-related avoidance and impairment. For clients who experienced early developmental trauma and have spent much of their life in Stage 1, this may be the first time they have ever reached this level of functioning. In these cases, treatment may include helping clients figure out new ways of living now that they are no longer in a constant state of crisis and instability. For clients who were reasonably well functioning prior to experiencing the trauma(s) that caused PTSD, this stage can be viewed as helping them to fully return to their pretrauma level of functioning. DBT may no longer be needed for many Stage 3 problems and other, less intensive treatments (e.g., cognitive-behavioral therapy or couples therapy) may be sufficient. For some clients, no further treatment may be needed at Stage 3 and they may instead rely on supportive people in their lives to process current problems.

Stage 4

At Stage 4, people are high functioning and do not have any mental health problems but may be wrestling with a more existential sense of incompleteness. Similar to the concept of self-actualization, the goal is to help these individuals achieve their full potential through increasing peak experiences and building the capacity for sustained joy and freedom. In some cases, this may include finding spiritual fulfillment. For clients with a history of trauma and PTSD, no trauma-related intervention is needed at this stage.

Linking Stages of Disorder to Eligibility Criteria for PTSD Treatments

The stages of disorder model is highly consistent with the eligibility criteria commonly used for trauma-focused treatments, such as PE (Foa et al., 2019), cognitive processing therapy (Resick, Monson, & Chard, 2017), and eye movement desensitization and reprocessing therapy (Shapiro,

2001). In particular, studies of these treatments use eligibility criteria that are designed to identify individuals who are ready to immediately begin trauma-focused treatment. In the stages of disorder model, these would correspond to individuals with a Stage 2 level of disorder. Accordingly, these treatments routinely exclude individuals with behaviors consistent with a Stage 1 level of disorder, including those that pose a significant threat to life (e.g., acute suicidality, recent suicidal or self-injurious behaviors), as well as those that are likely to interfere with PTSD treatment (e.g., severe dissociative disorders, ongoing trauma, substance dependence, active psychosis) (Bradley et al., 2005; Ronconi, Shiner, & Watts, 2014). In addition, these treatments often require PTSD to be the primary diagnosis (i.e., the most severe problem requiring treatment).

In contrast, studies of DBT + DBT PE have used eligibility criteria that are intended to identify individuals in need of stabilization prior to trauma-focused treatment—that is, those with a Stage 1 level of disorder. In my original efficacy studies, the inclusion criteria were selected to match the exclusion criteria for PE (Harned et al., 2012, 2014). In particular, clients were required to be at acute risk for suicide and/or have recent suicidal or serious nonsuicidal self-injurious behavior. Clients in those studies also met criteria for BPD as well as multiple other severe disorders. Subsequent effectiveness studies of DBT + DBT PE have utilized eligibility criteria designed to identify clients whose PTSD is not being addressed by standard treatments, including those who have been unable to complete trauma-focused treatments due to BPD-related problems (Meyers et al., 2017), as well as those who are receiving DBT and continue to have PTSD (Harned, Schmidt, et al., 2021).

Who Is Appropriate for DBT + DBT PE?

As described, the integrated DBT + DBT PE treatment is intended for individuals with PTSD and a Stage 1 level of disorder. With the exception of PTSD, clients are not required to have any specific disorder or problem behavior, but instead exhibit a combination of presenting problems that together indicate a Stage 1 level of disorder. Consequently, clients who are appropriate for DBT + DBT PE are a heterogeneous group. Although they share a common need for stabilization and skills acquisition prior to engaging in trauma-focused treatment, the exact problems that need stabilization vary by client. In this section, I describe the typical clinical presentation of clients who are appropriate for DBT + DBT PE in terms of their trauma histories, as well as the types of co-occurring problems they often exhibit (see Figure 2.1).

Posttraumatic Stress Disorder

According to the fifth edition of the *Diagnostic and Statistical Manual of Mental Disorders* (DSM-5; American Psychiatric Association, 2013), to be eligible to receive a PTSD diagnosis a person must have been directly, indirectly, or vicariously exposed to one or more events that involved actual or threatened death, serious injury, or sexual violence (Criterion A). The 20 PTSD symptom criteria are organized across four domains, including intrusive symptoms (e.g., recurrent nightmares, images, or thoughts about the trauma), avoidance symptoms (e.g., avoiding trauma-related thoughts, feelings, and situations), negative cognitions or mood (e.g., persistent negative emotional states and beliefs about the self and others, anhedonia, feelings of detachment), and increased arousal (e.g., insomnia, hypervigilance, exaggerated startle). Clients typically meet full diagnostic criteria for PTSD, but individuals with subthreshold PTSD,

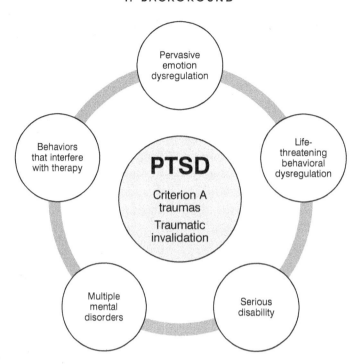

FIGURE 2.1. The target population for DBT + DBT PE.

as well as those who have PTSD symptoms in relation to non–Criterion A events, may also be appropriate if these symptoms are the source of significant distress or impairment. Of note, clients who receive DBT + DBT PE are also likely to meet the criteria for complex PTSD, although this is not required. Complex PTSD is currently included in the 11th edition of the *International Classification of Diseases* (ICD-11; World Health Organization, 2018), but not in DSM-5, and includes the same diagnostic criteria as PTSD plus three additional clusters of affect dysregulation, negative self-concept, and disturbances in relationships.

Trauma History

This treatment is intended to address any type of trauma that has led to significant PTSD symptoms, including events that do and do not meet Criterion A of the DSM-5 PTSD diagnosis.

Criterion A Traumas

Although DBT PE is appropriate for any type of Criterion A trauma, there are certain trauma types that are more likely to result in the severe impairment characteristic of individuals with a Stage 1 level of disorder and are thus more prevalent among clients receiving this treatment. In particular, early developmental trauma (e.g., child sexual and physical abuse), assaultive trauma (e.g., rape, physical assaults), and multiple (i.e., complex) traumas are associated with increased severity, complexity, and suicidality in individuals with PTSD (e.g., Briere, Kaltman, & Green, 2008; Cloitre et al., 2009; LeBouthillier, McMillan, Thibodeau, & Asmundson, 2015). Accordingly, clients in my original efficacy studies reported experiencing an average of 12 different types of Criterion A traumas that most often included intimate partner violence (74%), child sexual abuse (73%), being stalked (66%), adult sexual assault (62%), child physical abuse (59%), and witnessing family violence as a child (59%). When asked to identify an index (i.e., most distressing) trauma, the most common types were child sexual abuse (54%), adult rape (15%), child physical abuse (10%), and intimate partner violence (8%). These typical index traumas, including common themes, emotions, and beliefs that arise while processing them, are discussed in detail in Chapter 16.

Traumatic Invalidation

Most clients in need of DBT + DBT PE have also experienced severe and pervasive invalidation. Although invalidation is typically not a Criterion A trauma, these experiences can be traumatic when they are experienced as intensely emotionally and psychologically painful and have lasting adverse effects on the person's self-concept and functioning. In DBT, this is referred to as *traumatic invalidation*, which is defined as "extreme or repetitive invalidation of individuals' significant private experiences, characteristics identified as important aspects of themselves, or reactions to themselves or to the world" (Linehan, 2015, p. 304). Invalidating behaviors can take many forms but share a common feature of attacking the person's sense of self and personal validity by communicating that they are bad, wrong, unacceptable, and unwanted. Common examples of invalidation and the negative messages these behaviors convey are shown in Table 2.2 and discussed in more detail in Chapter 16. Traumatic invalidation can occur in the family of origin and in other important relationships, groups, or institutional contexts, as well as at the societal or cultural level for individuals from marginalized groups, such as racial, ethnic, sexual, and gender minorities (see Chapter 17). Often the person's responses to these invalidating behaviors are also invalidated, which further increases distress.

During the development of DBT PE, our clients very often told us that, of all the traumas they had experienced, traumatic invalidation was one of the most (if not *the* most) distressing. In addition, clients often reported PTSD symptoms in relation to these experiences, such as intrusive memories of past invalidation, persistent efforts to avoid thinking about these past invalidating experiences, distorted negative beliefs about themselves, frequent negative emotions (e.g., guilt, shame), and hypervigilance to subsequent invalidation. These PTSD symptoms were sometimes the result of a single extreme invalidating incident, such as a client I treated who was ignored by his parents, ridiculed by his siblings, and bullied by his peers after attempting suicide as a teenager. More often, however, PTSD symptoms were the cumulative effect of chronic, everyday invalidation, such as a client I worked with whose parents had been severely controlling, critical, and emotionally neglectful, and whose primarily White peers had often excluded her due to her Latinx ethnicity. Given the prevalence of these types of highly distressing experiences among our clients, it soon became clear that restricting treatment to focus only on Criterion A traumas would not only be missing a significant cause of PTSD symptoms for many clients but would also be contributing to further invalidation by communicating that their traumatic reactions to these events were not valid.

These clinical experiences are supported by research indicating that severe invalidation (often referred to as emotional or psychological abuse) by caregivers and intimate partners is as or more harmful than sexual and physical violence in terms of its impact on PTSD and other mental health outcomes (e.g., Mechanic, Weaver, & Resick, 2008; Spinazzola et al., 2014). Similarly, invalidation (e.g., discrimination, verbal harassment, exclusion) due to race/ethnicity, sexual orientation, and gender identity is associated with PTSD symptoms (e.g., Bandermann & Szymanski, 2014; Pieterse, Carter, Evans, & Walter, 2010; Reisner et al., 2016). Given this,

TABLE 2.2. Traumatic Invalidation

Type of invalidating behavior	Examples	Messages
Criticizing	Being insulted, put down, mocked, or called names. Others criticizing your behavior, appearance, emotions, or interests. People saying things intended to humiliate or belittle you.	You are bad. You are wrong.
Unequal treatment	Being treated as less than or different from others. Being treated unfairly compared to others. Being discriminated against based on your personal characteristics.	You are inferior. You are inadequate.
Ignoring	People acting like you are invisible. Others not paying attention to what you do or say. Being left alone for long periods of time.	You do not matter. You are not important.
Emotional neglect	Not receiving caring or loving responses from people. Others being indifferent to your suffering. Being told you are not supposed to feel or express distress.	You are unlovable. You do not deserve care.
Excluding	Being shunned by others. Being asked to leave or denied entry to valued social groups. Being excluded from important family, school, or professional activities.	You do not belong. You are unwanted.
Misinterpreting	Having your behavior misinterpreted in negative ways. Being assumed to have ill intentions. Being told you feel something that you do not feel.	You can't be trusted. You are harmful.
Controlling	Being told how you must behave. Not being allowed to engage in activities that you enjoy or value. Being treated like you are incapable of making wise decisions.	You are incompetent. You are unacceptable.
Blaming	Being blamed for things that are not your fault. Being wrongfully accused of problematic behavior. Being told you cause trouble for others.	You cause problems. You are a burden.
Denying reality	Being told your perceptions of basic facts are inaccurate. People denying they said or did something despite having proof. Being told you are making things up or overreacting.	You are crazy. You can't trust yourself.

experiences of traumatic invalidation that have resulted in PTSD symptoms are commonly treated in DBT PE. Indeed, failure to address these experiences, which have often been underrecognized and undertreated in PTSD treatments, is likely to limit the gains that clients who have suffered this type of trauma will make.

Pervasive Emotion Dysregulation

According to the biosocial theory, pervasive emotion dysregulation is the core problem of individuals with a Stage 1 level of disorder, which develops when an emotionally vulnerable individual is exposed to a chronically invalidating environment. Emotion dysregulation is the inability to influence the experience or expression of emotions in desired ways and is pervasive when it occurs across a wide range of emotions and situational contexts. The lives of individuals with PTSD and a Stage 1 level of disorder are dominated by frequent and intense painful emotions that they are often unable to understand, label, change, or tolerate. These emotions occur in response to a wide range of prompting events, many of which are related to the traumas they have experienced. In the presence of intense emotions, these individuals have limited access to adaptive emotion regulation strategies and instead frequently engage in behaviors that make things worse in the long run. As a result, they often view their emotions as dangerous, are not willing to experience them fully, and try to quickly suppress and escape them when they arise. However, these chronic efforts to avoid emotions only make them more intense and uncontrollable over time.

Severe Behavioral Dysregulation

To cope with pervasive emotion dysregulation, these individuals have learned to rely on fast-acting but ultimately damaging behaviors that provide short-term emotional relief at the expense of long-term suffering and life chaos. These typically include life-threatening behaviors as well as a variety of other impulsive and self-damaging behaviors.

Life-Threatening Behaviors

A hallmark feature of individuals with a Stage 1 level of disorder is the presence of severe, out-of-control behavior that causes significant threat to life or bodily harm. These behaviors may take many forms, but nearly always include recent and recurrent self-injurious behaviors (i.e., suicidal behavior and/or NSSI). Self-injurious behaviors may occur with or without suicidal intent but are done deliberately to cause bodily harm and result in injury. In addition, many clients are at acute risk of suicide (e.g., serious suicidal ideation with intent and a plan) and frequently engage in suicide crisis behaviors (e.g., suicide preparation, rehearsals, and communication). Self-injurious thoughts and behaviors are often functionally related to PTSD, exposure to trauma cues, and other trauma sequelae (e.g., dissociation). For example, among suicidal and self-injuring women with BPD and PTSD, episodes of self-injurious behavior often occur while the person is dissociated (67%), as well as in response to flashbacks or nightmares (44%), thoughts about sexual abuse or rape (30%), thoughts about physical abuse or assault (15%), talking to someone about sexual abuse or rape (11%), and talking to a therapist about sexual abuse or rape (4%; Harned, Rizvi, & Linehan, 2010).

Other Behavioral Dysregulation

Stage 1 clients also typically engage in other behaviors that are impulsive and self-destructive (e.g., excessive substance use, reckless driving, risky sex, binge eating), as well as behaviors that are potentially damaging to others (e.g., physical aggression, violent outbursts, threatening to harm others). Although these dysregulated behaviors may take many forms, they often share a common function of providing temporary relief from the intense negative emotions and cognitions associated with PTSD. Indeed, due to the high rate of overlap between PTSD and these types of behaviors, self-destructive and reckless behavior was added as a diagnostic criterion for PTSD in DSM-5. It is important to note, however, that to be considered to have a Stage 1 level of disorder these behaviors must be severe and uncontrolled enough to pose a significant danger to oneself or others and/or to cause serious instability and impairment.

Behaviors That Interfere with the Therapy Process

Individuals with a Stage 1 level of disorder typically also engage in a variety of behaviors that interfere with treatment, making it particularly difficult if not impossible to provide therapy. These may include nonattentive behaviors, such as frequently canceling or failing to attend therapy sessions, leaving sessions early, dropping out of therapy prematurely, and engaging in attention-interfering behaviors during sessions (e.g., dissociating, falling asleep, being under the influence of drugs or alcohol). In addition, Stage 1 clients may be noncollaborative during therapy sessions by, for example, refusing to speak, being argumentative and hostile, lying, providing intentionally vague answers to questions, and behaving in an inflexible or defiant manner. Finally, Stage 1 clients frequently exhibit a variety of noncompliant behaviors, such as refusing to engage in treatment tasks, failing to complete homework assignments, not keeping commitments, and violating treatment agreements. Taken together, these behaviors make Stage 1 clients particularly difficult to treat and are likely to significantly interfere with their ability to benefit from therapy.

Multiple Mental Disorders

Although a majority of individuals with PTSD have two or more comorbid diagnoses (Kessler, Sonnega, Bromet, Highes, & Nelson, 1995), the degree and type of diagnostic comorbidity present among individuals with a Stage 1 level of disorder make them particularly complex. It is common for Stage 1 clients to meet criteria for mood, anxiety, substance use, eating, dissociative, and personality disorders and for many of these disorders to be quite severe. In my original studies (Harned et al., 2012, 2014), clients receiving DBT + DBT PE met criteria for an average of seven current disorders, including PTSD (100%), BPD (100%), major depression (86–92%), social anxiety disorder (50–68%), panic disorder (45–58%), generalized anxiety disorder (42–59%), avoidant personality disorder (42–58%), substance use disorders (25–45%), paranoid personality disorder (17–21%), and eating disorders (14–25%). Although not formally diagnosed, 46–67% of clients were also above a clinical cutoff for dissociative disorders.

Often these comorbid disorders are functionally related to and exacerbated by PTSD. For example, a client I treated with severe combat-related PTSD became dependent on alcohol because it helped him cope with intrusive PTSD symptoms, developed panic disorder due to his efforts to avoid the intense physical sensations triggered by trauma cues, became depressed because PTSD-related behavioral avoidance severely limited his ability to engage in meaningful activities, and developed bulimia nervosa when he discovered that binge eating and purging helped to soothe his chronic hyperarousal. Importantly, this treatment is not designed for people with PTSD and another specific diagnosis or set of diagnoses, but rather is intended to be transdiagnostic and to address problems associated with multiple, co-occurring disorders. Although BPD and/or BPD traits have been used as inclusion criteria in several DBT + DBT PE studies, this has been done primarily to ensure a sufficiently complex sample, as well as to match the typical clinical populations included in DBT studies. A diagnosis of BPD, although common among people with PTSD and a Stage 1 level of disorder, is not required to be appropriate for this treatment.

Severe Disability

Individuals with a Stage 1 level of disorder typically exhibit severe levels of impairment in multiple domains of functioning that make it difficult to fulfill normative social roles. Their relationships are often characterized by conflict and instability, leaving them with few close friends and limited social support. This impaired interpersonal functioning is often due to patterns of relating to others that are linked to past trauma, such as being highly sensitive to rejection, having difficulty being assertive or accurately expressing needs, avoiding emotional intimacy, and being hostile or aggressive. In addition, Stage 1 clients often find it difficult to engage in productive activities, such as school and work. Adolescents may regularly skip school, fail to complete assignments, and exhibit behavior problems at school. Adults often impulsively quit jobs, are fired due to poor performance, or are chronically under- or unemployed. Many Stage 1 clients also have poor physical health, including frequent illness and chronic medical conditions. Taken together, these problems often result in significant hardship and disability, including insufficient money to meet their basic needs, unstable housing, and reliance on family or government financial assistance.

Who Is Not Appropriate for DBT + DBT PE?

The integrated DBT + DBT PE treatment is intended to be widely applicable to clients with PTSD whose overall clinical presentation is indicative of a Stage 1 level of disorder. Therefore, the primary reason to consider someone inappropriate for this treatment is if they have a Stage 2 level of disorder—that is, if they are stable enough to immediately begin trauma-focused treatment. Whenever possible, trauma-focused treatments should be the first-line approach to treating PTSD, as they provide clients with more rapid relief from trauma-related suffering and require significantly less time and resources to deliver. I often refer to DBT + DBT PE as the jackhammer of PTSD treatments. If a hammer tap is all that is needed to solve the problem, then by all means use this simpler and faster approach.

When clients have a Stage 1 level of disorder, there are few reasons to consider them inappropriate for this treatment. The most clear-cut reason is if a client endorses symptoms of PTSD but does not have at least some memory of a traumatic event that can be described in narrative form. Importantly, clients' trauma memories do not need to be fully elaborated or complete; many individuals who receive DBT PE have very fragmented trauma memories. However, if a person believes they have experienced trauma but has no memory of specific traumatic events, then this would preclude the use of imaginal exposure and would therefore make them inappropriate for this treatment. Second, there is no evidence to support (or refute) the use of DBT + DBT PE or standard PE with preadolescent children. Therefore, it is recommended that clinicians working with traumatized children utilize PTSD treatments with established empirical support for this age group.

Concluding Comments

In this chapter, I provided a conceptual framework based on DBT's stages of disorder model for identifying clients who are appropriate for the integrated DBT and DBT PE protocol treatment. As I described, this treatment is intended for individuals with a Stage 1 level of disorder who exhibit a constellation of severe and complex problems that make them unable to safely or effectively engage in trauma-focused treatment. At the same time, I am aware that this can be a challenging clinical decision and, in some cases, there may not be a clear "right" answer about whether DBT + DBT PE is the most appropriate treatment for a given individual. From a pragmatic perspective, what matters most is that clients who need PTSD treatment are able to receive it. If they have other problems that make trauma-focused treatment untenable, or they (or you) are simply unwilling to engage in such treatments without a prior stabilization or preparation phase, then we must find ways to make PTSD treatment accessible to them. PTSD is treatable even for our most high-risk and complex clients and does not need to cause lifelong suffering. Therefore, if DBT + DBT PE provides a way for clients to access and effectively engage in PTSD treatment, then that is what is ultimately most important.

STABILIZATION AND PREPARATION

CHAPTER 3

Setting the Stage for DBT PE in Pretreatment

Most evidence-based psychotherapies assume clients are ready and willing to start treatment immediately and therefore begin with active treatment in the first session. In contrast, in DBT it is assumed that clients may not have clearly defined treatment goals, DBT may not be appropriate for achieving these goals once they are determined, and clients may not be willing to engage in DBT even if it is a good fit. For clients with PTSD, it is also not assumed that they are interested in treating their PTSD or that they view DBT PE as an acceptable method of doing so. Thus, active treatment is not begun until clients have completed a pretreatment phase and it is clear that they are a good fit for and wish to engage in DBT. In this chapter, I provide a brief overview of DBT's standard pretreatment phase and discuss several additional pretreatment tasks that are specific to the integrated DBT and DBT PE treatment and are intended to set the stage for eventual PTSD treatment.

Overview of Pretreatment in DBT

DBT begins with a pretreatment phase designed to assess the client's treatment goals, orient the client to DBT, determine whether DBT is a good fit, and obtain a commitment to participate in treatment. This phase is often considered to be the "first four" sessions of treatment. However, the actual duration of pretreatment varies depending on each client's progression through the goals of this phase. For clients who are already well informed about DBT and are motivated for treatment, pretreatment may be a quick and straightforward process. Conversely, for clients who are ambivalent about treatment or have significant concerns about DBT's approach, pretreatment may be longer and more challenging. Either way, the goal is to begin active Stage 1 treatment as soon as possible for clients who are determined to be appropriate for DBT.

Assessing the Client's Treatment Goals

DBT is a client-centered treatment with therapists working on behalf of clients to help them achieve their self-defined goals. Accordingly, the first pretreatment session typically begins by asking clients about their treatment goals, which continue to be clarified throughout the pretreatment phase as part of getting to know the client and determining whether DBT is a good fit for their needs. For clients with a Stage 1 level of disorder, I often conceptualize these treatment goals as a "life-worth-living" list—that is, what would need to change in the client's life for them to want to be alive. You then work to get from general goals (e.g., "I want to have better relationships") to specific treatment targets that will need to either increase (e.g., participation in social activities) or decrease (e.g., avoidance of physical and emotional intimacy) for these goals to be achieved. In addition, you assess the overall behavioral patterns that are causing the client distress or impairment. This includes conducting a thorough assessment of self-injurious behaviors as well as other important problem behaviors and disorders. By the end of the pretreatment phase, the goal is to have a list of treatment targets that you and the client have identified as important for them to have a life they experience as worth living, as well as an initial plan about what is needed to achieve them.

Orienting to DBT

Another important goal of pretreatment is to orient clients to DBT so that they have the information they need to make an informed decision about whether to engage in the treatment. Therapists are expected to describe DBT's theoretical foundations, modes of treatment, skill-oriented focus, structure, rules, and requirements. These orienting tasks can be completed in any order over the course of the pretreatment sessions and are often woven into discussions in response to issues raised by the client. For example, as clients identify treatment goals (e.g., to be better able to control anger), you may orient them to relevant DBT skills modules (e.g., emotion regulation) as a way to build hope that DBT will be effective in helping them achieve their goals. The overall aim is to take the mystery out of treatment and ensure that clients have a reasonable understanding of what it means to "do DBT."

Determining Goodness of Fit

Once the client's treatment goals have been identified and DBT has been described, you and your client collaboratively decide whether DBT appears to be a good fit. A variety of issues may be considered when determining goodness of fit, such as the strength of the evidence base for DBT in treating the problems the client wishes to address, the intensity of treatment that is needed, the client's interest in DBT, and whether both of you believe you can work well together. If DBT is appropriate for the problems the client reports, the client wants to receive DBT from you, and you are willing to deliver it, then DBT is a "go."

Obtaining Commitments

Once DBT has been determined to be a good fit, then the client must make several commitments before progressing to the active treatment of Stage 1. First, clients must commit to the goal of reducing suicidal behavior. Ideally, this commitment includes an agreement to stay alive for the entire duration of treatment, but often shorter periods of time (e.g., a week or a month) are all that clients are initially willing to commit to. The principle here is that there needs to be some agreement that clients are working toward a goal that is compatible with life. However, treatment with acutely suicidal clients often begins with a rather tenuous or short-term commitment to staying alive, which is all that is needed to progress to Stage 1. Second, clients must commit to engaging in DBT, including attending both individual therapy and skills training group. Ideally, this commitment will also be for the entire duration of treatment but may be shortened if needed. Once these two commitments are obtained, they are strengthened (e.g., by using the devil's advocate technique to elicit change talk from clients) and troubleshot (e.g., by identifying and addressing potential obstacles to keeping these commitments).

Setting the Stage for DBT PE

When you intend to integrate DBT PE into DBT, you will complete the standard DBT pretreatment tasks just described, as well as several tasks specific to this treatment approach.

Assessing PTSD

Routine PTSD screening is essential to the successful implementation of the integrated DBT + DBT PE treatment. Ideally, this screening should occur at intake using a measure such as the PTSD Checklist for DSM-5 (PCL-5; Weathers et al., 2013) (see Appendix D) so that discussion of PTSD and its treatment can begin during the pretreatment phase of DBT. For clients who screen positive for PTSD, you should discuss it as a potential treatment target during pretreatment (see below). For clients who report a history of significant trauma and invalidation but are subthreshold for PTSD, it is often useful to ask follow-up questions to determine whether it may be a relevant treatment target. For some clients, PTSD may wax and wane based on overall levels of stress; proximity to anniversary dates or other reminders of trauma; and other factors, such as relationship status. In addition, some clients may underreport PTSD symptoms because they feel as if the traumas they have experienced "don't count" and therefore can't be considered as causes of PTSD. If this occurs, you can encourage clients to report on the PTSD symptoms they have regardless of the type of stressful event these symptoms are related to. In general, if PTSD is subthreshold but still causes significant impairment, or if there is reason to believe that it is likely to increase in certain contexts or as avoidance decreases, it may still be important to identify as a potential target of treatment.

Orienting to PTSD

For clients who screen positive for full or subthreshold PTSD, it is useful to spend time orienting them to this disorder during pretreatment (or whatever point in treatment it becomes clear that PTSD is a relevant treatment target). There are several general handouts for clients that can be used in this orienting process (see Appendix A). *General Handout 1 (What Is Posttraumatic Stress Disorder?)* is intended to provide clients with psychoeducational information about DSM-5 diagnostic criteria for PTSD and can be used to facilitate a discussion about PTSD and its impact on clients' lives. Typically, I describe each diagnostic criterion, ask clients whether they think it applies to them and, if it does, get examples of how that symptom shows up in their lives. For clients, this process can be incredibly informative as it is often the first time they have heard about the full range of PTSD symptoms. For many clients, their understanding of PTSD has previously been limited to symptoms that are clearly linked to past trauma, such as nightmares, flashbacks, and intrusive trauma memories. Many clients have not previously known that PTSD also includes many problems that are less clearly linked to past trauma, such as self-destructive behaviors, emotional numbness, feeling detached from people, extreme negative beliefs about oneself, intense shame, and poor concentration. This information often validates clients' experiences by helping them to more clearly understand that many of their problems are likely related to PTSD and past trauma and are not due to personal flaws or weaknesses.

For therapists, information obtained while orienting clients to PTSD can also be useful in understanding to what extent it is causing impairment, which specific symptoms are most intense, and how PTSD might be contributing to other problems the client is experiencing. For example, you may learn that a client often copes with flashbacks and intrusive trauma memories by self-injuring, avoids leaving the house alone, has high levels of trauma-related shame that makes them want to be dead, sleeps only 3–4 hours per night, regularly struggles with dissociation, and is often irritable with their partner. You can then use this information to help clients gain insight into the role of PTSD in maintaining their current problems and to reach a mutual understanding about the need to eventually treat PTSD in order to change these problems and improve many areas of the client's life.

When discussing PTSD with clients, it can also be useful to obtain basic information about the types of trauma they have experienced using self-report measures (see Appendix D) or informal assessment. It is important to note that clients are typically discouraged from going into detail about their trauma history, as this may be counterproductive at this stage of treatment. For now, it can be useful to have a general understanding of the most distressing types of trauma they have experienced—for example, that they experienced sexual or physical abuse in childhood, but without getting details about exactly what types of abusive behaviors occurred or who perpetrated them. It is also perfectly fine for clients to choose not to share anything about their trauma history if they prefer not to at this early point in treatment. When clients do share information about their trauma history, you should offer validation by, for example, highlighting that the types of trauma they have experienced are very common and cause PTSD for many people. Often clients have no knowledge of the prevalence of trauma and its impact, and this information alone can serve a normalizing function for clients who have previously thought that they were alone or abnormal in their experiences.

Pretreatment can also be a useful time to introduce the concept of traumatic invalidation to clients for whom this appears to be relevant. We often begin to learn about severe invalidation when orienting clients to the biosocial theory, and this can be a good segue into discussing the potential traumatic impact of such experiences for clients who screen positive for PTSD. *General Handout 2* (*What Is Traumatic Invalidation?*) provides examples of the types of invalidating behaviors that can be traumatic, as well as the common negative beliefs about the self that people develop as a result. *General Handout 3* (*The Impact of Traumatic Invalidation*) provides information about the typical outcomes of traumatic invalidation that include but are not limited to PTSD. For many clients, this information is profoundly validating as it gives them a framework for understanding their own experiences in a way that both acknowledges and normalizes the extremely damaging impact that severe invalidation can have. Thus, providing this psychoeducation early in treatment ensures these potentially traumatic experiences are not overlooked as possible contributors to PTSD symptoms.

Establishing Reducing PTSD as a Treatment Goal

Once PTSD has been identified as a problem that is causing distress and impairment, it is important to determine whether the client views treating PTSD as a relevant therapy goal. In my experience, it is rare for clients to specifically identify PTSD as a reason for seeking treatment, and those who do have typically been diagnosed with PTSD in the past and are aware that it is treatable. In these cases, it is a straightforward task to establish reducing PTSD as a goal of treatment. More often, however, clients are not familiar with PTSD and/or do not realize they have it. In these cases, it is first necessary to orient clients to PTSD before it can be considered as a potential treatment target. Once clients realize that they have PTSD, understand that it is likely contributing to their misery, and are told that it is treatable, most readily agree to make reducing PTSD a goal of treatment.

The more challenging situation is when clients know they have PTSD but are not interested in treating it. In these cases, the reasons clients do not want to treat it are often the same factors that are maintaining the disorder. For example, they may not view their traumatic experiences as "bad enough" to be considered trauma, their high guilt and shame about the trauma may make them feel they don't deserve to get relief from PTSD, or they may want to continue avoiding trauma-related situations and memories because they are painful. For these more hesitant clients, I often ask, "All things being equal, would you prefer to not have PTSD than to have PTSD?" I find that many ambivalent clients will answer "yes" to this question so that we can at least include reducing PTSD as a potential, if not definite, treatment goal. In all cases, but particularly with clients who are quite hesitant about treating their PTSD, it is important to emphasize that the list of treatment goals is not set in stone and that they get to decide which quality-of-life targets they want to address as treatment progresses. If they absolutely do not want to include reducing PTSD as a potential treatment goal, that is fine and there is no use in becoming polarized about this during pretreatment. In general, when clients express ambivalence about treating PTSD during pretreatment, this indicates that it will be important to further assess their concerns, and when PTSD truly is interfering with achieving the client's goals, work to build motivation to treat it as Stage 1 treatment continues (see Chapter 5).

Orienting to DBT PE

Once clients have been oriented to PTSD and have a clearer understanding of its impact on their lives, the conversation often naturally transitions into a discussion of how it can be treated. The goal of this discussion is not only to provide them with a general understanding of how PTSD is treated via DBT PE but also to build hope that their PTSD can be effectively treated. In addition, rather than framing treating PTSD as a "we'll talk about that later" issue, it is important to make completing DBT PE an explicit part of the treatment plan that is discussed during pretreatment. Indeed, in many cases, it is appropriate to frame treating PTSD as a "we will do this" issue and organize the entire treatment plan around the goal of being able to do so as soon as possible.

General Handout 4 (What Is DBT PE?) provides clients with a basic description of the rationale, procedures, and effectiveness of DBT PE. You can have clients read this handout before, during, and/or after orienting them to DBT PE in session. This initial orientation discussion is typically less detailed than the rationales that will eventually be provided during DBT PE. For now, the goal is to provide clients with enough information that they have a general understanding of how and why the treatment works (see Table 3.1 for a list of key points).

TABLE 3.1. Key Points in Orienting to the DBT PE Protocol in Pretreatment

1. Avoidance is a primary factor that maintains PTSD, including avoidance of trauma-related emotions, thoughts, and situations.

2. Although avoidance works in the short run to reduce distress, in the long run it maintains PTSD by preventing corrective learning.

3. DBT PE works by gradually approaching trauma memories and situations so that you can learn that they are safe and can be tolerated, which will make them less distressing.

4. DBT PE uses *in vivo* exposure (approaching avoided but safe situations in real life) and imaginal exposure (repeatedly telling the story of the trauma out loud) followed by processing (talking about and evaluating trauma-related beliefs and emotions) to treat PTSD.

5. DBT PE, and exposure therapy more broadly, is effective in reducing PTSD and improving overall functioning for most clients.

Overall, this initial foray into discussing DBT PE with a new client is best viewed as an opportunity to provide a "soft sell" of the treatment. Ideally, this discussion will begin to pique clients' interest in the treatment without being overly demanding in a way that makes them less willing to consider doing DBT PE in the long run. Of note, whereas clients are required to commit to engaging in DBT before progressing to Stage 1, they do not have to commit to engaging in DBT PE. Although some clients are clearly committed to receiving DBT PE from the beginning of treatment, for others this is a decision that is made over the course of Stage 1 treatment. Thus, no additional commitments beyond those required in standard DBT are needed before transitioning from pretreatment to Stage 1.

Case Example: Orienting to DBT PE in Pretreatment

Erica was a 52-year-old woman with PTSD and BPD who had experienced severe physical abuse and traumatic invalidation by her mother throughout her childhood, which led her to begin attempting suicide, self-injuring, using drugs, and shoplifting in her adolescence. She was also raped at age 23 by a coworker and physically abused by a boyfriend during their 10-year relationship, which had ended 2 years earlier. Erica sought treatment for chronic depression, constant suicidal thoughts, frequent NSSI (cutting, hitting herself), and difficulty managing anger. At intake, she was unemployed, receiving psychiatric disability benefits, and living in her car. The transcript below is from the third DBT pretreatment session. Erica had been given the *What Is DBT PE?* handout to read for homework so that she would be prepared to talk about the treatment in this session.

THERAPIST: I wanted to talk about the handout I gave you on DBT PE. Did you have any questions about what you read?

ERICA: So, I read it and the main things I had questions about were the *in vivo* exposure and imaginal exposure. Can you explain those to me?

THERAPIST: Yes, definitely. Those are two of the core treatment strategies of DBT PE. The main idea behind exposure therapy for PTSD is that we are trying to change the thing that is keeping it going, which is that people are avoiding things that remind them of their trauma.

ERICA: Oh yeah, that's right.

THERAPIST: Which makes sense, right? Thinking about your trauma or being near things that remind you of it is likely to be distressing, which is why people try to avoid them.

ERICA: Yes.

THERAPIST: For example, what happens when you see something that reminds you of your trauma and then you avoid it or walk away from it?

ERICA: I feel better.

THERAPIST: Yes, exactly. Avoidance works in the short run to reduce distress. However, the problem is that avoidance keeps PTSD around in the long run because it prevents people from learning anything new about the things they are avoiding.

ERICA: OK.

THERAPIST: What is something that you're avoiding because it reminds you of traumas you have experienced?

ERICA: I avoid being in small, enclosed spaces, especially if they have doors that lock, like public bathrooms. My mom used to lock me in my closet so I get panicky whenever I'm in a small space because it makes me afraid I won't be able to get out.

THERAPIST: That's a great example, and it makes a lot of sense why you would be afraid of small spaces given that history. So, let's say you avoid going into small spaces completely because you assume that you will get trapped in them. If you always avoid small spaces, then you won't have a chance to learn that in fact you don't get trapped and you are able to get out.

ERICA: But see, I'm afraid that's not going to happen and I'll end up getting stuck.

THERAPIST: Yes, and I can understand why. At the same time, those beliefs are part of what keeps PTSD going because they make you want to avoid things that may not actually be dangerous.

ERICA: OK.

THERAPIST: The idea behind exposure therapy is that you have to stop avoiding things that make you distressed so that you can learn something new about them, and *in vivo* exposure is one way to do that. *In vivo* means "in life" and involves putting you in contact with things in the world, like people, places, objects, and smells that bring up difficult emotions but that are not actually harmful. Just to be clear, I would never have you do *in vivo* exposure to anything that was unsafe. The goal is to have you approach things that remind you of your trauma over and over until you learn that they are not harmful and they no longer make you very distressed.

ERICA: You're not going to make me talk to my mom, are you?

THERAPIST: In general, I'm not going to make you do anything. You will choose what you want to do exposure to. And there may be some things that are wise for you to avoid, and your mom may be one of those things. Or you may decide that it's important to you to be able to talk to her. That will be up to you.

ERICA: OK, good.

THERAPIST: Great, so then let's talk about the imaginal exposure. Another thing that happens for people with PTSD is they not only avoid things in the world that remind them of their trauma but they also avoid their own thoughts and memories about past trauma.

ERICA: I definitely do that.

THERAPIST: Yes, everyone with PTSD does and it makes total sense why you would. The problem is that when you avoid thinking about your trauma, you never have a chance to process what happened to you and it continues to cause you a lot of distress. So, imaginal exposure helps you to process specific traumatic events by having you describe them out loud repeatedly in a very structured way that is under your control. After that, we will talk about the emotions and beliefs that this brings up for you and help you to get a new perspective on what happened.

ERICA: That sounds really hard!

THERAPIST: Oh, absolutely, it is really hard! It's probably one of the scariest things you could think of doing. However, it's an incredibly effective way to treat PTSD. About 70% of people who complete DBT PE experience a significant improvement in their PTSD.

ERICA: What if I can't remember things? Because I can remember some things, but some things I can't remember at all.

THERAPIST: It's really common for people to have gaps in their memories and to be unclear on some of the details. When people spend a lot of time and energy trying not to think about their trauma, those memories often get foggier.

ERICA: That's true for me.

THERAPIST: And if you allow yourself to think about it, it also makes sense that you may start to remember some of those details. Often what happens when people do imaginal exposure is that they remember more. And it's also totally fine if you don't, the treatment will still work.

ERICA: OK.

THERAPIST: So that's a quick overview of *in vivo* and imaginal exposure and how they work. Does that answer your questions?

ERICA: It does. I just think this is going to probably be the hardest thing I've ever done.

THERAPIST: It is going to be hard and it is going to be totally worthwhile.

ERICA: Yeah, it sounds like it's going to be really beneficial. But I can tell you I'm not looking forward to it at all.

THERAPIST: Of course not, I wouldn't be either if I were you. It's kind of like the saying "no pain, no gain," right? You have to know that there's going to be gain, and I'm telling you there is immense gain in this for you. But to get those gains you have to be willing to do this difficult treatment that will be painful in the short run and will improve your life in the long run.

ERICA: Well, maybe I had to get to be at this point in my life for this to work. I've done a lot of therapy in my life, but when I would get to those areas of remembering the traumas, I stopped. I need somebody to really be there and to say, "You can do this."

THERAPIST: I will be here to help you through this every step of the way. And I really believe you're going to be able to do this.

CASE EXAMPLE DISCUSSION

This example demonstrates how to provide a high-level orientation to the rationale and procedures of DBT PE during the pretreatment phase of DBT. This is not intended to be a script that you must follow, but rather to provide an example of how to discuss the key points listed

in Table 3.1 in a conversational and interactive manner. As this example illustrates, it is important to use language that is clear and understandable and to assess the client's comprehension
of the information being conveyed. Also, it is always useful to elicit client-relevant examples of
important constructs to help the client apply the information to their own experience. In this
example, Erica reported efforts to avoid small spaces, and this example was used to illustrate
the rationale for *in vivo* exposure.

Nearly all clients react to the initial description of DBT PE with fear and at least some
degree of ambivalence about the treatment. Erica was particularly worried about the difficulty
of the imaginal exposure and thought that overall DBT PE sounded like it would be incredibly
hard. As illustrated in this example, it is important that you both validate the difficulty of the
treatment and convey confidence in its effectiveness and the client's ability to do it. Therapists
who appear hesitant or anxious when discussing DBT PE are likely to create (more) hesitant
and anxious clients. Starting in pretreatment, it is therefore critical to use a matter-of-fact and
confident style when discussing the treatment that conveys that it is perfectly reasonable (and
perhaps expected) that clients will complete DBT PE as part of their treatment. As was done
here, it can also be helpful to provide specific data on the treatment's effectiveness in reducing
PTSD to build hope that it is quite likely to be beneficial. Consistent with a "soft-sell" approach,
it is typical to use more subtle persuasion techniques at this stage. This was done in this example
by repeatedly highlighting the benefits of the treatment without making any requests that Erica
commit to doing it.

During and after providing this initial orientation, it is also important to begin addressing
concerns the client may have about DBT PE in order to build motivation to do the treatment.
In this example, Erica expressed concern about whether she would be forced to contact her
mother, the perpetrator of her childhood trauma. In general, clients often assume that we are
going to force or badger them into doing exposure tasks. As was done in this example, it is often
useful to respond to these types of concerns by emphasizing that the selection of exposure tasks
is under the control of the client and that exposure will only be used to address things that
the client finds important. Erica also expressed concern about her inability to remember some
details of her past trauma, which was addressed by normalizing this experience, providing some
didactic information about the effects of chronic thought suppression on memory, and reassuring her that the treatment can still be effective even if she has gaps in her memories. In general,
responding to clients' concerns with validation, education, and cheerleading is often effective in
building motivation to do DBT PE and is discussed in more detail in Chapter 5. Overall, many
DBT strategies were utilized throughout this conversation to engage the client and increase her
motivation for treatment, including both acceptance- and change-based strategies and dialectical statements.

Clarifying the Contingencies for PTSD Treatment

Contingency clarification is typically used in DBT to highlight the "if–then" relationships
between clients' behaviors and relevant outcomes with the goal of increasing the likelihood of
adaptive behavior. In particular, if clients are aware of and able to predict the negative effects of
their problematic behaviors, then they may be more likely to choose adaptive behaviors instead.
In the present context, contingency clarification is used to highlight the problem behaviors
that, if not changed, will prevent the client from being able to receive DBT PE. I often begin
this discussion by reviewing the DBT target hierarchy (discussed in detail in Chapter 4), which

specifies that life-threatening behaviors must be addressed first, followed by therapy-interfering behaviors and behaviors that interfere with having a reasonable quality of life. Within this hierarchy, PTSD is viewed as a quality-of-life-interfering behavior that cannot be addressed until life-threatening and therapy-interfering behaviors are sufficiently controlled. Thus, the contingency to be clarified is *if* you stop life-threatening and serious therapy-interfering behaviors, *then* you will be able to receive treatment for your PTSD. In general, the goal is to establish receiving DBT PE as contingent upon positive behavior change.

It is also important to orient clients to the specific readiness criterion (discussed in detail in Chapter 6) that they must achieve a period of abstinence (at least 2 months in outpatient settings and 1 month in intensive or residential treatment settings) from all forms of suicidal and nonsuicidal self-injury before they can begin DBT PE. The rationale for clarifying this specific contingency during pretreatment is that it very often has the effect of increasing clients' motivation to quickly achieve control over life-threatening behaviors in order to be able to receive treatment for a problem (PTSD) they view as important. In other words, for most clients, DBT PE functions as a reinforcer for stopping life-threatening behaviors. However, the ability of any consequence to motivate behavior change is largely dependent on how much the person wants to receive the promised outcome. For clients who are less or perhaps not at all interested in treating their PTSD, it is still important to orient them to this readiness criterion even though it may not function as a reinforcer. For these clients it may also be useful to emphasize that they do not have to do DBT PE in order to mitigate against the possibility that they may continue to engage in life-threatening behaviors to avoid having to treat their PTSD.

Case Example: Clarifying the Contingencies for PTSD Treatment

The following transcript picks up from the point at which the earlier one left off when Erica had begun to express interest in and positive expectancies for DBT PE. Once this initial motivation to do DBT PE was in place, the therapist then moved into describing what she was going to need to do to be able to receive the treatment.

THERAPIST: From what you've told me so far, it really sounds like PTSD and the traumas you have experienced starting as a child are driving a lot of the problems in your life. Do you agree?

ERICA: Yes, this trauma stuff, it's why I've been so stuck in my life. Because when I would remember things, oh my gosh, that's when I'm a different person.

THERAPIST: So, I think it's going to be really critical that we treat your PTSD this year, don't you?

ERICA: Yes, I do.

THERAPIST: And I would love to treat your PTSD with you. I have every reason to think we can work together effectively and totally improve your life.

ERICA: Me too.

THERAPIST: But in order for us to be able to treat your PTSD, you're going to have to stop trying to kill yourself and self-injuring first.

ERICA: OK.

THERAPIST: Remember how I told you about the DBT target hierarchy?

ERICA: I think so.

THERAPIST: Well, the number one priority in DBT is to reduce suicidal behavior and self-injury. Basically, we can't focus on anything else until you are safe from imminent harm.

ERICA: Right.

THERAPIST: After life-threatening behaviors, the next priority is to reduce any behaviors that interfere with you engaging in therapy. The third priority is to target any problems that are significantly reducing your quality of life. PTSD falls into this last category, which means we can't treat it until life-threatening behaviors and therapy-interfering behaviors are under control. What do you think about that?

ERICA: That seems reasonable.

THERAPIST: Good. There is one specific requirement you should know about, which is that we can't treat your PTSD until you have gone at least 2 months without attempting suicide or self-injuring. So, the sooner you take suicide and self-injury off the table, the sooner we'll be able to treat your PTSD.

ERICA: You know what? You're probably not going to believe this, but I think I can stop the self-injury.

THERAPIST: You do?

ERICA: Because I don't do it as much as I used to.

THERAPIST: OK.

ERICA: Like yesterday, I was thinking I'm just getting so old and I'm really going to hurt myself. And I don't want this extra scarring.

THERAPIST: That makes sense.

ERICA: I think I can stop the self-injury. I think I can do that.

THERAPIST: That's fantastic! But why would you want to stop? It seems like it would be a hard thing to give up.

ERICA: It's important to me to not have scars, and it's not working the same way. I hit myself a lot because I'm so angry, you know? But I don't want to do it. It's almost like I am tired of it, it's not effective anymore. I think I can stop it, I really do.

THERAPIST: I love this! I mean, I love the fact that self-injury is not really working for you anymore because that's going to make it not as hard to give up.

ERICA: That's what I mean, I think I can stop that. But the suicidal part is going to be harder. Whatever that little thread to stay alive is, I worry about that thread.

THERAPIST: Yes, we've got to make sure that stays solid and we've got to turn it into a rope.

ERICA: I'm worried I'm not going to be able to do all this in a year of treatment. I've got so much trauma to cover!

THERAPIST: Well, if you keep self-injuring and trying to kill yourself, we may not have enough time to treat your PTSD. But if you stop those behaviors quickly, then we will.

ERICA: Right, that's why I need to take the harmful behavior off the table, because that's going to open up time for me to work on my trauma

THERAPIST: Exactly. That's going to give us space to treat your PTSD, which is going to be really important for you to be able to have the life you want to have.

ERICA: I agree.

CASE EXAMPLE DISCUSSION

This case example illustrates the process of clarifying the "if–then" relationship between clients' problem behaviors and their ability to receive DBT PE. In particular, it is important for clients to understand that *if* they continue to engage in life-threatening or serious therapy-interfering behaviors, *then* they will not be able to receive DBT PE. The goal is to increase the likelihood of adaptive behavior by increasing the client's awareness of the contingencies operating in therapy. In Erica's case, learning that she would not be able to receive DBT PE until she stopped engaging in life-threatening behaviors clearly had the effect of increasing her motivation to quickly gain control over these behaviors. This is true for most clients with PTSD and therefore establishing this contingency during pretreatment has proven to be a critical strategy for helping clients to rapidly achieve behavioral control—the primary goal of Stage 1.

This case example also illustrates a variety of additional strategies intended to build motivation to stop life-threatening behaviors. One strategy is called the "yes set" technique, which is often used in sales and is designed to get a person to agree with you for several statements so that it becomes more difficult for them to disagree with the next thing you say. In this example, Erica agreed with the therapist three times before she was presented with the more difficult contingency about stopping suicidal and self-injurious behaviors in order to receive DBT PE. Building up this "yes" momentum may make it easier for clients to agree to make these hard but necessary behavior changes. In addition, the foot-in-the-door technique was used to first get her buy-in to the more vague goals outlined by the target hierarchy before presenting her with the specific requirement of 2 months of abstinence from all life-threatening behaviors. Notably, prior to this session Erica had been unwilling to commit to stay alive for longer than a month. However, after this discussion she committed to stay alive and not self-injure for the entire year of treatment. As this example illustrates, linking these standard DBT commitments to being able to treat PTSD is often quite effective in increasing motivation to stop these higher-priority behaviors.

Concluding Comments

Although treatment doesn't technically start until Stage 1 begins, the pretreatment phase is critical in setting the stage for treatment, including both DBT and DBT PE. Ideally, by the end of pretreatment, PTSD will be established as an important treatment goal, clients will have hope that they can receive an effective treatment for PTSD as part of DBT, and it will be clear that this is contingent on achieving control over life-threatening and other higher-priority behaviors.

CHAPTER 4

Achieving Safety, Stability, and Skills in Stage 1

Once the pretreatment goals of commitment and orientation have been completed, active treatment begins with Stage 1 DBT focused on decreasing life-threatening and other problematic behaviors by increasing the use of skills. Helping clients to achieve behavioral control is DBT's wheelhouse as extensive research indicates that Stage 1 DBT is highly effective in reducing the acute behaviors of high-risk and multiproblem clients. However, the goal of behavioral control is not simply behavioral control. Rather, it is *achieving behavioral control in order to be able to treat the core problems causing emotional misery*. For clients with PTSD, achieving behavioral control is specifically in the service of being able to engage in treatment for PTSD that will lead to resolution of trauma-related suffering. Thus, achieving safety and behavioral stability is viewed as a necessary but unlikely a sufficient step toward building a life worth living. Adopting this mindset about Stage 1 DBT means that therapists must no longer view PTSD as a "maybe" or "not me" problem to be addressed in a faraway second stage of treatment. Instead, Stage 1 DBT is delivered as briefly and efficiently as possible to minimize the delay until PTSD can be treated.

I assume that readers are already familiar with standard Stage 1 DBT, which is delivered without adaptation according to the treatment manuals (Linehan, 1993, 2015). In this chapter, I focus primarily on how this stage of treatment is applied to help clients with PTSD prepare for DBT PE. To provide a framework for this work, I first discuss several dialectical tensions that underlie this stage of treatment with clients with PTSD before illustrating how Stage 1 targets are selected and addressed using DBT's core problem-solving strategies.

Common Dialectical Tensions in Stage 1

For clients with PTSD, three common dialectical tensions arise during Stage 1 DBT related to the degree to which trauma-related cues are avoided versus approached both in and outside of therapy sessions. Clients often begin treatment at the extreme avoidance end of these dialectics and progress during Stage 1 is evidenced by an increasing ability to intentionally incorporate aspects of the opposing approach pole into their behavioral repertoire.

Emotional Avoidance versus Emotional Exposure

The primary dialectic in Stage 1 treatment with clients with PTSD involves finding an effective balance between the extremes of emotional avoidance and emotional exposure. We do not want clients to always push emotions away or distract from them, nor do we want them to experience unrelenting emotional pain without any opportunity for escape. Instead, the goal is to help clients flexibly meet the demands of specific situations by skillfully utilizing both emotional avoidance and emotional exposure strategies when needed. Overall, Stage 1 treatment can be conceptualized as helping clients to achieve enough mastery over emotional experiencing to be able to effectively complete DBT PE in Stage 2.

Most clients begin Stage 1 on the extreme emotional avoidance end of this dialectic. Their lives are typically structured to minimize exposure to emotion-eliciting events by, for example, limiting the activities they engage in, not allowing themselves to talk or think about painful events, and reducing contact with people likely to cue emotional responses. However, these chronic efforts to avoid emotions are bound to fail and, when they do, clients rapidly and uncontrollably swing to the other end of this dialectic and become overwhelmed by intense emotions. Although these extreme emotions sometimes last for long periods of time, often clients stay on the emotional exposure end of the pole only briefly before they engage in maladaptive behaviors to escape from these emotions and return to their default position of emotional avoidance. Indeed, the primary target behaviors of Stage 1 can often be conceptualized as effective but maladaptive emotional avoidance strategies. Given this, Stage 1 typically begins by teaching clients how to replace problematic emotional avoidance strategies with skillful ways of avoiding emotions, such as DBT's crisis survival skills.

Stage 1 treatment, however, cannot only focus on increasing skillful emotional avoidance. Throughout Stage 1, you must actively work to help clients learn how to experience emotions effectively and without immediately avoiding. I often use a metaphor with clients of Stage 1 DBT being like training for a marathon. DBT PE is the marathon, as it requires clients to experience intense and painful emotions for extended periods of time without avoiding. In Stage 1, clients must strengthen their muscles and build their endurance by engaging in training runs of increasing lengths. Many clients begin Stage 1 treatment with the ability to experience an emotion for only a few seconds before switching to avoidance. Over the course of Stage 1, the length of time that clients can experience an emotion without avoiding will need to increase significantly for the formal exposure strategies of DBT PE to be effective.

Present Focus versus Past Focus

A second dialectical tension in Stage 1 with clients with PTSD is the degree to which treatment focuses on present problems in the client's life versus past traumatic events that may have caused these problems to develop. In general, Stage 1 DBT is a present-focused treatment that aims to help clients solve problems by addressing the current factors that maintain these problems—not by discussing their etiology. This present-focused approach can be particularly hard to maintain with clients with PTSD for whom memories of past trauma are frequently intruding in the present and are functionally related to life-threatening and other maladaptive behaviors. For example, intrusive PTSD symptoms are often on the chain of events leading to Stage 1 target behaviors. However, these trauma-related antecedents of behavioral dyscontrol are addressed in the same way as any other type of prompting event—by teaching clients skills to cope with them more effectively—a task that can be accomplished without discussing the details of the trauma itself. At the same time, past trauma is not ignored if the client brings it up. Rather, the degree to which you respond by redirecting to the present versus allowing the client to focus on the past (and for how long) will vary depending on the client's ability to cope effectively with these discussions. The overarching principle is that we do not want clients focusing on past trauma at a level of detail or intensity that exceeds their capability to effectively manage the painful emotions this will elicit.

At the beginning of Stage 1, clients typically have little to no desire to talk about the details of past trauma due to their high levels of shame and tendency to avoid trauma-related thoughts and emotions. In other words, the very things that are maintaining their PTSD often function to keep them silent about the traumas they have suffered. In most cases, this desire to avoid is adaptive (although the strategies used to avoid often are not), as clients do not yet possess the skills necessary to approach trauma cues without loss of behavioral control. For these clients, you can validate the wisdom of waiting to discuss trauma in detail until they gain the behavioral skills necessary to do so safely. At the same time, it is important to be clear that avoiding discussing trauma is a temporary strategy that, over time, will need to shift to approaching trauma if they are going to get relief from their PTSD.

In contrast, some clients enter Stage 1 at the approach end of this dialectic and express a clear desire to talk about their traumas in detail. For these clients, attempting to completely block discussions of past trauma is likely to be both invalidating and unrealistic. Moreover, adopting a rigid stance that any discussion of past trauma must be avoided in Stage 1 has the potential to reinforce problematic beliefs that maintain PTSD, such as that trauma memories are dangerous and must be hidden from others. For clients who view it as important to talk about past trauma, you might initially respond by validating why this is understandable and orienting clients to the stage model of treatment. It is important that you reassure clients that you want to hear about the details of past trauma, but not until they have the skills to effectively manage the emotions likely to result from such a discussion. In the meantime, you and the client can collaboratively decide whether to engage in brief discussions about past trauma, for what purposes, and at what level of detail.

It is also important to note that some clients vacillate between these extremes, at times plunging into talking about their traumas in detail, getting overwhelmed, and then retreating to the avoidance end of the pole. In general, the goal is to help clients find an effective middle path between these two extremes. This includes being able to fluidly and intentionally shift back and forth from present to past (e.g., thinking about past trauma for a period of time and then redirecting attention back to the present), as well as finding a synthesis between these two approaches (e.g., remaining grounded in the present while focusing on past trauma). To that end, as Stage 1 treatment progresses you may strategically begin to ask clients to share some information about their traumatic experiences or allow clients who naturally bring up trauma to continue to discuss it for a period of time. The goal is to allow clients to dip their toes in the water of trauma-focused discussions without fully immersing themselves in imaginal exposure. Beginning to discuss trauma in some amount of detail is often a useful strategy to assess clients' readiness for DBT PE, increase their confidence in their ability to do the treatment, and make the transition to the heavily past-focused strategies of Stage 2 less jarring.

Accept PTSD versus Change PTSD

A final dialectical tension in Stage 1 treatment with clients with PTSD relates to the degree to which acceptance versus change strategies are used to address PTSD and other painful trauma sequelae. Given that detailed trauma processing does not occur until Stage 2, the primary focus of Stage 1 is on learning to accept and cope effectively with PTSD without treating the underlying disorder. Similar to people with chronic medical conditions, such as diabetes, clients in Stage 1 must learn how to live with PTSD while reducing the harm that it causes. For example, clients are taught skills to cope effectively with flashbacks, distract from intrusive trauma memories, reduce the intensity of physiological reactions to trauma cues, and increase effective expression of anger. However, PTSD is difficult to accept not only because it is incredibly painful but also because it is treatable. Once clients know that they don't have to live forever with PTSD, some will want to move more rapidly than would be effective into targeted PTSD treatment. In these cases, working to accept and tolerate these painful symptoms until they can be safely and effectively treated is a particularly challenging task.

At the same time, you should help clients to change specific PTSD symptoms during Stage 1 that can be treated without trauma processing, such as reducing nightmares and improving sleep. In addition, other trauma sequelae, such as dissociation, intense shame, and interpersonal problems, can often be improved but not eliminated in Stage 1. The goal is to treat whatever can be treated while PTSD remains active and to reduce the intensity of trauma-related problems to levels that are both more tolerable and less likely to interfere with later DBT PE. However, for many problems that are functionally related to PTSD and past trauma, there is a limit to how much they can improve until PTSD is treated. For example, although clients typically develop skills to better control dissociation so that it is no longer severely impairing, they often continue to experience low to moderate levels of dissociation throughout Stage 1. Thus, the task becomes finding a balance between accepting PTSD and other trauma-related problems that cannot be fully treated during Stage 1 and changing what can be treated without engaging in detailed trauma processing.

Treatment Targets

When working with clients with PTSD and a Stage 1 level of disorder, you face the difficult task of determining which problems should be addressed (and in what order) prior to treating PTSD. To help with this task, Stage 1 DBT structures individual therapy sessions in terms of a hierarchy of primary behavioral targets. Within this general target hierarchy, the specific behaviors that are addressed vary for each client depending on the problems they exhibit, the interrelationships among these problems, and the client's treatment goals. The target selection process in Stage 1 is therefore both idiographic and principle driven, and decisions about which targets to address when are made collaboratively based on continuous assessment of the client's progress and goals.

Primary Behavioral Targets

Individual sessions in Stage 1 DBT are organized based on a hierarchy that specifies the following order of targets: (1) decreasing life-threatening behaviors (i.e., behaviors that cause an immediate risk to life and/or physical injury), (2) decreasing therapy-interfering behaviors (i.e., behaviors that interfere with the client's ability to engage in or receive effective therapy), and (3) decreasing quality-of-life-interfering behaviors (i.e., behaviors that cause serious distress and impairment that significantly reduce the client's quality of life). The rationale for this hierarchy is that clients must be alive and reasonably engaged in therapy before problems contributing to a poor quality of life can be addressed effectively. Throughout this process, clients are taught behavioral skills to help them decrease these primary behavioral targets and remediate key areas of skills deficits. Table 4.1 includes common examples of the types of problems exhibited by Stage 1 clients with PTSD in each target domain.

Selecting Primary Targets for Clients with PTSD

For clients with PTSD, the target selection process in Stage 1 uses the general framework of the DBT target hierarchy while also taking into account the behaviors and skills deficits that, if not addressed, are likely to reduce the effectiveness of DBT PE in Stage 2. The specific criteria that are used to determine readiness to start DBT PE are described in detail in Chapter 6—for now, it is important to understand the principles underlying the Stage 1 target selection process.

TABLE 4.1. Common Primary Targets in Stage 1 DBT with Clients with PTSD

1. Life-threatening behaviors

- Suicide attempts (i.e., intentional self-injury with suicidal intent)
- Suicide crisis behaviors (i.e., behaviors indicative of acute suicide risk, such as suicide planning, preparation, rehearsals, intent, and communication)
- Nonsuicidal self-injury (i.e., intentional self-injury without suicidal intent)

2. Therapy-interfering behaviors

- Nonattentive behaviors (e.g., not attending sessions or dropping out; distraction, dissociation, falling asleep, intoxication during sessions)
- Noncollaborative behaviors (e.g., hostility, argumentativeness, nonresponsiveness, lying during sessions)
- Noncompliant behaviors (e.g., not completing homework, not keeping commitments, refusal to engage in treatment tasks or agree to treatment goals)

3. Decreasing quality-of-life-interfering behaviors

- PTSD and trauma sequelae (e.g., dissociation, self-hatred, intense shame, sexual problems)
- Other mental disorders (e.g., mood, anxiety, eating, substance use, dissociative, and personality disorders)
- Impulsive, self-damaging behaviors (e.g., substance use, binge eating, unsafe sexual behavior, gambling, reckless driving, shoplifting)
- Dysfunctional interpersonal behaviors (e.g., extreme rejection sensitivity, isolation, ending relationships abruptly, involvement with abusive partners, pervasive mistrust, aggressiveness)
- Employment- or school-related problems (e.g., getting fired, frequent conflict with coworkers, unemployment, detentions and suspensions, poor grades, nonattendance)
- Serious financial problems (e.g., inability to afford basic needs of self or family, excessive spending, extreme debt, bankruptcy, inability to pay for treatment)
- Housing instability (e.g., homelessness, living in shelters or transitional housing, moving repeatedly, frequent evictions)
- Serious medical conditions (e.g., chronic pain, fibromyalgia, chronic fatigue, STIs/STDs)
- Mental health service use problems (e.g., repeated psychiatric hospitalizations and ER visits, frequent provider changes, demanding or receiving inappropriate treatments)

Note. STIs/STDs, sexually transmitted infections/sexually transmitted diseases; ER, emergency room.

In the DBT target hierarchy, PTSD is considered a quality-of-life-interfering behavior that cannot be addressed until the higher-priority targets of life-threatening and serious therapy-interfering behaviors have decreased. In addition, within the quality-of-life domain there may be other problems that are a higher priority than PTSD. According to the DBT manual, quality-of-life-interfering behaviors should be prioritized as follows: (1) behaviors causing immediate crises (e.g., homelessness, ongoing abuse), (2) easy-to-change over difficult-to-change behaviors (e.g., problems that can be solved reasonably quickly), and (3) behaviors functionally related to higher-order targets (e.g., behaviors that commonly precede life-threatening behaviors). Using these guidelines, PTSD may be considered a reasonably easy-to-change problem (given that DBT PE usually lasts 3–4 months) and it is almost always functionally related to higher-priority targets. Given this, PTSD is likely to be among the most important quality-of-life targets for most clients with this diagnosis. However, whereas therapists dictate that life-threatening and therapy-interfering behaviors must be addressed before anything else, the client's goals and preferences are given priority when deciding which quality-of-life problems to target. Therefore, although we offer guidance about which quality-of-life problems seem most important to address, these decisions are ultimately made by clients.

Case Example: Target Selection

Natalie was a 30-year-old woman with PTSD related to child sexual abuse by her father, witnessing domestic violence while growing up, and a rape as an adolescent by a male peer. She also met criteria for major depressive disorder, social anxiety disorder, binge eating disorder, and BPD. Natalie sought treatment due to being "very irritable, I can't seem to get emotions under control, and will snap without warning." Her problems regulating anger began when she was being sexually abused and led to frequent aggression toward peers and adults in elementary and middle school. At intake, she reported regularly getting angry at her girlfriend with whom she had frequent verbal conflicts that at times escalated to physical aggression. She also had episodes of "road rage" in which she would follow drivers who made her angry and cut them off while driving at high speeds.

At intake, Natalie was engaging in NSSI by cutting her arms and legs two to three times per month, a behavior that had started when she was 12. She had also attempted suicide three times in her life, all by overdose, with the first attempt occurring at age 16. Her most recent suicide attempt had occurred 1 month prior to treatment in the context of a fight with her girlfriend and had resulted in psychiatric hospitalization. She had been psychiatrically hospitalized five other times since age 16 due to suicidal and self-injurious behaviors, as well as threatening to kill herself. Natalie had worked briefly in her early 20s but was currently unemployed and experiencing considerable financial hardship. She lived with her girlfriend but otherwise had no close friends and rarely left the house or interacted with anyone besides her mother. Her sleep was very disrupted, which resulted in extreme fatigue that often made it difficult for her to concentrate during therapy sessions. In addition, she missed about one out of every three sessions and rarely completed homework assignments outside of session. Natalie's target hierarchy is shown in Table 4.2.

As with most Stage 1 clients, Natalie had multiple problems in each of DBT's three target domains. Within each domain, these behaviors are ordered in terms of priority. For life-threatening behaviors, priorities were based on the potential lethality of the behavior, whereas therapy-interfering behaviors were prioritized based on the degree to which they were likely

TABLE 4.2. Natalie's Target Hierarchy

I. Life-threatening behaviors

1. Recent and repeated suicide attempts (three lifetime, most recent 1 month ago)
2. Nonsuicidal self-injury (cutting arms and legs two to three times/month)
3. Suicide communication (telling others she is going to kill herself)

II. Therapy-interfering behaviors

1. Inconsistent attendance
2. Fatigue during sessions
3. Homework noncompletion

III. Quality-of-life-interfering behaviors

1. Pervasive emotion dysregulation (particularly anger)
2. Verbal and physical aggression
3. PTSD
4. Impulsive, self-damaging behaviors (binge eating, reckless driving)
5. Depression
6. Social anxiety
7. Unemployment and financial hardship
8. Repeated psychiatric hospitalizations

to make treatment ineffective. Quality-of-life problems were prioritized in terms of Natalie's treatment goals, the severity of distress and impairment they were causing, and whether they would be likely to interfere with DBT PE. In Natalie's case, her pervasive anger and verbal and physical aggression took priority over PTSD because they (1) were her primary treatment goals, (2) caused frequent crises (e.g., threats of being kicked out of her house), (3) often preceded episodes of life-threatening behavior, and (4) were likely to interfere with DBT PE (e.g., if anger prevented her from experiencing other emotions, such as fear, guilt, and sadness). Natalie identified PTSD as her next most important problem given that she viewed many of the behaviors she struggled with (in all target domains) as stemming from her past trauma. Thus, she and her therapist believed that treating PTSD would be likely to improve many of the other quality-of-life problems she was experiencing.

Treatment Strategies

The target selection process provides a general road map of what needs to change during Stage 1, but how exactly are these targets addressed? The short and extraordinarily simplified answer is by doing DBT. DBT includes within it many strategies that are balanced across the paradigms of change, acceptance, and dialectics. For the present purposes, I focus on describing DBT's core problem-solving strategies of chain analysis and solution analysis, with a particular emphasis on how these core strategies are commonly applied to address the higher-priority targets of Stage 1 clients with PTSD.

Chain Analysis

The first step in the problem-solving process is to clearly define the target behavior and assess the factors that are maintaining it. In DBT, this is most often done by conducting a chain analysis, or a detailed assessment of the chain of internal and external events that led up to and followed a specific episode of a target behavior. Chain analyses can be conducted for any type of target behavior with the goal of identifying specific points of intervention (i.e., controlling variables) that, if altered, might prevent the behavior from occurring again.

Chain analyses typically include six elements. *Prompting events* precede the target behavior and are internal or external events that most clearly caused the behavior to occur. For people with PTSD, prompting events are often trauma related and frequently include specific PTSD symptoms (e.g., intrusive trauma memories) or exposure to a trauma-related cue (e.g., a person who resembles a perpetrator). *Vulnerability factors* are variables that increased the person's likelihood of responding to the prompting event with the target behavior and often explain why the same prompting event (e.g., interpersonal conflict) led to the target behavior (e.g., self-injury) on one day but not another. Generally speaking, vulnerability factors are things that occur within hours or days of the prompting event and are modifiable (e.g., being hungover) as opposed to distal and static (e.g., trauma history). For clients with PTSD, common vulnerability factors are poor sleep, high anxiety, and elevated arousal. The *links* between the prompting event and the target behavior are the final element of the "front end" of the chain (i.e., the things that occurred before the target behavior). These links may include emotions, thoughts, and behaviors (of oneself or others) and, for clients with PTSD, these links are often trauma related. For example, the prompting event often cues PTSD symptoms (e.g., flashbacks, dissociation) or other trauma-related emotions (e.g., fear, shame), thoughts (e.g., "I'm disgusting," "I'm unsafe"), and behaviors (e.g., fight, flight, or freeze responses).

The next element of the chain is the *target behavior* itself. This includes a behaviorally specific description of the type, severity, duration, and topography of the behavior. It is not enough, for example, to simply know that self-injury occurred. Instead, we must know what type of self-injury (e.g., burning), the method that was used (e.g., a cigarette), where on the body the injury was located (e.g., the upper leg), how much and for how long it occurred (e.g., twice over a period of 5 minutes), and how severe it was (e.g., the degree of tissue damage). These details are necessary to provide a comprehensive understanding of exactly what the behavior was and how it was enacted, which often provides useful information for intervention.

Finally, it is also critical to assess the "back end" of the chain (i.e., the things that occurred after the target behavior). *Short-term consequences* are the immediate aftereffects of the target behavior, which often increase the likelihood of the behavior occurring again. These may include internal events (e.g., changes in emotions, thoughts, and physical sensations) and external events (e.g., responses from people in the environment). For clients with PTSD, problem behaviors very often function to provide immediate relief from PTSD symptoms. For example, cutting may be used to stop dissociation, suicidal ideation may provide an escape from painful trauma-related memories, and substance use may function to reduce hyperarousal. In addition, target behaviors can have an interpersonal function. For example, many clients with PTSD struggle to ask for help because they do not believe they deserve to have their needs met. Target behaviors, such as suicidal and self-injurious behaviors, may at times serve a help-seeking function if they lead others to increase care and support, decrease demands, and/or give the person something they want.

Whereas the short-term consequences of target behaviors often include some positive (reinforcing) outcome, the *long-term consequences* of target behaviors are predominantly negative. A primary negative long-term consequence for clients with PTSD is that many of these target behaviors contribute to the maintenance of PTSD and trauma-related suffering in the long run. In particular, target behaviors very often function to avoid prolonged contact with trauma-related stimuli and this avoidance is a primary factor that maintains their PTSD over time. The long-term consequences of target behaviors also often include various psychosocial problems that increase instability and hardship in the client's life. For example, target behaviors often contribute to relationship ruptures, housing instability, financial hardship, repeated hospitalizations, and legal problems. These negative long-term consequences often lead clients to experience guilt, shame, and regret for engaging in the behavior, which often contributes to increasing self-hatred and self-loathing over time.

Case Example: Chain Analysis

This chain analysis was conducted in Natalie's eighth week of treatment. At the beginning of the session, review of Natalie's diary card indicated that she had self-injured and had high urges to kill herself (five out of five) on the same day. Natalie also told her therapist that she had spent 2 days in a psychiatric inpatient unit as a result of this episode. The following chain analysis was conducted to assess the episode of self-injury and high suicide urges, and the DBT strategies that were used during this chain are specified in parentheses. In addition, the complete chain analysis is illustrated in Figure 4.1 on page 55.

THERAPIST: Let's talk about last Thursday. What happened first, the self-injury or the high suicide urges? (*clarifying timeline*)

NATALIE: The self-injury.

THERAPIST: What time did the self-injury happen? (*clarifying timeline*)

NATALIE: It was probably about 8:30 at night.

THERAPIST: OK, so when did the thought of self-injury first enter your mind that day? (*beginning to assess for the prompting event*)

NATALIE: I don't really know what exactly happened. My girlfriend wasn't being nice and we were arguing. She was saying mean things like "get the hell out of my house" and I was threatening her back, saying she couldn't use my car to get to work anymore.

THERAPIST: OK, back me up to the beginning here. How did this fight start? (*clarifying details of prompting event*)

NATALIE: I had been at my mom's house all day and had come home to watch a movie with her. But when I got home she was asleep, which made me really irritated because it was early.

THERAPIST: What time was it? (*clarifying timeline*)

NATALIE: Around 8:00 P.M. And usually we stay up really late, like as late as 5:00 in the morning sometimes.

THERAPIST: What did you think and feel about the fact that she had gone to bed so early? (*assessing cognitions and emotions about prompting event*)

NATALIE: It made me feel hurt and like she didn't really love me. So, I tried to wake her up by jumping up and down on the bed. That's what she does to me when I don't feel well and am in bed, so I wanted to do it to her.

THERAPIST: OK, so it sounds like you interpreted her being asleep as meaning something negative about you and you wanted to get back at her for this. Do you still think that? (*validation level 2, identifying potential cognitive distortion to address in solution analysis*)

NATALIE: Yeah, I mean she would have stayed up if I really mattered to her.

THERAPIST: Hmm, we're going to have to check the facts about that in a bit. (*preview of solution analysis*) For now, though, tell me what happened next.

NATALIE: I was bouncing up and down on the bed to try to wake her up and after a little while she said, "You're f---ing rude!" and she got out of bed and went into the living room.

THERAPIST: Had self-injury come into your mind at this point yet? (*clarifying details*)

NATALIE: Not yet. I followed her in there and we were yelling at each other. That's when she threatened to kick me out of the house and I said she couldn't drive my car anymore.

THERAPIST: This conflict sounds more intense than usual. Was there something different on this day that made it worse? (*assessing potential vulnerability factors*)

NATALIE: I hadn't taken my medications for about 3 days, so I was just feeling really irritable.

THERAPIST: Oh no, that's a problem! Why hadn't you taken your medications? (*direct confrontation, identifying potential problem to address during solution analysis*)

NATALIE: I kept forgetting to take them before I went to bed and then I didn't want to get out of bed to take them because I was too tired.

THERAPIST: OK, we'll figure out what to do about that later. (*preview of solution analysis*) For now, let's get back to what happened on Thursday. So, you're yelling at each other and she threatened to kick you out of the house and you threatened her back about the car. Then what?

NATALIE: After she threatened to kick me out of the house, I got really mad and I hit her.

THERAPIST: Oh no! Why did you hit her in that moment? (*clarifying controlling variable*)

NATALIE: It reminded me of my dad who always used to threaten to throw my mom and me out on the street. I just didn't want her to have that kind of power over me.

THERAPIST: OK, so that was a trauma reminder. What sensations did you notice in your body in that moment right before you hit her? (*assessing links*)

NATALIE: I felt really hot and tense, and my heart was racing.

THERAPIST: OK, those sound like important warning signs that you are about to become physically aggressive. Where did you hit her? (*highlighting pattern, clarifying details*)

NATALIE: On her shoulder. I guess it was pretty hard because she said, "Ow, that hurt!" But it's like I didn't know what I was doing until I already did it.

THERAPIST: What happened after you hit her? Did your emotions or sensations change? (*assessing links*)

NATALIE: I felt even more angry, almost enraged. I felt like I was going to explode.

THERAPIST: So, hitting her actually made your anger worse. (*clarifying contingencies, increasing insight*)

NATALIE: Yeah, and then I also felt sad and upset that I hit her. I don't want to be a person who hits.

THERAPIST: Well, I'm glad to hear that. Were you feeling guilty? (*hypothesis testing*)

NATALIE: Very guilty.

THERAPIST: So, you're feeling enraged, sad, and guilty. It sounds like you were overflowing with emotions at that point. What happened next? (*validation level 2*)

NATALIE: I told her I was going to kill myself. She said she was going to call the police, and then I cut.

THERAPIST: Was it her saying she was going to call the police that made you want to cut? (*clarifying controlling variable*)

NATALIE: Yes, I just didn't want her to control me. So, I went to the kitchen to get the knives.

THERAPIST: As you were walking to the kitchen, did you have any thoughts about reasons not to cut? Or did you try at all to stop yourself from doing it? (*assessing potential problems for solution analysis*)

NATALIE: No, I just went straight to the kitchen and cut. It happened really fast after she said she was going to call the police, like maybe only a minute later.

THERAPIST: Was your girlfriend in the kitchen with you when you cut? (*clarifying details*)

NATALIE: No, she stayed in the living room.

THERAPIST: What did you do when you cut? (*getting details about the target behavior*)

NATALIE: I used a kitchen knife and made a bunch of little cuts on my upper arm, maybe 10. They were bleeding, but not that deep.

THERAPIST: What were you feeling after you cut? (*assessing short-term emotional consequence*)

NATALIE: Really bad.

THERAPIST: What does that mean? (*getting specificity about emotions*)

NATALIE: Sad, hopeless.

THERAPIST: Did it do anything positive for you? (*assessing potential reinforcers*)

NATALIE: My anger came down and I felt less like I was going to explode, but I actually felt worse overall.

THERAPIST: Well, that's good news! So, cutting is actually increasing your misery now. It seems like there's really no good reason for you to do it anymore. (*irreverence, clarifying contingencies, increasing insight*)

NATALIE: Yeah.

THERAPIST: After you cut, what were you thinking about? (*assessing short-term cognitive consequences*)

NATALIE: I was thinking about killing myself.

THERAPIST: Was this when your urges to kill yourself got to a five out of five? (*assessing details*)

NATALIE: Yes, the urges got worse after I cut. I just wanted to be dead.

THERAPIST: OK, well that's another reason to stop self-injuring. What were you thinking about doing to kill yourself? (*clarifying contingencies, assessing details*)

NATALIE: I was thinking about overdosing, but I couldn't because you had made me give my medications to my girlfriend to lock up.

THERAPIST: Thank goodness I did that! What happened next? (*irreverence, assessing details*)

NATALIE: Then my girlfriend came into the kitchen and started trying to coach me to use skills, like telling me to breathe and use ice and stuff, which was really annoying. I told her to leave me alone, but she wouldn't, so I got even more mad.

THERAPIST: Wait, let's back up for a second. What made you angry about her trying to help you use skills? (*clarifying details*)

NATALIE: I don't like being told what to do when I'm angry. It just makes me want to attack the person.

THERAPIST: It sounds like there were several points in this episode when you felt like she was trying to control you and this made you angry and want to do something destructive. It makes sense that you don't want to be controlled, I don't like being controlled either. However, we're going to have to find less destructive ways for you to respond when you are feeling controlled. So what happened next? (*highlighting patterns, validation level 5, direct confrontation, preview of solution analysis*)

NATALIE: I yelled, "Leave me alone or I'm going to hit you again!" Then I started to chase her. So she ran and locked herself in the bedroom.

THERAPIST: Oh my god, what a disaster! (*direct confrontation*)

NATALIE: I started crying and saying I was sorry. I kept begging her to open the door, but she was mad and she wouldn't come out. I told her I wanted to kill myself for hurting her. Then she told me if I put the knives away that she would come out. When I did, she unlocked the door and told me it was going to be OK and that we would work it out.

THERAPIST: Was she kind of soothing you at that point? (*assessing potentially reinforcing consequences*)

NATALIE: Yeah. I told her I was really scared because it was like I was in a zone or something and couldn't stop myself. I was really scared of losing control again and killing myself or hurting her.

THERAPIST: So how much time had passed by this point, from when you first got home at 8:00 P.M. until the fight was over? (*clarifying duration*)

NATALIE: I think about an hour.

THERAPIST: OK. And how did you end up in the hospital? (*details of long-term consequences*)

NATALIE: When I said I was scared I wasn't going to be able to control myself, she called my mom and they decided that I should go to the ER and I agreed. She drove me to the ER and my mom met us there. I told the social worker that I was afraid I was going to kill myself and that's how I ended up being hospitalized.

THERAPIST: Were you glad to be hospitalized? (*assessing potentially reinforcing consequences*)

NATALIE: Not really, I just wanted to be safe and I felt safe there. But being in the hospital isn't fun.

THERAPIST: Well, I'm glad to hear you didn't enjoy it. That seems like a good reason to prevent this type of behavior in the future. Were there any other negative consequences of this whole incident for you? (*clarifying contingencies, assessing long-term consequences*)

NATALIE: Yeah, I mean I put my girlfriend through a lot and this is really hard on her. I feel really ashamed about that. If this keeps happening, she may actually kick me out of the house.

THERAPIST: I agree that this must be putting quite a strain on your relationship. I imagine she could eventually burn out and ask you to leave if this continues. Also, a lot of the reason you get so angry like this is because of your PTSD, and we're not going to be able to treat it if these kinds of behaviors are still going on. So, let's get to work on figuring out how to prevent this from happening again. (*matter-of-fact, clarifying contingencies, building motivation to change*)

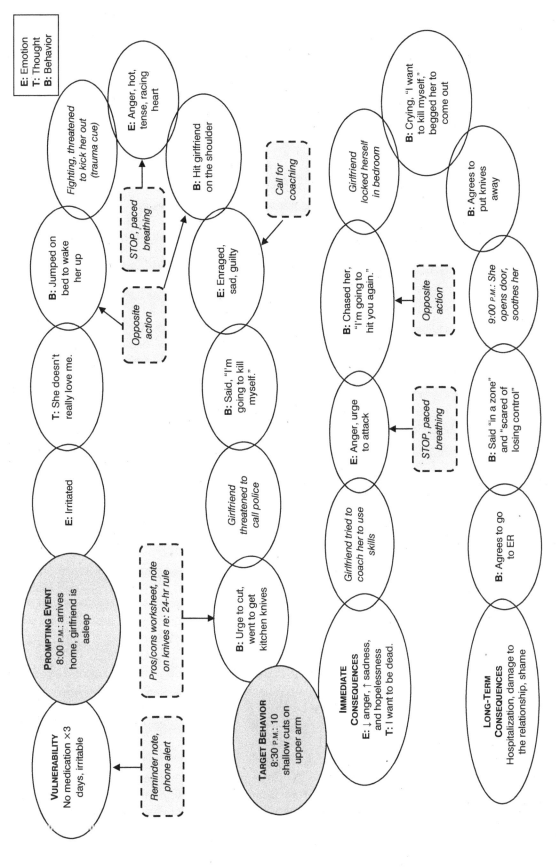

FIGURE 4.1. Natalie's chain and solution analyses.

E: Emotion
T: Thought
B: Behavior

VULNERABILITY
No medication ×3 days, irritable

Reminder note, phone alert

PROMPTING EVENT
8:00 P.M.: arrives home, girlfriend is asleep

E: Irritated

T: She doesn't really love me.

B: Jumped on bed to wake her up

Fighting, threatened to kick her out (trauma cue)

E: Anger, hot, tense, racing heart

Opposite action

STOP, paced breathing

B: Hit girlfriend on the shoulder

E: Enraged, sad, guilty

Call for coaching

B: Said, "I'm going to kill myself."

Girlfriend threatened to call police

Pros/cons worksheet, note on knives re: 24-hr rule

B: Urge to cut, went to get kitchen knives

TARGET BEHAVIOR
8:30 P.M.: 10 shallow cuts on upper arm

IMMEDIATE CONSEQUENCES
E: ↓ anger, ↑ sadness, and hopelessness
T: I want to be dead.

Girlfriend tried to coach her to use skills

E: Anger, urge to attack

STOP, paced breathing

B: Chased her, "I'm going to hit you again."

Opposite action

Girlfriend locked herself in bedroom

B: Crying, "I want to kill myself," begged her to come out

B: Agrees to put knives away

9:00 P.M.: She opens door, soothes her

B: Said "in a zone" and "scared of losing control"

B: Agrees to go to ER

LONG-TERM CONSEQUENCES
Hospitalization, damage to the relationship, shame

CASE EXAMPLE DISCUSSION

This illustration provides an example of how to conduct a chain analysis that assesses each of the six elements of the chain while incorporating a variety of DBT strategies. We see validation being used to balance the heavy change focus of chain analysis and keep the client engaged. A variety of assessment strategies are used, including asking relevant questions, testing hypotheses, eliciting behaviorally specific descriptions, and highlighting patterns. There is also an effort to build insight and clarify the contingencies of Natalie's problematic behaviors, which is intended to increase motivation to change. In addition, the therapist's communication style balances change-based irreverence (e.g., direct confrontation, matter-of-fact approach) with acceptance-based reciprocity (e.g., remaining nonjudgmental, self-disclosure). All of this is done while maintaining a laser focus on understanding the exact chain of events that occurred.

As is typical for many clients, Natalie's chain analysis included a series of interrelated problem behaviors. While the primary target behavior was NSSI, multiple other dysfunctional behaviors also occurred, including hitting her girlfriend, threatening to kill herself, and suicidal urges. A key vulnerability factor was her failure to take her psychotropic medications for several days prior to this episode. The initial prompting event was that her girlfriend had gone to bed early, which made her feel both angry and unloved. Key links between this event and the primary target behavior (cutting herself) included her girlfriend's threats to kick her out of the house and call the police. These external events elicited a series of internal experiences for Natalie, including memories of her abusive father, anger, intense sensations, thoughts about not wanting to be controlled, and urges to engage in destructive behaviors that led quickly and impulsively to the problem behaviors themselves. The immediate consequences of cutting included some relief from anger but were otherwise negative, including feeling sad, hopeless, and wanting to be dead, which quickly spiraled her into another episode of behavioral dyscontrol in which she threatened to hit her girlfriend after she tried to coach her to use skills. The potential positive consequences of these behaviors were that they stopped her girlfriend from following through on her threats and eventually elicited soothing from her. The long-term consequences were uniformly negative, including psychiatric hospitalization, damage to the relationship, and increased shame.

Given Natalie's trauma history and PTSD, it is not surprising that several trauma-related factors influenced the occurrence of these problem behaviors. Natalie's irritability and aggressive behavior are a symptom of PTSD that played a major role in this entire sequence of events. Notably, the intense anger was triggered by threats from her girlfriend, which were reminders of her father's abusive behavior. For Natalie, exposure to trauma reminders nearly always elicited a fight response, which in this episode took the form of verbal and physical aggression. Another PTSD symptom evident in this chain was Natalie's overly negative beliefs about herself, which led her to interpret the fact that her girlfriend was asleep as meaning that she did not matter. A final notable element of Natalie's chain is her description of dissociation—namely, she reported being unaware of her behavior until it had already happened and feeling like she was "in a zone" and unable to control her actions. As is typical in Stage 1, a general link between this episode of problem behavior and Natalie's PTSD was made, with the goal of building motivation to gain behavioral control so that this underlying problem can be treated.

It is also important to note that, although no direct effort was made during this chain analysis to teach Natalie new skills, the entire exercise functioned as an opportunity for her to practice mindfulness skills in the context of informal exposure to emotion. Natalie began the chain by saying she didn't really know what had happened. This lack of awareness of the factors leading up to and following problem behaviors is very common, and chain analysis requires clients to counteract this by mindfully observing and describing the internal and external details of a specific past event in a manner very similar to imaginal exposure. In addition, chain analysis very often elicits uncomfortable emotions that are associated with the episode of problem behavior. In Natalie's case, she felt sadness, guilt, and shame while engaged in this chain analysis. Thus, chain analysis, although primarily a behavioral assessment tool, can also serve as a valuable opportunity to build clients' capacity to mindfully narrate a specific past event while experiencing the emotions this elicits—skills that are essential to the success of DBT PE.

Solution Analysis

The goal of conducting a chain analysis is to increase understanding about what the problem is and what factors may be controlling its occurrence. Once this understanding is achieved, you and the client clarify the goals (e.g., behaviors to increase or decrease) and then work to identify adaptive behaviors that could have been employed at different points in the chain to achieve these goals. This solution analysis can be done once the entire chain analysis is complete, or it can be woven into the chain analysis by identifying interventions as it is being conducted. As discussed below, there are four types of solutions that are utilized in DBT: skills training, exposure, cognitive modification, and contingency management. Solutions may be generated from one or more of these categories depending on what is likely to be most effective and pragmatic for the specific client and situation. Once solutions are selected, clients are oriented to the solutions (e.g., by clarifying and role playing exactly what they will be expected to do), a commitment to implement the solutions is obtained, and troubleshooting of potential interfering factors is completed.

Common Solutions for Clients with PTSD

SKILLS TRAINING

DBT is a heavily skills-focused treatment and skills training is commonly utilized as a solution when clients lack the capability to engage in more adaptive behavior. This is often the case, as many clients have never been taught or exposed to skillful ways of coping. Instead, the invalidating and abusive environments in which they have lived have often modeled and reinforced dysfunctional ways of coping. To address these skills deficits, DBT teaches clients skills in four key areas that are balanced in terms of their focus on acceptance (mindfulness, distress tolerance) and change (emotion regulation, interpersonal effectiveness). These skills are first acquired via direct instruction and modeling, then strengthened through rehearsal and coaching, and ultimately generalized to ensure they can be implemented in a variety of situations in which skilled responses are needed. The overall goal is to teach clients skillful behavior to replace problem behavior in all relevant contexts. Clients with PTSD are likely to benefit from all of the DBT skills—I provide some examples in Table 4.3 of how skills are commonly applied for clients with PTSD.

EXPOSURE

DBT utilizes both informal and formal exposure as solutions when intense emotions automatically elicit emotional avoidance or maladaptive behavior. In Stage 1, informal exposure is most often used to help clients with PTSD build the capacity to experience emotions without

TABLE 4.3. Applying DBT Skills to Cope with PTSD and Trauma-Related Problems

DBT skills modules	Example applications
Mindfulness Goal: to increase awareness of the present moment without judgment	• Observe and describe the current environment to reduce dissociation and feel grounded in the present • Increase awareness of trauma cues and associated reactions to decrease impulsive responses to these cues • Use wise mind to decide whether to avoid or approach feared situations • Practice being nonjudgmental of self and others
Distress tolerance Goal: to survive crises without making them worse and accept reality as it is	• Paced breathing to reduce intense arousal after a flashback • Tip the temperature with ice water to stop dissociation • Distract from intrusive trauma memories with activities • Self-soothe to tolerate painful trauma-related emotions • Imagery to create a "safe place" in times of high anxiety • Radical acceptance of past trauma and PTSD • Mindfulness of current thoughts about past trauma
Emotion regulation Goal: to understand emotions, reduce emotional vulnerability, and change unwanted emotions	• Identify and label trauma-related emotions • PLEASE skills to reduce vulnerability to negative emotions • Cope ahead to plan and rehearse skillful responses to situations likely to prompt PTSD symptoms • Nightmare and sleep hygiene protocols to improve sleep • Check the facts about distorted trauma-related beliefs • Opposite action to reduce trauma-related emotions • Problem solving to reduce contact with trauma cues • Mindfulness of current emotions to increase the ability to experience intense emotions without avoiding
Interpersonal effectiveness Goal: to get what you want from others, improve relationships, and maintain self-respect	• DEAR MAN to say "no" to things that cross one's limits rather than tolerating mistreatment • GIVE to behave in ways that make people like you rather than being irritable or detached • FAST to increase self-respect in relationships • End destructive relationships and build new ones

Note. Readers who are unfamiliar with any of these skills are encouraged to review the *DBT Skills Training Manual* (Linehan, 2015).

avoiding, which is necessary for the formal exposure procedures of DBT PE to work. Informal exposure is generally unplanned and occurs spontaneously when therapists detect emotional avoidance occurring in session. For example, a client may start to feel ashamed and hide her face when talking about a recent interaction with a friend and then abruptly change the topic. Informal exposure in this case could involve directing the client to return her attention to the cue that prompted the shame while attending to the body sensations this elicits. This exposure to emotion may only last a few minutes, as this may be all that is needed to achieve the goal of breaking the habit of automatic emotional avoidance. Often these brief informal exposure practices are interwoven throughout therapy sessions as therapists repeatedly highlight and block emotional avoidance when it occurs.

Informal exposure may also be used when a specific emotion regularly prompts maladaptive behavior. For example, I once treated a client for whom intense sadness almost always led her to drink alcohol, which then greatly increased her risk of attempting suicide. To break this conditioned association between sadness and drinking, we used informal exposure to approach cues that elicited sadness (e.g., watching sad movies, looking at photos of her deceased mother).

Once sadness was present, she used the DBT skills of mindfulness of current emotion and urge surfing to focus on the emotion while letting the urge to drink come and go. Over time, these types of informal exposure practices made it so that she was able to experience intense sadness without drinking. As discussed more in Chapter 6, these types of emotional exposure tasks are often conducted toward the end of Stage 1 to evaluate clients' ability to experience intense emotions without escaping or engaging in maladaptive behaviors, an important indicator of readiness to move on to Stage 2 PTSD treatment.

COGNITIVE MODIFICATION

In DBT, cognitive modification strategies are used as solutions when distorted beliefs interfere with using skillful behavior. Clients with PTSD have many problematic trauma-related beliefs that lead them to interpret present-day events in self-critical ways or in ways that assume danger or hostile intentions on the part of others. These faulty interpretations (e.g., "I'm stupid") often prompt intense emotions (e.g., shame) and urges to engage in problematic behaviors (e.g., self-injury). You may use cognitive restructuring to help clients observe, evaluate, and challenge the problematic thoughts that contribute to dysfunctional behavior. This may be done using logic, behavioral experiments, strategies to access wise mind, and direct suggestions of more adaptive ways of thinking. Of note, many clients with PTSD find it very difficult to generate or believe challenges to their trauma-related beliefs, particularly negative core beliefs about themselves (e.g., "I am bad"). In these cases, it may be more useful to focus on whether the beliefs are effective in helping the client reach their goals, rather than on whether they are accurate. Clients can be coached to use the acceptance-based skill of mindfulness of current thoughts to avoid getting attached to ineffective trauma-related beliefs rather than trying to challenge their validity.

DBT's cognitive modification strategies also include contingency clarification, which typically involves highlighting the consequences of a client's behaviors to increase insight and motivation for change. For clients with PTSD, contingency clarification is often used to build motivation to gain control over Stage 1 behaviors in order to be able to engage in DBT PE. For example, when life-threatening behavior occurs, you can highlight that continuing to engage in these behaviors will delay their ability to receive PTSD treatment. Therapists also commonly work to increase clients' awareness of the negative consequences of avoidance by, for example, highlighting that avoidance of emotions, thoughts, and trauma cues may reduce distress in the short run, but will prolong suffering, including PTSD, in the long run.

CONTINGENCY MANAGEMENT

DBT utilizes contingency management as the solution when a problem behavior is being reinforced or an adaptive behavior is being punished. Contingency management is rooted in operant conditioning theory and involves using reinforcement (i.e., anything that increases the likelihood of a behavior) and punishment (i.e., anything that decreases the likelihood of a behavior) to change behavior. Contingency management is most often used informally during therapy sessions and involves therapists modulating their in-the-moment responses to either reinforce or punish the client's behavior. For example, when a client is engaging in adaptive behavior (e.g., collaboratively engaging in problem solving, committing to stop target behaviors), therapists may respond in ways likely to be reinforcing (e.g., smiling, praising, leaning forward). In contrast, when clients are engaging in dysfunctional behaviors (e.g., yelling, refusing to engage in treatment tasks), therapists may respond in ways likely to be aversive (e.g., reducing warmth, expressing irritation, crossing arms).

Contingency management strategies can also be applied in formal, structured ways. For example, formal contingency management is commonly used to change environmental responses that may be contributing to problem behaviors, such as when family members or friends are responding in reinforcing ways to life-threatening behavior. In such cases, therapists may coach clients to ask the other person to change their responses to be less reinforcing and/or they may hold joint or family sessions with the other person. Formal contingency management can also be used to target specific problem behaviors by rewarding desired behavior and, less often, punishing undesired behavior. For example, formal contingency management can be used to target severe dissociation when less intensive interventions (e.g., DBT skills) have not been sufficiently effective (see Chapter 14).

Case Example: Solution Analysis

After completing the chain analysis, Natalie's therapist asked her what she would have liked to have done differently in this situation. Consistent with their previously identified treatment goals, she said that she would have wanted to not self-injure or threaten to kill herself, not be physically aggressive toward her girlfriend, and not be psychiatrically hospitalized. She also said she generally wished she had been better able to control her anger. With these goals in place, Natalie and her therapist began to generate a variety of potential solutions to address the critical points on the chain. Her therapist started by asking her what she thought she could have done differently to be better able to reach her goals. Her primary solution focused on the need to reduce vulnerability factors for anger by taking her psychotropic medications regularly (PLEASE skill) and she generated several ways to remind herself to do so, including putting a note by her toothbrush and setting a daily alert on her phone. Her therapist immediately gave her a sticky note to write down the reminder to put in her bathroom and had her set her phone alert.

Natalie also suggested paced breathing (TIP skill) as a potential solution, as she had previously had success using this skill to reduce intense anger. Her therapist then worked to clarify exactly when and how this skill could be used. Since paced breathing is a distress tolerance skill designed for managing crisis situations involving extreme emotions, Natalie decided she would use it once her anger reached a 6 out of 10 or if she had urges to threaten or hit her girlfriend. Her therapist suggested that she would first need to use the STOP skill to freeze when she noticed the physical sensations associated with urges to be aggressive, take a step back, observe that her anger had become extreme, and then proceed mindfully to use paced breathing. Natalie agreed that she would go to (or ask to be left alone in) her bedroom so she could lie down on the bed and do paced breathing until her anger reduced to at least a 4. Her therapist then had her engage in the cope ahead skill by having her imagine freezing, taking a step back, and then going to her bedroom and practicing paced breathing in response to her girlfriend threatening to kick her out of the house. As Natalie imagined doing this, she began to feel both sad and angry and then abruptly stopped and said she didn't want to think about it anymore. Her therapist then used informal exposure by coaching her to go back to imagining coping effectively with this scenario while allowing herself to experience the emotions this elicited. Natalie was able to do this in the session, which provided a useful opportunity to practice experiencing rather than avoiding the emotions that had contributed to this event.

After practicing the cope ahead skill, Natalie and her therapist began to generate some solutions that focused on reducing ineffective anger before it became extreme. Her therapist suggested the check the facts skill to generate alternative interpretations to her girlfriend being asleep that might be less likely to prompt anger. Natalie was able to come up with the interpretation of "she was really tired because she had worked several long shifts in a row" and noted that this made her feel more compassionate and less angry. However, she expressed some doubt that she would be able to generate this more adaptive way of thinking when she was angry. Her therapist then suggested the opposite action skill to use once anger was present, including gently avoiding her girlfriend (e.g., not going into the bedroom, not chasing her when she left the kitchen) and being kind (e.g., letting her sleep rather than jumping on the bed, not making threats). Natalie thought she would be more likely to be able to act opposite to anger, but that this would still be hard to do. Her therapist then suggested phone coaching as a solution. Natalie agreed and thought this would be particularly helpful if she was feeling unable to control her anger.

Her therapist also expressed concern about the fact that Natalie had not made any effort to stop herself from cutting and that this self-injury had occurred without any consideration of the negative consequences. The therapist reminded her about the DBT *pros and cons* worksheet she had previously completed that led her to decide that the negative consequences of cutting outweighed the potential benefits. Natalie agreed that this was now even more true given that cutting had only made things worse in this episode. To increase awareness of the negative consequences of cutting, Natalie agreed to hang the pros and cons worksheet on her refrigerator (*contingency clarification*). She also reported that one of the main negative consequences of cutting was that, because of DBT's 24-hour rule, she would not be able to call her therapist for skills coaching for 24 hours afterward (*contingency management*). Since she found skills coaching helpful and did not want to lose the ability to call her therapist, she thought that it would help to put a note by the kitchen knives reminding her of this. Her therapist then had her write out the note in the session.

After generating a variety of solutions, they then evaluated them and selected the specific solutions Natalie was going to implement in the coming week. Natalie believed it would be most realistic for her to use the following solutions, which she wrote down on her diary card and are shown in the dashed boxes in Figure 4.1:

1. Put the reminder note about taking her medications by her toothbrush.
2. Use the STOP skill as soon as she notices urges to be physically aggressive.
3. Practice paced breathing alone in her bedroom three times when not angry and any time anger becomes intense (6+ out of 10).
4. Use opposite action to gently avoid her girlfriend when anger leads to urges to be verbally or physically aggressive.
5. Put her worksheet on the pros and cons of cutting on the refrigerator.
6. Put the reminder note about the 24-hour rule by the kitchen knives.
7. Call for skills coaching if she is unable to control her anger.

After obtaining commitments to complete these tasks, her therapist then engaged in troubleshooting by asking Natalie what might get in the way of implementing these solutions. She said the main barrier was that she may not want to call for coaching because she was worried about being a burden. Her therapist assured her that it would be less burdensome to help her in the moment to prevent these kinds of high-risk behaviors from occurring than to have to spend their entire session focused on what had gone wrong without having any opportunity to intervene. Natalie said that this helped her to feel more comfortable calling for skills coaching and could not identify other barriers to implementing the agreed-upon solutions.

CASE EXAMPLE DISCUSSION

This example illustrates the key steps of solution analysis, including clarifying goals for a specific episode of problem behavior(s), and then generating, evaluating, and selecting solutions to achieve these goals. In this case, Natalie's goals spanned several domains of the Stage 1 target hierarchy, including stopping life-threatening behaviors (self-injury and suicide crisis behaviors), decreasing quality-of-life-interfering behaviors (physical aggression and hospitalization), and increasing behavioral skills (ability to regulate anger). Solutions were generated to address multiple elements from the chain analysis that were contributing to these problem behaviors, including vulnerability factors (failure to take medications), controlling variables (e.g., her girlfriend threatening to kick her out), other links (e.g., distorted beliefs, anger), and consequences of the problem behavior (e.g., inability to utilize phone coaching). The process of solution generation was done in a manner likely to increase the client's problem-solving skills over time, by asking her to self-generate solutions as much as possible and only offering solutions when needed to supplement her suggestions. At several points in this process, new behavior was activated that was consistent with the proposed solutions, including asking Natalie to write down reminders, set her phone alert, and practice the cope ahead skill. In addition, informal exposure was used in session to help Natalie practice experiencing the emotions that had contributed to this episode of problem behavior without avoiding. The identified solutions were then evaluated in terms of their feasibility. Seven specific solutions were selected that were both adaptive and did not exceed the client's current abilities, and a commitment to implement these solutions was obtained and troubleshot.

This example also highlights that a multipronged approach is often used to change Stage 1 target behaviors with multiple solutions being generated and implemented at once. In this example, solutions were generated from three of the four core types of solutions, including skills training, cognitive modification, and contingency management. Consistent with DBT's dialectical approach, the solutions were balanced in terms of acceptance and change. This was most evident in the solutions for Natalie's anger, which included strategies for tolerating extreme anger without engaging in problem behaviors (STOP, paced breathing) and strategies for changing anger before it becomes extreme (opposite action). It is also important to note that there are many additional solutions that could have been generated to address the problems that occurred in this episode. For example, the therapist did not attempt to address the possibility that her life-threatening behaviors were being reinforced by the concerned and soothing responses of her girlfriend. In general, there is often no clear "right" answer to solving these Stage 1 target behaviors and treatment typically involves a trial-and-error process in which multiple solutions are implemented until one or more are found to be effective.

Finally, it is important to highlight that several solutions were generated to address the PTSD symptoms that played a role in this episode. In Natalie's case, the most prominent PTSD symptom was her persistent anger and irritability, and solutions focused on decreasing her vulnerability to anger, changing ineffective anger once it starts, and managing extreme anger without loss of behavioral control. In addition, Natalie's extreme anger was prompted by exposure to a reminder of her abusive father, and she was asked to use the cope ahead skill to mentally rehearse coping effectively with this type of trauma cue in the future while experiencing the emotions this elicited. As is typical of Stage 1 DBT, these solutions were generated using a present-focused approach that did not require Natalie to engage in any kind of detailed discussion of her past trauma. At the same time, it is not expected that these PTSD symptoms will be fully resolved until it is treated in Stage 2. Rather, the goal is to help clients to cope effectively with trauma-related problems so that PTSD can be treated.

Concluding Comments

In the integrated DBT and DBT PE treatment, Stage 1 DBT is a means to an end, with the end being enabling clients to receive treatment for PTSD. Stage 1 DBT is delivered without adaptation, but with an explicit focus on preparing clients for DBT PE. Throughout Stage 1, therapists doggedly target higher-priority behaviors using chain and solution analyses while infusing this work with a trauma focus. The relationships between current problems and PTSD are highlighted, the importance of treating PTSD is stressed, and progress toward desired behaviors is linked to the goal of being able to receive PTSD treatment. It still never ceases to amaze me how often clients are motivated to change long-standing patterns of maladaptive behavior in order to access effective treatment for PTSD. More than anything, this speaks to the intensity of their trauma-related suffering and underscores the importance of delivering Stage 1 DBT as efficiently and effectively as possible to minimize the delay before PTSD is treated.

CHAPTER 5

Building Motivation for DBT PE

Asking our emotionally and behaviorally dysregulated clients to engage in an exposure-based treatment for PTSD is like asking a cat to swim—it runs completely counter to what they believe is appropriate and necessary for their survival. Therefore, it is to be expected that clients will initially express hesitation or even unwillingness to engage in DBT PE. Although most clients will express concerns about DBT PE, they vary widely in the intensity of their concerns, with some raising only a few questions before committing to doing the treatment and others vehemently refusing to even consider it. You should expect rather than be disarmed by this ambivalence and be prepared to steadfastly continue to work to build your clients' motivation in the face of it. I can tell you with certainty that a great many clients will absolutely, if not always immediately, choose to engage in DBT PE despite its challenges. Why? Because it is likely to be effective in reducing their trauma-related suffering, and to do so reasonably quickly. How do they know this? Most often it is because we have actively worked to "sell" DBT PE to them rather than passively sitting back and hoping they choose to do it. In this chapter, I discuss strategies for building clients' motivation for DBT PE and, ideally, obtaining a commitment from them to participate in the treatment.

Presenting DBT PE as a Choice

Although clients are usually told about the option of receiving DBT PE during pretreatment, the process of deciding whether they wish to engage in it typically occurs in Stage 1. A necessary first step in this process is to ensure that clients recognize that there is a decision to be made. Thus, it is important that you continue to raise the topic of DBT PE as a treatment option during Stage 1 and do not assume that clients will remember this or will think about it on their own without prompting. We often remind clients about the option of receiving DBT PE as we learn more about how PTSD is contributing to their problems. For example, if you learn that nightmares are regularly disrupting your client's sleep or that trauma-related self-hatred is driving their desire to be dead, you can suggest DBT PE as a solution to these problems and remind clients of this treatment option. Essentially, the goal is to make it clear to clients that there is a choice to be made about whether they want to treat their PTSD and, specifically, whether they wish to receive DBT with or without DBT PE.

Providing Information about DBT PE

To help clients make this decision, you must provide them with clear and practical information about DBT PE and what it entails. In particular, it is important that clients understand how DBT PE works, what they will be expected to do, its effectiveness, and potential risks and benefits. This information is included in *General Handout 4 (What Is DBT PE?)* in Appendix A, which can be reviewed and discussed with clients. In addition, you can provide clients with other resources to review, such as the DBT PE website (*www.dbtpe.org*), which includes written information about the treatment, as well as podcasts, webinars, client testimonials, and videos. Clients should be given time to study this information on their own and to share it with trusted people in their lives if they would like. This informational material is often quite persuasive to clients and begins to shift their intentions in the direction of doing DBT PE. For example, studies have shown that a majority of DBT clients with PTSD report a preference for the combined DBT and DBT PE treatment over either DBT or PE alone after reading a written description of the treatment (74%; Harned et al., 2013) or learning about DBT PE in focus groups (90%; Harned & Schmidt, 2019).

In general, providing clients with psychoeducational information about the rationale for and effectiveness of exposure-based treatments for PTSD is associated with high receptivity for these treatments (e.g., Feeny, Zoellner, Mavissakalian, & Roy-Byrne, 2009; Kehle-Forbes, Polusny, Erbes, & Gerould, 2014). Therefore, you should ensure that your clients clearly understand both how DBT PE works and what outcomes they can expect if they choose to do it. The amount of information that is provided is often determined by the questions clients ask and can range from a general overview (see Chapter 3) to the more detailed treatment rationales that are typically provided in Sessions 1–3 of DBT PE. The manner in which you provide information about DBT PE is as important as the information itself—in particular, it is critical that you appear confident and competent. If you seem unconvinced about the potential benefits of DBT PE, unsure about your own skills, or doubtful that clients will be able to complete it, then your clients are likely to be less interested in receiving it. In contrast, if you instill hope that DBT PE is likely to improve your clients' lives, act confident in your ability to provide it, and inspire clients to believe they will eventually be able to do it, then your clients are more likely to be receptive to the treatment.

Addressing Concerns about DBT PE

During the process of providing clients with information about DBT PE, they are likely to express a variety of concerns about the treatment, which is both understandable and a positive sign that they are an active and engaged consumer of mental health services. In my experience, clients who have fully expressed their concerns and had them addressed prior to choosing to do DBT PE are likely to have a stronger and more lasting commitment to the treatment than those who quickly agree to it without giving it much thought. In addition, the concerns expressed by clients often provide important insights into the problematic beliefs and emotions that are maintaining their PTSD that will need to be targeted during DBT PE. When clients express concerns, your task is to respond in a manner that balances validation and change and will ideally move clients closer to being willing to do the treatment. The following four-step model provides a useful approach for addressing clients' concerns about DBT PE.

Step 1. Assess

To effectively address a concern, it is critical that you understand exactly what the client is concerned about. Often clients initially express somewhat vague concerns, such as "I'm worried that DBT PE will make me worse." In this example, you would need to understand exactly how the client thinks the treatment will make them worse. Is it that they think it will cause an increase in PTSD symptoms? Or that it will make them unable to function well enough to go to school or work? Or that it will lead them to kill themselves? This level of specificity is necessary to be sure your response is effectively tailored to the client's core concern. Below I describe some of the most common concerns raised by clients.

- *"It sounds really hard!"* When DBT PE is first described to clients, their immediate response is nearly always that it sounds hard. Some clients will say that they think DBT PE would be so hard that it would actually be retraumatizing or equivalent to experiencing the trauma all over again. In general, people with PTSD have often designed their lives to avoid doing exactly what DBT PE would require them to do, and the idea of shifting their way of being in the world from avoiding to approaching is both hard to imagine and terrifying.
- *"I won't be able to tolerate the distress."* Many clients believe that DBT PE will be so hard, painful, or overwhelming that they won't be able to tolerate it. This often means that they believe the intense emotions elicited by exposure will cause them to fall apart or break down. Clients often predict that, once started, these painful emotions are likely to last for hours or days and that they will not be able to withstand them. Other times clients believe that they simply don't have the ability to experience an emotion at a high intensity for long and that they will quickly shut the emotion off.
- *"It will make me worse."* Nearly all clients worry that DBT PE will make them worse rather than better. For Stage 1 clients, this often means that they think the emotions elicited by exposure would cause them to kill themselves or self-injure. Most clients also fear that DBT PE will cause them to engage in a variety of other impulsive, destructive behaviors (e.g., substance use, physical aggression), lead to increases in mental health problems (e.g., depression, dissociation), and/or impair their ability to function in their lives.
- *"I don't want to stop avoiding."* Some clients will insist that they are not interested in changing their avoidant approach to coping with their trauma. For example, they may say that they don't want to think about the trauma, feel emotions related to it, or approach things that remind them of it. These clients may argue the merits of avoidance, suggesting that it is an effective coping strategy that has enabled them to remain at least somewhat functional in their daily lives. Similarly, clients may say that they do not mind, are willing to accept, or even prefer the limitations that avoidance has placed on their lives.
- *"I don't think the treatment will work."* Some clients will report that they do not believe DBT PE will work or that exposure is an effective method of treating PTSD. For example, clients may say that they think about their trauma all the time and it hasn't helped to improve their PTSD. Other clients will say that they believe DBT PE is likely to be effective for most people,

but not for them. They may think that they possess specific characteristics that make them a poor fit for DBT PE, or they may believe they are permanently damaged.

- *"You will think I'm bad."* Many clients will express concerns about how you will react to learning about the details of their traumatic experiences. Clients typically hold many self-critical beliefs about their trauma and assume that you will view them similarly. For example, they may worry that you will think it was their fault or that they are repulsive. To avoid these predicted negative interpersonal consequences, clients may say that they do not want to disclose their traumas and that they prefer to keep them secret.

- *"It will take too much time."* Finally, some clients will express pragmatic concerns about the extra time it will take to do DBT PE, including longer or more frequent sessions, as well as large amounts of homework. The added session time may also be cost prohibitive for some clients.

Step 2. Validate

Once a client's concern is clearly defined, you should validate how the concern makes sense. In DBT, validation is used to balance change and often helps to make change possible. In the present context, clients are likely to be more receptive to your attempts to challenge a concern if they first feel as if you have made an effort to understand and validate it. When validating clients' concerns about DBT PE, I recommend relying primarily on validation levels 4, 5, and 6.

Validation Level 4

It is almost always possible and often helpful to validate clients' concerns in terms of their past learning, particularly the learning that resulted from past trauma. Validation level 4 (V4) is often my go-to strategy for validating client concerns about DBT PE that accurately reflect past experiences but not present circumstances. For example, when clients express concerns that *in vivo* exposure will be dangerous, this is almost always because the situations they are avoiding (or similar situations) were in fact unsafe at some point in their past. V4 could involve saying things such as "It is completely understandable that you believe that all parking garages are dangerous given that you were raped in a parking garage." Similarly, concerns that DBT PE will lead to worsening can also be validated in terms of clients' past experiences. For example, you might say, "Of course you're afraid you will kill yourself! There have been times in the past that thinking about your trauma has led you to attempt suicide." Similarly, clients who are afraid you will reject them can be validated by saying things like "It makes sense that you're worried about how I'll react given that in the past important people in your life have reacted poorly to learning about your trauma." As these examples illustrate, V4 provides you with a way to communicate that unrealistic or excessive fears make sense based on the past without suggesting they are accurate in the present.

Validation Level 5

Validation level 5 (V5) is often the most powerful type of validation you can offer, as it communicates that the client's concern is normal, understandable, and makes sense in the current context. In contrast to V4, which focuses on how concerns make sense based on past learning (and often implicitly communicates that they don't make sense in the present), V5 wholly embraces the client's concern as a valid response to the present situation. A critical function of V5 is normalization—that is, communicating that the concern is common and the client is not crazy or pathological for having it. Nearly all concerns can be normalized in comparison to other clients considering DBT PE by saying things like "Many clients who do DBT PE have that concern." Other concerns can be normalized in terms of people with PTSD. For example, you might say, "Most people with PTSD don't want to think about their trauma—that's completely normal." It can also be helpful to validate clients' concerns as normative for non–mental health populations by making comparisons to other groups to which they belong. For example, if a client is concerned that DBT PE will make them unable to control their emotions around their children, you might say, "You're not alone in that. Lots of parents find it important to hide their emotional distress from their children." When possible, it can be particularly powerful to normalize a concern as being typical for humans in general, including you. For example, if a client expresses a concern that approaching feared situations will be really hard, you might respond with "Of course! It's human nature to not want to approach things that terrify us. I would find this really hard too."

V5 is also a useful strategy when clients express concerns that accurately reflect the present reality, including the reality of what DBT PE will entail. This can include concerns such as DBT PE being likely to cause intense emotions, take a lot of time and effort, and require clients to share trauma details that cause them to feel shame. When clients raise these kinds of concerns, V5 essentially involves communicating that the client's concern is correct and that you share their view of reality. This can be achieved by saying things like "You're absolutely right, doing exposure is going to cause you to experience distressing emotions in the short term." Therapists often feel reticent to validate the accuracy of a concern due to fear that it will make it more likely to become a barrier to engaging in DBT PE. However, communicating that a concern accurately reflects the facts does not mean that you agree that it is an insurmountable barrier and, if anything, acknowledging the reality of the concern can help to set the stage for active problem solving about how to address it.

Validation Level 6

Validation level 6 (V6) involves being radically genuine with clients. I often think of this type of validation as meaning that I should strive to behave with my clients in the same way I behave with friends and family. How would you respond if a friend told you that they are terrified they will break down if they talk about a trauma they experienced? Chances are you wouldn't say stereotypical therapist things like "What I hear you saying is that you are really afraid right now," and instead would respond genuinely with something like "Of course you are! Oh my god, I would be too!" In general, the goal is for therapists to be themselves and respond naturally to clients' concerns rather than putting up a professional facade. This type of genuine reaction can help clients to feel more comfortable sharing their concerns, as well as to trust that you will be transparent and truthful in your response.

V6 also involves responding to the client as a person of equal status. Rather than assuming the position of the expert who unequivocally knows what is best for the client, you should instead respond to clients as equal partners who have valuable expertise to offer about how to make DBT PE work best for them. This can include highlighting the wisdom in clients' concerns and being open to influence about when and how to do the treatment. In addition, you may respond to clients' concerns by matching with your own vulnerability. When it is believed to be helpful to the client, this may include disclosure of your personal efforts to cope with similar problems. For example, I often share information about my own past phobias with clients and talk about the pervasiveness of my avoidance, the intensity of my anxiety, and how difficult, but ultimately effective, it was for me to do exposure. This type of genuine response conveys not only that the client's concern is understandable but that we are subject to the same laws of the universe as they are and are in this with them as one human to another.

Step 3. Educate and/or Problem-Solve

After validating a client's concern, you typically move to figuring out how to address it. Although the emphasis shifts to change at this point, you should continue to provide validation as needed. The goal is to communicate both that the client's concern is understandable and that it can be addressed so that DBT PE can still be possible. The determination of how to address a concern largely depends on its accuracy and/or the degree to which it reflects the client's wise mind. If a concern is inaccurate or unwise, then your response is typically to provide information that challenges the concern with the goal of helping the client to modify their faulty understanding and/or shift to a perspective that is more effective for their personal goals. On the other hand, if a concern does accurately fit the facts and is consistent with the client's wise mind, then your response is generally to help the client problem-solve if or how DBT PE could be possible despite this reality. Therefore, a necessary first step is to determine whether a client's concern is accurate and/or wise.

A concern may be inaccurate if it reflects a straightforward factual error. For example, clients' concerns are often based on a misunderstanding of the procedures and goals of DBT PE. Clients may believe that you will make them do exposure against their will, approach objectively dangerous situations, or interact with the perpetrators of their trauma. Similarly, clients may believe that the goal of exposure is to make them have no emotions about their trauma or to think that what they experienced was not a big deal. When clients express these types of misunderstandings, they can usually be readily resolved by providing them with psychoeducation about how DBT PE works and what they will be expected to do. Many times, however, clients' concerns are harder to dispel because they reflect predictions about what they believe will happen in the future as a result of engaging in DBT PE (e.g., that they will get worse and become nonfunctional). We often challenge these predictions by appealing to reason, using logical argument, or presenting scientific evidence. Although this type of factual information may help some clients to adjust their expectations, others will find it difficult to believe or may think it doesn't apply to them. As many clients will highlight, there is no way for you to know for sure what will or will not happen in the future. When this type of impasse occurs, it can be useful to frame the client's prediction as a hypothesis to be tested and to highlight that, although there is good reason to think it will not be true, the only way to find out for sure is by doing the treatment.

When challenging clients' concerns, it may also be useful to discuss whether the concern accurately reflects the client's wise mind. In DBT, wise mind refers to the inner wisdom that each one of us has. When we are in wise mind, emotion and reason are integrated to reach an effective decision that is most likely to help us reach our goals. Many concerns that clients raise about DBT PE are coming from emotion mind—that is, they reflect emotion-driven urges, thoughts, and behaviors and ignore reason or logic. For example, concerns that DBT PE will be too hard or intolerable are often driven by a desire to avoid the painful emotions that will be elicited by exposure, even though clients may recognize that continued avoidance is likely to make things worse in the long run. When clients' concerns are being driven by emotion, it can be helpful to explicitly work with clients to activate their wise mind by searching for a balanced perspective that integrates reason and is more likely to help them reach their goals.

On the other hand, when clients express concerns that fit the facts and/or are consistent with their wise mind, we rely primarily on problem solving to determine whether or how these barriers can be overcome. Examples of these types of concerns may include that exposure may cause temporary increases in distress before things improve, that thinking about a trauma may result in new details being remembered, and that it may be difficult to find time to do exposure homework. When these kinds of concerns arise, it can be helpful to brainstorm solutions about how clients can prepare for these outcomes in advance, cope effectively with them if they occur, and minimize the potential negative impact they will have. Ultimately, when concerns are realistic, clients must decide whether the positives of moving forward with DBT PE outweigh these negatives. Table 5.1 includes examples of ways to respond to the common client concerns described above.

Step 4. Cheerlead

Clients with a Stage 1 level of disorder are often quick to become hopeless, feel discouraged about their ability to do things, and doubt that they will ever be able to overcome their difficulties. The more challenging the task, the more likely it is that clients will believe they are incapable of doing it. When considering the possibility of doing DBT PE, many clients will therefore express concerns about their ability to do the treatment, be convinced that they are too dysfunctional to benefit from it, and doubt that they will be able to make the changes necessary to receive it. When responding to clients' concerns about DBT PE, you must not only address them with pragmatic information and solutions, you must also—and perhaps even more critically—inspire clients to believe they can overcome them. This is achieved by cheerleading—that is, offering encouragement, instilling hope, and remaining steadfast about clients' ability to do DBT PE. You may highlight clients' inherent abilities that will help them to do DBT PE effectively, such as their determination to get better and willingness to do hard things, while remaining realistic about areas that need to be expanded and strengthened, such as their ability to regulate and tolerate emotions without self-injuring. Even when clients are not yet capable of doing DBT PE safely or effectively, we provide encouragement that they can and will get there. Overall, the goal is to express confidence that clients will be able to succeed at DBT PE eventually, if not now, and to convey "I believe in you."

Obtaining a Commitment to DBT PE

Once clients' concerns have been addressed and they have the information they need to make a decision, you will work to obtain a commitment from clients to engage in DBT PE. This is done using DBT's commitment strategies, which are designed to obtain and strengthen commitments from clients to complete difficult tasks that they may not want to do. These tasks range from the mundane, such as choosing to get out of bed in the morning despite being depressed, to life-and-death issues, such as choosing to stay alive despite wanting to be dead. The more effortful the task is, the more difficult it is likely to be to elicit a commitment to do it—and there is no doubt that doing DBT PE requires great effort on the part of clients. Encouragingly, relatively few therapists trained in DBT PE (14–16%) report that lack of client interest is a significant

TABLE 5.1. Example Responses to Common Concerns about DBT PE

Concern	Example responses
"It sounds really hard!"	• The treatment is typically hardest in the first few imaginal exposure sessions and then starts to get easier after that. • Thinking about your trauma is not the same as being retraumatized. In fact, imaginal exposure will help you learn that thinking about your trauma is not dangerous and is not the same as having the trauma happen again. • *In vivo* exposure will start by having you do things that feel hard but manageable. • A benefit of doing DBT PE is that it will help you feel more confident in your ability to do hard things. • It is not easy and it is effective. If you stick with it through the hard parts, your life will be easier in the long run.
"I won't be able to tolerate the distress."	• One of the things DBT PE will help you to learn is that you can tolerate intense emotions and don't need to be so afraid of them. • Emotions can be uncomfortable and they are not dangerous. • Before we start DBT PE, we will make sure you have the skills you need to experience and tolerate intense emotions. • At the beginning of DBT PE, we will create a DBT skills plan for you to use to manage intense emotions or urges that may arise as a result of exposure.
"It will make me worse."	• If PTSD is not treated, it is unlikely to go away on its own and is likely to get worse over time. • There is no evidence that DBT PE makes people worse. People who receive DBT PE usually have better outcomes than people who receive DBT alone. • Research suggests that clients who receive DBT PE are less likely to attempt suicide and self-injure during treatment than clients who receive DBT alone. • At the beginning of DBT PE, some clients experience a temporary increase in certain symptoms, such as PTSD, depression, and dissociation. If this occurs, it usually lasts no more than a few weeks before things begin to improve. • By the end of treatment, about 70% of clients who complete DBT PE report a significant improvement in PTSD. Clients who complete DBT PE are twice as likely to no longer have PTSD as clients who receive DBT alone. • DBT PE is also associated with significant improvements in other areas, such as depression, dissociation, shame, emotion dysregulation, and difficulty functioning in daily life, and these changes are larger than in DBT alone.
"I don't want to stop avoiding."	• Avoidance is keeping your PTSD going and preventing you from recovering. • Although avoidance may make you feel better in the moment, in the long run it makes things worse and starts to control your life. • Trying to avoid thoughts and feelings about your trauma makes them come up more often and get more intense over time. • Avoiding situations, activities, and things that remind you of your trauma makes those things more distressing and harder to do over time. • Although thinking about your trauma and approaching things that remind you of it will be hard in the short run, it is a much more effective strategy in the long run for helping you to gain control over your memories and your life.

(continued)

TABLE 5.1. *(continued)*

Concern	Example responses
"I don't think it will work."	• DBT PE is effective for most clients, including people who have many of the same types of problems as you.
	• One of the reasons we do DBT first is to work on changing behaviors that are likely to make DBT PE less effective. Our goal is to set you up for success by addressing problems that may interfere with DBT PE before we start.
	• It's true that you often think about your trauma and your PTSD has not gone away. However, imaginal exposure is different because you will think about the trauma in more detail and without pushing it away, which is more effective for improving PTSD.
	• Fortunately, you don't have to believe DBT PE will work for it to be effective. You just need to do the treatment all the way and it is likely to work.
	• I can't promise it will work if you do it, but I can promise it won't work if you don't do it. The only way to know for sure is to do it and see what happens.
"You will think I'm bad."	• I know you believe that what happened to you makes you a bad person, but that is not how I think about people who have experienced trauma.
	• These types of negative beliefs about yourself are a symptom of PTSD that DBT PE will help to change.
	• Sharing your trauma with people who you trust can be a really helpful way to learn that others don't share your negative views about yourself and are not going to judge or reject you for what happened to you.
	• If you choose to talk about your trauma with me, I will be happy to share my genuine reactions with you so that you don't have to guess what I'm thinking.
	• When people share trauma information with me, it usually makes me admire them even more because I understand better what they have been through.
"It will take too much time."	• DBT PE typically takes about 12–16 sessions and during those 3–4 months you should expect to spend more time than usual in therapy and doing homework.
	• We can be flexible about how we structure the sessions in terms of frequency and length, and we will try to figure out an option that works best for you.
	• *In vivo* exposure often involves doing things that people want or need to be doing anyway but are avoiding, so it may make you more productive.
	• It may be helpful to plan to start DBT PE when you have more time available, like a school break or when family is around to help out.
	• Putting time into doing DBT PE now will pay off later by making you more able to participate in and enjoy activities that are important to you.

barrier to delivering the treatment (Harned, Ritschel, et al., 2021). In my view, this is unlikely to be a sign that DBT clients are unusually eager to engage in trauma-focused treatment, but rather that DBT therapists are particularly effective at obtaining commitments from clients to engage in this treatment despite its difficulty.

Timing and Levels of Commitment

Although there is no specific point in Stage 1 that you should ask for a commitment from clients to engage in DBT PE, it is recommended that you do so as early as possible in treatment.

Ideally, you will obtain this commitment within the first few months of Stage 1, which is usually well before clients have achieved the behavioral stability and skills necessary to actually start DBT PE. This initial commitment typically focuses on getting an agreement that the client will engage in DBT PE at some future, unspecified point in treatment. By getting this agreement in place early, it sets the stage for clients to immediately begin preparing for the treatment by working to change behaviors that would make DBT PE unsafe or ineffective (these are described in detail in Chapter 6). Throughout Stage 1, this initial commitment is regularly revisited, strengthened, and remade when motivation wanes or behaviors such as self-injury are occurring that are incompatible with doing DBT PE. In addition, the commitment is refined and becomes more detailed over the course of Stage 1, shifting from a vague commitment to do DBT PE to a specific commitment to start on a certain date. As in DBT more broadly, there are a variety of strategies that can be used to obtain and strengthen these commitments and recommitments to engage in DBT PE.

Evaluating the Pros and Cons

People are much more likely to commit to something they view as beneficial to them, particularly when the potential advantages are believed to outweigh the disadvantages. The pros and cons skill from DBT offers a useful method of helping clients reach a wise mind decision about engaging in DBT PE by considering this choice from four possible perspectives. In terms of the *pros of engaging in DBT PE*, the most obvious advantage is that it is very likely to lead to improvements in PTSD, including whichever symptoms are most distressing or impairing for a given client. In addition, by improving PTSD, clients are often more able to achieve other important life goals, such as having more friends, doing well in school, being in a romantic relationship, getting and maintaining a job, or being a patient and loving parent. Similarly, when PTSD contributes to other problems, such as substance use, disordered eating, dissociation, and depression, getting treatment for PTSD is likely to lead to improvements in these other problems as well. Other advantages of treating PTSD may include positive changes in the client's self-concept, such as greater self-compassion, an increased sense of competence, and less self-hatred. Another way to identify the potential benefits of the treatment is to have clients evaluate the *cons of not engaging in DBT PE*. These often include continuing to live a life that is both dominated and restricted by PTSD and the problems it causes. In addition, many clients indicate that choosing not to do DBT PE could result in later feelings of regret for not having taken full advantage of the treatment that was available to them.

It is also important for clients to consider the potential *cons of engaging in DBT PE*. These typically include realistic concerns about the difficulty of the treatment, such as that they will experience painful emotions, the homework will be time intensive, and they may experience increased distress early in treatment before they begin to feel better. Similarly, *pros of not engaging in DBT PE* often include the realistic short-term benefits of continued avoidance, such as not having to talk about the details of one's trauma, approach distressing trauma-related cues, or experience the intense emotions that will be elicited by exposure. However, the perceived cons of doing DBT PE often initially include unrealistic concerns, such as fear that the treatment will make them worse or will be unsafe. Similarly, the assumed pros of not doing DBT PE often include emotion-driven concerns, such as not having to experience the predicted negative outcomes of exposure (e.g., being retraumatized, loss of control). When the perceived disadvantages of DBT PE include concerns that do not fit the facts, it is important to help clients develop more accurate expectations on which to base their decision. Overall, thinking through the pros and cons of DBT PE can help clients to access wise mind, which often increases the likelihood they will decide to do DBT PE despite its challenges.

Foot-in-the-Door and Door-in-the-Face

DBT commitment strategies also include two methods of increasing compliance with requests that are based in social psychology. The *foot-in-the-door* technique involves making an initial small request, and when the person says yes, asking for something more difficult. When working to obtain a commitment to engage in DBT PE, you can first ask clients to engage in smaller tasks that are compatible with doing DBT PE even if they have not yet committed to doing the treatment. These could include things such as asking clients to consider doing the treatment (e.g., to not unequivocally say "no"); to read handouts or watch videos that provide psychoeducation about the treatment; and to complete mildly distressing, non-trauma-related exposure tasks. Another way to use foot-in-the-door is to first describe DBT PE in a somewhat vague yet very positive manner without mentioning how challenging it is. For example, you might say that the treatment focuses on processing past trauma and is very effective in reducing PTSD. When clients indicate that they are interested in the treatment, then you may begin to provide more information about it, including some acknowledgment of how hard it can be. At each step, you can elicit a commitment before "upping the ante" and eventually reaching a detailed description of the rationale and procedures of DBT PE and presenting it as quite challenging to complete.

The opposite approach is the *door-in-the-face* technique, which involves asking for something much more difficult than is actually needed, and when the person says no, scaling back the request to something easier. This approach can be useful when selecting a target start date for DBT PE. For example, you might ask a client to commit to starting DBT PE very early in treatment (e.g., after 8 weeks of DBT), and then relax this to something less difficult (e.g., by Month 6 of DBT).

Highlighting the Freedom to Choose and the Absence of Alternatives

People are also more likely to commit to doing something difficult if they feel in control of the choice and believe there is no other way to achieve their goals. Although we often feel strongly that clients should do DBT PE, it is critical that we make it clear that the client gets to make this choice. This dialectical balance can be achieved by saying things like "I really believe doing DBT PE will change your life and it's completely up to you if you decide to do it." In addition to highlighting clients' freedom to choose not to do DBT PE, you must also stress that they need to be prepared to accept the natural consequences of this choice. For example, you could paint a vivid picture of what a life with PTSD would look like, such as "If you choose not to treat your PTSD, we'll have to figure out how to accept that your life will be dominated by nightmares, intrusive trauma memories, high anxiety, and avoidance that limits what you can do." Similarly, you may highlight that if your client chooses not to treat PTSD, they will need to accept that it may be impossible to achieve some of their life-worth-living goals. For example, you may say, "If you do not treat your PTSD, it may not be possible to improve your marriage as much as you would like." This strategy of highlighting the absence of alternatives can also be useful when clients express a desire to continue avoiding trauma-related memories and situations. When this occurs, you may say things like "You can absolutely choose to continue avoiding, although you should be aware that if you do, your PTSD is not going to improve and may even get worse."

Ultimately, you want to strive to make clients feel free to make the choice to not do DBT PE, while at the same time making it as difficult as possible to view this as an effective choice.

Devil's Advocate

Once an initial commitment to DBT PE has been obtained, it is important to strengthen it by using the devil's advocate strategy to argue against it in a way that leads the client to argue more strongly in favor of it. For example, you might say, "Are you sure you really want to do this treatment? It's going to be a lot of work and you're going to have to feel a lot of painful emotions." The goal is for this to elicit from the client reasons why they think it will be beneficial to do DBT PE despite its challenges. For clients who buy in to the rationale of needing to stop avoidance to reduce PTSD, devil's advocate may include arguing for the benefits of avoidance. For example, you could suggest, "Maybe avoidance isn't such a bad thing. I mean, avoiding situations that remind you of your trauma works well to reduce your distress in the moment." Ideally clients will respond to these types of suggestions with counterarguments that highlight that avoidance works only as a short-term strategy, that having to avoid all the time is really limiting their lives in ways they don't like, and that they remain haunted by trauma memories despite efforts to push those thoughts away.

The trick with devil's advocate is to be sure that your arguments against DBT PE are not stronger than the client's current motivation to do it. For clients who are more ambivalent about doing DBT PE, I might make my arguments against DBT PE more extreme such that it would be nearly impossible for the client to agree with them. For example, I might suggest that rather than doing DBT PE, our time would be better spent figuring out how to make them feel good rather than miserable about having constant nightmares, flashbacks, and intrusive trauma memories. Essentially, the strategy here is to suggest that maybe it would be tolerable to continue living with PTSD while at the same time highlighting how intolerable it would be. I might also suggest that rather than treating their PTSD we could figure out how to make them an expert avoider. For example, I might suggest that the client adopt extreme avoidance strategies, such as enlisting others to do any tasks that require them to leave the house, finding a job that allows them to never have to interact with people, and ridding their house of all reminders of their past. Typically, you can find at least some arguments against DBT PE that the client will disagree with, and the experience of arguing for the merits of DBT PE will help to strengthen the client's resolve to do the treatment. However, if this strategy backfires and leads the client to retract their earlier commitment, then you can similarly retract your counterargument, remind the client of the reasons why they committed to doing DBT PE, and work to find a more effective devil's advocate position.

Connecting to Prior Commitments

It is also to be expected that clients' commitment to DBT PE may waver over the course of Stage 1 and they may at times return to expressing uncertainty about whether they wish to do the treatment. In this situation, you may remind the client that they had previously committed to doing DBT PE and encourage them to stick with this prior commitment. It can also be helpful in these moments to remind clients of the reasons they initially committed to doing DBT PE by saying, for example, "I thought it was really important to you to no longer be haunted by memories of your trauma?" The strategy of highlighting a prior commitment can also be useful if clients are engaging in behaviors that would make them unable to start DBT PE. For example, if a client who has made a commitment to doing DBT PE calls you in a crisis and says they are planning to kill themselves, you might respond with "But I thought you agreed to stay alive so that we can treat your PTSD and help you build a life that you want to be alive for?" The goal here is to encourage clients to stick with their prior commitment to doing DBT PE, even when they may feel hopeless, tired, willful, or dysregulated.

Balancing Pushing for Commitment and Enhancing Control

One of my greatest challenges in working to motivate clients to do DBT PE is accepting that I cannot ultimately control whether they choose to do the treatment. I believe so strongly in DBT PE and the enormous changes that can result from it, that I can at times push more than is effective to get clients to agree to do it. When clients feel pressured to do something they don't want to do, particularly something as instinctively terrifying as trauma-focused exposure, there is a risk that they will dig in their heels and become even more determined not to do it. Alternatively, if clients agree to do DBT PE to get us or someone else to stop badgering them about it, they may be less likely to engage in the treatment fully or effectively. Therefore, my advice is to adopt the role of a consultant by providing clients with honest and accurate information about DBT PE, making recommendations, and offering encouragement, while clearly leaving the decision in their hands. In this process, you must be nonjudgmental about the possibility that your clients may choose not to do DBT PE, and search for and validate the wisdom in this potential decision. Overall, the goal is for clients to take ownership over the decision to do or not do DBT PE, which is likely to increase their commitment to the treatment if they choose to do it.

Concluding Comments

Having to sell clients with PTSD on the idea of actively approaching trauma memories and reminders can be a daunting task. Indeed, I have not met a client who did not initially have concerns about doing DBT PE, and often the clients who need the treatment the most are the most hesitant to do it. You must be prepared for clients to be ambivalent and to respond thoughtfully and in a balanced manner to their concerns. The decision to do DBT PE is almost always a gradual one that is fostered by our active efforts to build motivation for the treatment, as well as our steadfast belief in DBT PE and the client's ability to do the treatment. Indeed, it is often our passion for the treatment that is most persuasive to clients. Therefore, my advice to you is to wholeheartedly sell the treatment with confidence and optimism, and then step back and let the client decide whether they wish to do it. Our clients are amazingly courageous people and most will eventually, if not immediately, be willing to take the leap of faith that is required to engage in this challenging treatment in the hope that it will change their lives.

CHAPTER 6

Determining Readiness for DBT PE

When I first began developing DBT PE, the most challenging question I faced was: When are high-risk, complex, and multidiagnostic clients stable enough to begin PTSD treatment? It did not seem hyperbolic to say that finding the "right" answer could literally mean life or death for these vulnerable clients. My search for an answer began by having discussions with Marsha Linehan and other DBT experts about how best to differentiate between clients with a Stage 1 and Stage 2 level of disorder, and I soon realized that there was much uncertainty and some disagreement about this issue in DBT. Similarly, I spoke with Edna Foa and other PTSD treatment experts about how they decide which clients are appropriate for trauma-focused treatment, and I discovered that there was no clear expert consensus on this topic either. A scientist at heart, I turned to the empirical literature to determine whether research had succeeded in identifying factors that clearly predicted treatment response in psychotherapies for PTSD. This search yielded a variety of potential prognostic factors, many of which had mixed evidence, and nearly all of which were derived from clinical samples that excluded individuals with the types of high-risk and severe problems typical of clients with a Stage 1 level of disorder. In short, no clear answer existed to this difficult question.

Faced with the task of having to develop my own criteria for determining client readiness to begin DBT PE, my overarching goal was to enable clients to get relief from the suffering caused by PTSD as rapidly as possible without compromising their safety or setting them up for failure. To that end, I sought to identify readiness criteria that would maximize the likelihood that clients would complete DBT PE safely (i.e., without engaging in life-threatening behaviors) and effectively (i.e., in a manner that resulted in clinically significant improvement in PTSD). The readiness criteria that are now used in DBT PE are the result of years of treatment development during which various criteria derived from research and expert opinion were implemented with clients and then refined based on the outcomes achieved. As reviewed in Chapter 1, research has shown that these readiness criteria appear to not only be attainable for most Stage 1 clients who complete DBT but also to reasonably define the tipping point at which PTSD treatment is likely to be both safe and effective. In this chapter, I begin by discussing conceptual issues related to determining client readiness for PTSD treatment, as well as the principles underlying this determination. I then review the specific readiness criteria for DBT PE and common challenges that arise in deciding whether clients are ready to start.

Conceptual Issues in Determining Client Readiness

In many ways, describing clients as "ready" for DBT PE falsely implies there is a clear demarcation between clients who are ready versus not ready to engage in trauma-focused treatment. Instead, I would argue that client readiness is best conceptualized as existing on a continuum, with few clients falling on the extreme ends of being unequivocally ready or not ready and most clients exhibiting varying degrees of readiness. DBT PE is typically initiated with clients who are "ready enough"—that is, when the evidence suggesting they will be able to safely and effectively navigate the rigors of the treatment outweighs the evidence suggesting they will not. In addition, readiness is not always a stable state and clients' degree of readiness may wax and wane with periods of progress interrupted by periods of regression into old problem behaviors. Accordingly, the decision that a client is sufficiently ready to begin DBT PE is not a permanent or irreversible one, and once started, the protocol may be paused if clients show serious or persistent signs of no longer being ready for the treatment. In this way, clients may progress through treatment nonlinearly, with multiple transitions in and out of DBT PE depending on fluctuations in their degree of readiness for PTSD treatment over time.

Another false dichotomy that can arise when making decisions about client readiness is the idea that delivering DBT PE will either be "risky" or "not risky." In particular, therapists often express a desire to delay starting PTSD treatment until it will be a risk-free endeavor. I hate to be the bearer of bad news, but this moment in time does not exist. In general, treating clients at high risk for suicide is a risky endeavor. When you add to this high baseline level of risk the fact that DBT PE is a trauma-focused treatment that is intended to elicit intense distress, you can give up now on the idea that risk can ever be fully eliminated. This is particularly true when you consider that there is also risk associated with *not* providing PTSD treatment to these high-risk clients. Indeed, as reviewed in Chapter 1, high-risk clients with PTSD who receive DBT without DBT PE are likely to have *higher* rates of suicide attempts and self-injury than those who receive both treatments. These findings indicate both that treating PTSD is likely to be less risky than not treating PTSD, and that any treatment with this client population will involve some level of risk. Thus, the decision to start DBT PE may best be viewed as a calculated risk that you and your client, in consultation with your DBT team, have agreed to take together.

The real dilemma in determining client readiness for DBT PE lies in finding an effective balance between the extremes of starting too soon versus excessively delaying PTSD treatment. While it is clear that the goal is to provide Stage 1 DBT as briefly and efficiently as possible, it is less clear how long this stabilization period should last. Unlike some stage-based treatments for PTSD in which the length of the initial skill-building phase is predetermined, in DBT + DBT PE the amount of time spent in Stage 1 is based on each client's progress toward individualized readiness goals. Some clients achieve these readiness goals within weeks or months, whereas others may take a year or more. In my efficacy studies, actively suicidal and self-injuring clients required an average of 20 weeks of Stage 1 DBT to achieve the stability necessary to begin DBT PE. However, deciding exactly when to start DBT PE can be a challenging task.

On the one hand, there is valid reason to be concerned about engaging in DBT PE with a high-risk client who does not yet have the ability to cope effectively with the intense emotions this treatment will elicit. Although there have been no studies indicating that DBT PE or PE are associated with an increased risk of life-threatening behavior, these treatments have not been researched among clients with acute suicidality or recent/ongoing suicidal or self-injurious behaviors. However, any therapist who has delivered DBT to Stage 1 clients with PTSD can attest to the fact that trauma cues and the emotions they elicit are common links in the chain of events leading to suicide attempts, self-injury, and other problem behaviors. Given this, it seems clinically wise to assume that premature initiation of DBT PE with a high-risk client could increase the risk of serious behavioral dyscontrol. In my experience, this is the most common concern expressed by new DBT PE therapists—namely, that they will start the treatment too soon and their clients will die or seriously deteriorate as a result. Because of this, it is uncommon for the treatment to be started prematurely and, when this happens, it is typically because the client and/or therapist are particularly eager to engage in DBT PE or there is pressure to accelerate the timeline due to practical constraints on the length of treatment.

The much more common problem is that therapists excessively delay starting DBT PE. This is often because therapists and/or clients are anxious about undertaking PTSD treatment and repeatedly find (often compelling) reasons to avoid starting. The danger on this side of the dialectic is that excessive caution will not only prolong suffering caused by PTSD but will also increase the risk of other adverse outcomes over time, including suicide. When PTSD remains untreated, clients may have difficulty maintaining the gains they make in Stage 1 (e.g., stopping suicidal and self-injurious behaviors) and the risk of relapse is likely to increase the longer they are required to wait. Clients with PTSD may also be unable to achieve significant improvements in some areas that are integrally tied to their trauma (e.g., self-hatred, relationship problems) and that increase their long-term suicide risk.

DBT with DBT PE attempts to reach a "both–and" synthesis for this dilemma by making treating PTSD a clear part of the treatment plan beginning in pretreatment, actively working to prepare and build motivation for PTSD treatment throughout Stage 1, being clear and resolute about the readiness goals that must be achieved, and beginning DBT PE as soon as these goals have been reached. To mitigate against the possibility of starting DBT PE too soon or too late, you should regularly discuss your clients' degree of readiness with your DBT consultation team. Ideally, the decision to start DBT PE is a collaborative one in which you, the client, and the consultation team have weighed the pros and cons of starting now versus waiting, and a wise mind consensus to move forward has been reached.

The Principles Underlying the Readiness Criteria

A significant dilemma I encountered when developing the readiness criteria was how much to make them rule-based versus principle-driven. On the one hand, having a set of clear and straightforward rules would make it easier for therapists to determine when their clients are ready to start. For example, DBT PE cannot be started until Behavior 1 is absent for X weeks and Behavior 2 is reduced to no more than Y times per week. On the other hand, DBT is a principle-driven treatment that requires therapists to make clinical decisions based on the theories underlying the treatment and the needs of the client in front of them. As a result, DBT rarely relies on universal or inflexible rules and the two rules that do exist—the 24-hour rule and the four-miss rule—are principle-driven in that they function as contingency management strategies that often increase clients' motivation to prevent problem behaviors from occurring in the first place. Ultimately, I opted to use a similar approach by creating readiness criteria for DBT PE that are principle-driven, including the one criterion that is a specific rule. Thus, as in DBT more broadly, it is important that therapists understand the principles underlying the readiness criteria so that they can make effective clinical decisions when applying them.

Principle 1: Contingency Management

The primary principle underlying the readiness criteria is contingency management. Contingency management involves using consequences to either increase adaptive behavior or decrease maladaptive behavior. Since most clients view being able to treat their PTSD as a desired outcome, the entire endeavor of "getting ready" for DBT PE can be viewed as a formal contingency management plan in which the readiness criteria specify the behaviors that must be increased or decreased to earn the reward of DBT PE. Accordingly, the readiness criteria often function to motivate clients to more rapidly change their behavior during Stage 1.

Principle 2: Risk Management

A second principle underlying the determination of readiness for DBT PE is that we must prioritize the management of suicide risk. Consistent with the DBT target hierarchy, if a client is at acute risk of suicide or engaging in suicidal or self-injurious behaviors, this must be the number one priority of treatment. Therefore, DBT PE is not started until life-threatening behaviors have been eliminated. At the same time, it is important to maintain a dialectical stance in managing risk: we must stay vigilant to the potential risk of suicidal and self-injurious behaviors and take reasonable precautions to not unduly exacerbate risk while at the same time not allowing fears about risk to lead us to become overly cautious about initiating DBT PE.

Principle 3: Outcome Optimization

The final guiding principle is that we want to maximize the likelihood that the treatment will be successful in reducing PTSD. Although trauma-focused treatments for PTSD are effective for most clients, they do not work for everyone. Research has identified a variety of factors that predict nonresponse to PTSD treatments and, when these prognostic factors are malleable, they should be targeted first in Stage 1 with the goal of optimizing the outcomes of subsequent DBT PE.

DBT PE Protocol Readiness Criteria

Six principle-driven criteria are used to determine readiness to start DBT PE (see Table 6.1). These readiness criteria align with DBT's target hierarchy: The first three address life-threatening behaviors, the fourth pertains to therapy-interfering behaviors, and the fifth and sixth relate to behaviors that interfere with quality of life.

1. Not at Imminent Risk of Suicide

Consistent with other PTSD treatments, DBT PE is not initiated with clients who are believed to be at imminent risk of suicide. Importantly, the emphasis is on *imminent*, which means there is reason to believe a client is at high risk of dying by suicide within the next several days or weeks. Clients who have a high chronic risk of suicide or who may be at high risk for suicide

TABLE 6.1. Readiness Criteria for Starting DBT PE

1. Not at imminent risk of suicide.
2. No recent suicidal or nonsuicidal self-injurious behavior.
3. Able to control suicidal and nonsuicidal self-injurious behaviors in the presence of cues for those behaviors.
4. No serious therapy-interfering behaviors.
5. PTSD is the client's highest-priority quality-of-life target.
6. Ability and willingness to experience intense emotion without escaping.

at some specific point in the future (e.g., "if treatment doesn't work") would not be considered at imminent risk. Unfortunately, determining a client's level of imminent suicide risk is not a precise science and can be particularly challenging with clients who are chronically suicidal and may experience rapid changes in their level of acute risk. As in DBT more broadly, you are expected to conduct thorough suicide risk assessments to evaluate empirically derived risk and protective factors for suicide and to use this information to inform your clinical determination of a client's level of imminent suicide risk.

In addition, clients are typically required to demonstrate behaviorally that they are not or are unlikely to be at imminent risk of suicide. Behavioral indicators of reduced risk should be based on a case formulation of the factors that are most likely to prompt or prevent suicidal behavior for a given client. For example, if a client's past suicide attempts have always occurred in the context of alcohol intoxication, you might require the client to stop drinking to reduce the acute risk of suicide. In addition, clients are typically required to be firmly committed to staying alive for the duration of DBT PE. In line with this commitment, clients are also expected to not be actively preparing to kill themselves, as indicated by behaviors such as acquiring the means to kill themselves, making a specific suicide plan, or writing a suicide note. Given that risk levels can fluctuate rapidly, and suicide attempts often occur impulsively, clients are also expected to have disposed of or restricted their access to lethal means, especially their preferred methods of killing themselves. Finally, it is also important to consider the client's willingness and ability to follow established crisis plans, including contacting you for skills coaching in the event that suicide urges increase.

Importantly, suicidal ideation—even when it is frequent and intense—is not by itself viewed as an indicator of imminent suicide risk. Indeed, ongoing suicidal thoughts and urges are to be expected at the start of DBT PE given that PTSD and trauma-related suffering, which often fuel these thoughts, remain untreated. Therefore, suicidal ideation would not preclude us from starting DBT PE as long as clients have no intent or plans to act on these thoughts. Indeed, most clients who engage in DBT PE continue to have suicidal urges and thoughts, which are likely to decrease as treatment progresses and PTSD improves.

2. No Recent Suicidal or Nonsuicidal Self-Injurious Behavior

The one clear readiness rule is that clients are required to be abstinent from suicidal and non-suicidal self-injury for a period of 2 months in outpatient settings or 1 month in intensive treatment settings (e.g., intensive outpatient, partial hospital, residential). This requirement applies to any type of self-injurious behavior regardless of its severity or suicidal intent and is primarily intended to function as a contingency management strategy—namely, it is intended to motivate clients to stop these behaviors and/or to not engage in them in the first place. It is quite common for clients in Stage 1 to report that, in the context of high suicide or self-injury urges, they chose not to act on these urges because they knew that engaging in these behaviors would delay their ability to start DBT PE. Establishing and maintaining this contingency is therefore often a highly effective strategy for helping clients to more rapidly eliminate self-injurious behaviors during Stage 1. From a contingency management perspective, allowing clients to continue to engage in some forms of self-injury (e.g., low-lethality behaviors) and still receive DBT PE would be much less effective in getting these behaviors to stop. Therefore, this requirement of total abstinence is both consistent with DBT's general stance that clients must stop all forms of self-injurious behavior, as well as a strategic therapeutic move.

To maximize the effectiveness of this rule as a contingency management strategy, it was also necessary to clearly specify an amount of time that abstinence from self-injurious behaviors must be maintained. The standard 2-month time period used in outpatient settings was selected through an iterative process of treatment development in which we began by requiring 4 months of abstinence and, based on the low rate of relapse of self-injurious behaviors during DBT PE, progressively reduced this to 2 months. The decision to further reduce the required period of abstinence to 1 month in intensive treatment settings was largely a pragmatic one. In particular, because these settings typically provide shorter-term treatment, requiring 2 months of abstinence may leave insufficient time to complete DBT PE for clients engaging in self-injurious behaviors at treatment start. Additionally, the shorter period of abstinence is offset by an increased ability of milieu staff to monitor client safety, provide in-person skills coaching, and intervene to prevent escalation of life-threatening behavior.

A second reason for requiring abstinence from self-injurious behaviors is related to the principle of outcome optimization. From a theoretical perspective, self-injurious behaviors that occur during DBT PE, particularly when these behaviors occur shortly before, during, or after exposure tasks, are likely to decrease the effectiveness of the treatment by interfering with corrective learning. For example, many clients believe that approaching trauma-related cues will lead them to kill or injure themselves and these beliefs contribute to the avoidance that maintains PTSD. In such cases, self-injurious behaviors that occur during DBT PE would reinforce rather than disconfirm these PTSD-maintaining beliefs. In addition, self-injurious behaviors that occur in close proximity to exposure tasks are likely to artificially reduce the intensity or duration of emotions elicited by these tasks, thereby interfering with clients' ability to learn that they can tolerate these emotions until they naturally decrease. From an empirical standpoint, the impact of active self-injurious behaviors on PTSD treatment outcomes is unknown as studies to date have only evaluated a prior history of these behaviors as potential predictors of outcome with mixed results (e.g., Ehlers et al., 2013; Krüger et al., 2014; Tarrier, Sommerfield, Pilgrim, & Faragher, 2000).

Finally, the requirement of abstinence from self-injurious behaviors is also influenced by the principle of risk management, which specifies that the reduction of potentially life-threatening behaviors must take priority over all else. Recent and/or ongoing suicidal behavior or NSSI not only poses a clear risk of harm but also often indicates that clients do not yet have sufficient behavioral skills to cope safely with intense emotion. Given that DBT PE is designed to elicit intense emotions, it seems probable that self-injurious behaviors that are active when DBT PE is started are likely to continue, and perhaps even worsen, during the treatment, which may make the treatment unsafe.

Of note, DBT PE's requirement of 1–2 months of abstinence from suicidal behavior and NSSI is more liberal than the eligibility criteria for most PTSD treatments, which typically exclude clients with suicide attempts or NSSI in the past 3 months (e.g., Foa et al., 2019; Resick et al., 2017). However, this requirement is more conservative than several PTSD treatments that exclude clients with suicidal or life-threatening behaviors in the past 2–3 months, but include clients with recent NSSI (Bohus et al., 2013, 2020) or recent NSSI that did not require medical treatment (Cloitre et al., 2014).

3. Able to Control Suicidal and Nonsuicidal Self-Injurious Behaviors in the Presence of Cues for Those Behaviors

Clients are also expected to demonstrate the ability to come into contact with internal and external cues that elicit urges to engage in suicidal behavior and NSSI without engaging in those behaviors. This requirement is designed to ensure that clients have not achieved abstinence from self-injurious behaviors solely by avoiding the cues that typically prompt them. The assumption here is both that these cues cannot be completely avoided, and that PTSD treatment is likely to involve coming into contact with a number of these cues (e.g., trauma memories, feared situations, intense shame, self-critical thoughts). For example, an adolescent with a history of repeated suicidal behavior may not have attempted suicide for several months and appear to be quite stable. However, upon closer examination, it is determined that conflict with his mother has typically been the prompting event for his past suicide attempts, and he has recently been minimizing his interactions with his mother (with whom he lives) as a way to avoid conflict. In this case, the therapist (and client) would need to feel confident that he could interact and potentially have conflict with his mother and still not attempt suicide.

To evaluate readiness in this domain, it is often useful to conduct behavioral tests of clients' ability to skillfully cope with urges to engage in self-injurious behaviors when presented with cues, particularly those that are likely to be present during DBT PE. The typical cues for these behaviors are usually identified through chain analyses and are often linked by a common emotion (e.g., shame) or thought (e.g., "I am disgusting") that they elicit. Thus, behavioral tests often involve exposure-like exercises to non-trauma-related cues that are designed to evoke specific emotions (e.g., inducing shame by sharing a perceived flaw with a trusted other) or thoughts (e.g., prompting self-judgmental thoughts by looking at a photo of oneself) after which clients are expected to demonstrate their ability to cope with the emotions and urges these cues elicit without engaging in self-injurious behaviors.

4. No Serious Therapy-Interfering Behaviors

Consistent with the DBT target hierarchy, clients are also required to not exhibit serious therapy-interfering behaviors. The primary principle underlying this criterion is that of outcome optimization—that is, clients need to have demonstrated the ability to engage in therapy in such a way that DBT PE is likely to be effective. The decision about whether a therapy-interfering behavior is serious enough to make DBT PE unlikely to work is determined by several principle-driven questions.

First, it is important to consider whether the behavior will prevent the client from receiving a sufficient dose of DBT PE. This concern is based on research indicating that positive outcomes in PTSD treatments are strongly predicted by consistent treatment attendance and higher adherence to homework (e.g., Cooper et al., 2017; Tarrier et al., 2000). Essentially, clients must reliably attend treatment and complete exposure tasks both in and outside of sessions for the treatment to work. I often talk to clients about this as being similar to having to take the full dose of an antibiotic for an infection to be effectively treated. If you stop taking the antibiotic, take it inconsistently, or take a lower dose than prescribed, your infection is not likely to go away and may even get worse. Thus, a client who routinely misses therapy sessions, arrives at sessions late or leaves early, fails to complete homework assignments, or engages in any behavior during therapy sessions (e.g., frequent arguments, refusing to speak, dissociating) that makes it difficult or impossible to complete therapy tasks is likely to be considered not yet ready to begin DBT PE.

A second issue to consider is whether the behavior is likely to interfere with the mechanisms of action in DBT PE. In particular, clients need to able to attend to, take in, and retain corrective information present during exposure and processing in order for beliefs to change and emotions to decrease in intensity over time. Thus, behaviors that significantly interfere with attention and/or information processing during therapy sessions and homework tasks are likely to reduce the effectiveness of DBT PE. For example, clients with high state dissociation during therapy sessions show less improvement in PTSD after trauma-focused treatment (Kleindienst et al., 2016). Other behaviors that are likely to interfere with the ability to learn during exposure are things such as intoxication, extreme fatigue, or severe malnourishment.

Another potential factor to consider is the strength of the therapeutic alliance. Several studies have shown that poorer alliance and more unrepaired ruptures in the therapy relationship predict worse outcomes in PTSD treatments (Cloitre et al., 2002; McLaughlin, Keller, Feeny, Youngstrom, & Zoellner, 2014). In DBT PE, having strong rapport increases our ability to strategically use ourselves as a reinforcer to help clients engage in the treatment effectively. This may be particularly important for clients who are believed to be at high (but not imminent) risk for suicide and for whom having a strong attachment to the therapist is often a primary reason for staying alive during times of increased stress. If there is frequent conflict in the therapy relationship or a significant relationship rupture has recently occurred, it may be wise to delay initiating DBT PE until the relationship is stronger.

Importantly, we routinely begin DBT PE with clients who continue to exhibit mild to moderate therapy-interfering behaviors (e.g., who sometimes miss sessions, do not always complete homework, or who dissociate intermittently during therapy sessions) and who may be only somewhat attached to us. To make a client ineligible to begin DBT PE, the therapy-interfering behavior must be severe enough that the client's willingness and/or ability to engage in treatment in an effective manner is seriously in doubt.

5. PTSD Is the Client's Highest-Priority Quality-of-Life Target

Once treatment is focused on quality-of-life issues, the selection of treatment targets is largely determined by the client's preferences and goals. Accordingly, to begin DBT PE, PTSD must be the client's highest-priority target and it must be the client's goal to treat PTSD now. For some clients, PTSD may not initially be their highest-priority target and they may elect to address other quality-of-life issues prior to addressing PTSD. Other clients may view PTSD as their highest priority but may not be interested in treating it now. It is also the case that some clients may never view PTSD as an important treatment target. Our role is not to dictate what clients should do, but rather to serve as a consultant in helping them decide their treatment priorities and reach a wise mind decision about whether and when to treat PTSD.

It is also important to highlight that nearly all clients who begin DBT PE continue to exhibit multiple problems in addition to PTSD that fall within DBT's quality-of-life interfering behavior domain. If clients have other problems that are causing immediate crises (e.g., criminal behavior), significant life instability (e.g., bankruptcy, homelessness), and/or pose a high risk of serious harm (e.g., ongoing physical abuse, accidental drug overdoses), these problems may require priority treatment over PTSD. In addition, if other quality-of-life behaviors (e.g., substance use, dissociation, food restriction) are likely to significantly interfere with therapy (Criterion 4) or clients' ability to experience emotions without escaping (Criterion 6), then they will need to be addressed prior to starting DBT PE. At the same time, because many quality-of-life problems are maintained or exacerbated by PTSD, they are unlikely to fully improve until PTSD is treated. Therefore, the goal is often to reduce the severity of these problems to a level where they are not causing crises or likely to significantly interfere with PTSD treatment, but not to require complete control or cessation before initiating DBT PE.

As a general guideline, clients are typically expected to be able to refrain from escape-related quality-of-life interfering behaviors immediately before, during, and for about 2 hours after any exposure task. Prior to starting DBT PE, this is often evaluated by asking clients to demonstrate the ability to not engage in these behaviors for several hours at a time, including when intense emotions are present. For example, clients who are abusing substances may be asked to come to therapy sessions sober and to refrain from substance use for at least 2 hours after a session. The same expectation can be set for other quality-of-life interfering behaviors (e.g., binge eating, impulsive sex, gambling) likely to disrupt emotional experiencing or confirm rather than violate clients' expectancies about the likely outcomes of exposure. The goal here is to ensure that clients will be able to create sufficient windows of learning during which they approach avoided cues, experience emotions, and process corrective information without engaging in problematic escape behaviors likely to interfere with or undo this learning.

6. Ability and Willingness to Experience Intense Emotions without Escaping

For exposure to be effective, emotions must be activated and experienced without engaging in escape strategies to reduce their intensity, shorten their duration, or stop them altogether. This readiness criterion is therefore intended to optimize outcomes by ensuring that clients have the capacity to experience emotions effectively. In particular, clients must be able and willing to tolerate intense emotions without significant avoidance for the length of a typical exposure trial (about 30 minutes), and to skillfully regulate emotions afterward. Importantly, clients must have demonstrated these abilities with a range of emotions. For example, clients who only allow themselves to feel anger, and routinely suppress other emotions, are unlikely to be viewed as ready for DBT PE.

It is therefore important to evaluate clients' ability and willingness to experience intense emotions prior to beginning DBT PE. This may be accomplished by observing clients' responses to naturally occurring emotions during therapy sessions. For example, when clients experience sadness in session, do they allow themselves to cry and remain focused on the cause of the sadness, or do they immediately shut down or distract? When intense shame occurs in a session, can clients stay engaged and talk about what prompted the shame, or do they withdraw and become nonresponsive? Over the course of Stage 1, you may increasingly use informal exposure when emotions naturally arise during sessions to encourage clients to actively attend to and experience the emotion rather than avoid it.

In addition, you can plan and conduct emotion exposure tasks to behaviorally test the client's ability to experience and regulate emotions. Examples of these types of tasks include:

- Describe a painful (nontraumatic) past event out loud using emotion words.
- Read about a scary event in the news and focus on physical sensations.

- Watch "tearjerker" movies and allow yourself to cry.
- Listen to music that elicits an emotion and practice mindfulness of the emotion.
- Write about something you are ashamed of for 20 minutes.

Importantly, whatever emotion-induction tasks are used, clients are expected to demonstrate the ability to allow emotions during the task, as well as to regulate emotions effectively after the task, without immediately engaging in problem behaviors (see Criterion 5 above).

Orienting Clients to the Readiness Criteria

In order for the readiness criteria to function as a contingency management strategy that motivates behavior change, clients must be oriented to the criteria and the specific behaviors they will need to change to be eligible to receive DBT PE. As previously described, this orientation begins during pretreatment with a general overview of how PTSD factors into the DBT target hierarchy, along with a clear description of the amount of time that clients must be abstinent from suicidal and nonsuicidal self-injury before DBT PE can be started. As Stage 1 progresses, you should provide a detailed orientation to all six readiness criteria and work with clients to shape these criteria into an individualized treatment plan. The timing of this detailed readiness discussion varies, but generally occurs after clients have begun to express interest in receiving DBT PE. Although the timing varies, it is critical that clients are oriented to the readiness criteria while there is still sufficient time left in treatment both to make the required behavior changes and complete DBT PE.

When orienting clients to the readiness criteria, the goal is to collaboratively and clearly define the behaviors that must be increased or decreased to receive DBT PE. *General Handout 5* (*Getting Ready to Start DBT PE*) in Appendix A is used to translate each of the readiness criteria into individualized and behaviorally specific targets for each client. Examples of the types of behavioral targets that are commonly used to determine readiness in each criterion domain are provided in Table 6.2. These are not intended to be an exhaustive or required list of targets, and these potential indicators of readiness need to be specifically defined to match the behaviors relevant to each client. For example, what are the specific cues that elicit urges for suicide and self-injury that a client needs to show that they can cope effectively with (Criterion 3)? What specific behaviors does the client engage in during sessions that interfere with therapy (Criterion 4)? Ideally, these specific targets are generated collaboratively with your client. For example, you may ask, "What do you think will need to change so that we can be confident that you are no longer at imminent risk of killing yourself?" In this way, establishing the readiness goals become less likely to be experienced as a rigid or punitive procedure that is being forced on the client, and more likely to be experienced as a motivation-enhancing strategy that clearly aligns with the client's own goals.

When Clients Do Not Achieve Readiness Goals

Once clients are oriented to the readiness criteria and the behavioral targets that must change to begin DBT PE have been clearly defined, it is important to apply this plan consistently during treatment. In general, contingency management plans are less likely to motivate behavior change if the requirements specified in the plan change over time or exceptions are made. It is

TABLE 6.2. Translating the Readiness Criteria into Behaviorally Specific Goals

Readiness criteria	Example behavioral indicators of readiness
1. Not at imminent risk of suicide.	• No current suicidal intent, planning, or preparation • Strong commitment to stay alive • Restricted access to lethal means • Willing to follow the established crisis plan
2. No recent suicidal or nonsuicidal self-injurious behaviors.	• Abstinence from suicide attempts and nonsuicidal self-injury for at least 2 months (outpatient) or 1 month (intensive treatment settings)
3. Able to control suicidal and nonsuicidal self-injurious behaviors in the presence of cues for those behaviors.	• Able to tolerate urges to attempt suicide and self-injure without acting on them • Able to use DBT skills to cope effectively with specific cues for these behaviors (e.g., flashbacks, intense shame, interpersonal conflict)
4. No serious therapy-interfering behaviors.	• Consistent attendance at therapy sessions and completion of homework • Able to maintain attention during therapy sessions • Willing to engage in treatment tasks
5. PTSD is the client's highest-priority quality-of-life target.	• It is the client's goal to treat their PTSD now • Other quality-of-life problems are not causing crises or a higher degree of impairment than PTSD • Other quality-of-life problems can be controlled enough that they will be unlikely to occur before, during, or immediately after exposure tasks
6. Ability and willingness to experience intense emotion without escaping.	• Consistent willingness to experience and express emotions during therapy sessions • Able to practice mindfulness of current emotion for ~30 minutes without significant avoidance • Able to talk about distressing situations while effectively emotionally engaged

therefore important to set clear readiness targets and stick to them using a benevolently demanding approach that balances encouraging and supporting clients to reach the goals and remaining resolute that the goals must be met. Adhering to the plan can be particularly challenging when clients are making slow or insufficient progress, which may lead you and/or your clients to want to deviate from the plan and begin DBT PE despite not having made the required behavior changes. This may occur when, for example, a client has reduced the frequency of NSSI but has not completely stopped engaging in this behavior. Or a client may now be attending treatment consistently, but still rarely completes homework. In such cases, you should obtain consultation from your team to address urges to deviate from the plan. In general, it is recommended that you adopt the standard readiness criteria to maximize your fidelity to the research-tested model. Decisions to adapt the readiness criteria and/or modify the specific readiness requirements that were originally established for a client should be rare and occur only after careful consideration of the following issues:

1. *Would initiating DBT PE reinforce the problem behavior that has interfered with achieving readiness?* A primary concern about deviating from an established contingency management plan is that this is likely to reinforce maladaptive behavior. For example, if a client

was initially told that they could not receive DBT PE if they were actively self-injuring, and in response to ongoing self-injury you remove this contingency and allow them to start the treatment, there is a risk that the client's self-injury may be reinforced by this deviation. Therefore, when a behavior targeted for change as part of the readiness plan is not sufficiently improving, you should carefully consider whether the behavior is likely to be reinforced by making the established readiness plan more lenient to accommodate it.

2. *Would continuing to withhold DBT PE be likely to change the problem behavior?* Making the start of DBT PE contingent on changing other higher-priority problem behaviors is intended in large part to motivate clients to change these behaviors. Given this, the more a client wants to receive DBT PE, the more likely it is that withholding it will help to motivate behavior change and the less likely it is that we would deviate from an established readiness plan when a problem behavior is not sufficiently changing. On the other hand, in cases where withholding DBT PE is unlikely to impact the behavior (e.g., because treating PTSD is not a reinforcer for a particular client), we might be more likely to consider starting DBT PE even though the behavior has not sufficiently changed.

3. *Has the behavior persisted despite both the therapist and client making substantial and competent efforts to get the behavior to stop?* Another important issue to consider is how effectively and/or comprehensively the problem behavior has been targeted. Have treatment strategies been implemented to address the primary controlling variables for the problem behavior? Have multiple treatment strategies been tried over a sufficient duration of time? Has the client demonstrated significant motivation to change the behaviors, and worked to implement the potential solutions that have been generated? If the answers to these questions are "yes," then we would be more likely to consider beginning DBT PE despite an ongoing problem behavior. In contrast, if the behavior has not been comprehensively or effectively addressed (by either you or the client), then DBT PE would likely continue to be postponed.

4. *Is the behavior functionally related to PTSD?* One potential reason that a problem behavior may persist despite wholehearted efforts to prevent it is that it is functionally related to ongoing PTSD symptoms. For example, dissociation may have decreased from severe episodes lasting multiple hours to briefer episodes lasting up to 30 minutes, including sometimes during therapy sessions. Similarly, a client whose hyperarousal includes frequent anger outbursts may have stopped punching walls and breaking objects but may continue to yell and make verbal threats when angry. In cases in which problem behaviors that are functionally related to PTSD have not improved as much as desired, then it may be both appropriate and necessary to begin PTSD treatment to get these behaviors to more fully resolve. In contrast, if the behavior is not typically linked to PTSD (e.g., it occurs in response to unrelated life stressors), then beginning DBT PE may not be an effective strategy for getting the behavior to change.

5. *Has new information emerged that suggests the behavior is not as problematic as once believed?* In some cases, a behavior that was targeted for change prior to starting DBT PE is determined to be less worrisome than originally thought. For example, a client who regularly misses therapy sessions due to transportation problems may demonstrate that they are able to complete homework assignments, stay in contact with the therapist as needed, and generally make progress in treatment despite not being able to reliably attend. In some cases, a behavior may persist but its function may change over the course of treatment in ways that make it less likely to interfere with DBT PE. For example, a goal may have been set for a client to abstain from alcohol use for at least a month prior to starting DBT PE because in the past alcohol had primarily been used to reduce his inhibitions about killing himself. However, as treatment

progresses and the client becomes less suicidal, alcohol stops functioning to increase his capacity for suicide and instead begins to have a social function (e.g., as a social activity engaged in with friends). In cases where new information about the problem behavior reduces concerns that it is likely to interfere with DBT PE, it may be reasonable to deviate from the original readiness goal.

6. *Is there sufficient time left in treatment to delay beginning DBT PE?* This issue is purely pragmatic—namely, if DBT PE is not started now, will there still be sufficient time to implement it later in the treatment? For example, in a 1-year treatment, clients need to begin DBT PE by approximately the eighth month of treatment to allow sufficient time to complete it. Thus, if a client is continuing to engage in a targeted problem behavior by the eighth month, we would be more likely to consider starting DBT PE than for a client who is at an earlier point in treatment.

Concluding Comments

While I have often wished there was a measurable set of characteristics whose presence clearly indicates readiness for PTSD treatment, in reality this determination lies somewhere in the murky middle ground between the subjectivity of a Ouija board and the objectivity of a biomarker test. For better or worse, this reflects much of the practice of psychotherapy, in which decisions about when and with whom to apply evidence-based treatments is ultimately a clinical judgment. At the same time, these clinical decisions should be based on the best available empirical evidence and the principles underlying the treatment. In DBT PE, decisions about readiness to start the treatment should be guided by the principles of contingency management, risk management, and outcome optimization, and made collaboratively with the client and your consultation team. Overall, the goal is to enable clients to receive DBT PE as soon as it is believed to be both safe and effective to do so, and to avoid either prematurely initiating or excessively delaying the treatment.

CHAPTER 7

Preparing to Start DBT PE

In the weeks leading up to starting DBT PE, therapists and clients typically engage in several final preparatory tasks that range from the purely logistical to the clinically critical. You and your client need to make decisions about how to structure the treatment, monitor progress, and record sessions; discuss relevant ethical and legal issues; and create an initial DBT PE case formulation to guide treatment planning. The common thread among these tasks is that they will help to ensure that you both arrive at Session 1 as prepared as possible to succeed.

Structuring Treatment

Before starting DBT PE, there are several important decisions to be made about how to structure the treatment. When making these implementation decisions, therapists are often faced with the dilemma of whether to adopt or adapt the standard treatment structure. As with any research-tested intervention, it is generally recommended that you adopt the model that has been used in the research trials that support DBT PE's efficacy. This "adopt" approach ensures that you are providing the most adherent care possible, therefore increasing the likelihood that comparable outcomes will be achieved. In addition, adhering to a validated treatment model may reduce the risk and legal liability that is a common worry when working with populations at high risk for suicide.

On the other hand, it is also true that the standard structure of the integrated DBT + DBT PE treatment may be incompatible with the needs and constraints of some treatment settings and clients. For example, the longer or more frequent individual therapy sessions typically used in DBT PE may be cost-prohibitive for some clients or require too much time for some therapists. When these types of real-world constraints are present, it may be necessary to adapt the standard treatment structure. In this section, I offer suggestions for potential adaptations that are based on surveys of and consultation with therapists delivering DBT PE in a wide variety of routine practice settings. I encourage you to approach the dilemma of adopting versus adapting thoughtfully and work to find a solution that adheres as closely as possible to the standard model while also being feasible to implement.

Structuring Individual Therapy

Standard Session Formats

The DBT PE protocol is intended to be integrated into DBT individual therapy sessions during ongoing delivery of standard DBT. To achieve this integration, you need to decide how to structure individual therapy sessions to enable the client to receive both DBT and DBT PE. In my original efficacy studies (Harned et al., 2012, 2014), there were two options for structuring individual therapy sessions, and therapists and clients collaboratively decided which option to use. Consistent with the session format prescribed in the PE manual (Foa et al., 2019), both options include 90 minutes for DBT PE, but vary in the amount of time allotted for DBT (30 vs. 60 minutes).

STANDARD OPTION 1

This option involves two sessions per week: one 90-minute DBT PE session and one 60-minute DBT session, totaling 2.5 hours of individual therapy. This session structure is likely to be preferable for clients with multiple or severe problems that need to be treated in addition to PTSD and/or whose lives are characterized by a high degree of chaos or instability. These clients may continue to require a standard 60-minute DBT individual therapy session each week to have sufficient time to address their complex co-occurring problems. When considering this more intensive treatment format, both you and your client need to determine whether temporarily increasing to two sessions per week is feasible. In some cases, this more intensive treatment format may be preferable from a clinical perspective, but infeasible from a pragmatic one, in which case a less intensive format may be necessary.

STANDARD OPTION 2

This option combines DBT PE (90 minutes) and DBT (30 minutes) into a single 2-hour weekly session. This somewhat less intensive session structure is most suitable for clients whose remaining co-occurring problems are relatively few or nonsevere and whose lives are reasonably stable. For these clients, 30 minutes of DBT may be sufficient to address other problems that exist beyond PTSD. If this session structure is chosen, you and your client need to decide whether to conduct the 30 minutes of DBT before or after DBT PE. Starting the session with DBT is recommended for clients who are likely to find it difficult to engage productively in DBT after completing DBT PE. For example, some clients feel particularly exhausted after completing imaginal exposure and processing, and this can limit their ability to engage effectively in subsequent DBT treatment tasks. If the session starts with DBT, the main thing to be careful about is potentially extending DBT longer than 30 minutes and running out of time for DBT PE. Alternatively, the session may begin with 90 minutes of DBT PE and end with 30 minutes of DBT. This session structure can be useful for clients who prefer to have more time with you to regulate after completing imaginal exposure and processing. For these clients, ending the session with 30 minutes of DBT can function as an extended wind-down period that enables them to refocus their attention on topics other than trauma before the session ends. It may be hard to predict in advance which order of treatments within the session is likely to be most effective, in which case both configurations can be tried before choosing the one that works best for the client.

Alternative Session Formats

In some settings, these standard session formats may not be possible due to productivity demands, lack of insurance reimbursement, or other pragmatic barriers. Indeed, in studies of DBT PE in community practice settings, only 28–46% of therapists reported using one of the standard session formats (Harned, Ritschel, et al., 2021; Harned, Schmidt, et al., 2021). Other common session formats were one 90-minute combined DBT + DBT PE session per week or two separate 60-minute sessions for DBT and DBT PE per week. Given that clients in these studies typically showed improvements in PTSD, it is possible that DBT PE may be effective when delivered in sessions of varying lengths and frequencies, although more research is needed to rigorously evaluate this. Encouragingly, studies of PE have compared 60- versus 90-minute sessions and found that both session lengths yield equivalent outcomes (Nacasch et al., 2015; van Minnen & Foa, 2006). Therefore, when significant barriers make it infeasible to utilize the more intensive standard session formats, it may be reasonable to utilize an alternative format that includes a minimum of 60 minutes for DBT PE and may better fit the constraints of your setting.

CLINICAL TIP

Can DBT PE Be Delivered Using a More Intensive Session Format?

The session formats described above each include one DBT PE session per week. Several studies support the use of more intensive session formats to deliver PTSD treatments, including DBT PE. In a study of DBT PE for veterans, DBT PE sessions occurred twice weekly for 6 weeks of a 12-week intensive outpatient program (Meyers et al., 2017). Similarly, several RCTs of standard PE have used a twice-weekly session format in which clients received two 90-minute PE sessions per week for 5 weeks (nine sessions total; Foa et al., 1991; Foa, Dancu, et al., 1999). One RCT has tested an even more intensive treatment format and found that massed PE (10 sessions over 2 weeks) was comparable to spaced PE (10 sessions over 8 weeks; Foa et al., 2018). Taken together, these findings suggest that it is reasonable to increase the frequency of DBT PE sessions to two to five times per week in settings where a more intensive session format is possible or preferred.

CLINICAL TIP

Can Different Therapists Deliver DBT and DBT PE to the Same Client?

In research trials, DBT PE has been delivered by the DBT individual therapist. The primary advantage of this approach is that the therapist and client are already well acquainted before they begin DBT PE. For therapists, this makes it easier to develop a case formulation, predict and respond to potential difficulties that may arise, and leverage the relationship to increase effective engagement in DBT PE. For clients, the fact that they already know and trust their therapist often increases their willingness to engage in DBT PE, including sharing sensitive details of their trauma history. However, in some cases it may be necessary to have separate DBT and DBT PE therapists, such as in DBT teams where only some therapists are trained to deliver DBT PE. When this treatment structure is used, there are three key issues to consider:

1. *Who is the primary therapist?* Consistent with the standard hierarchy of treatment providers in DBT, the DBT individual therapist is typically the primary therapist and the DBT PE therapist is secondary. This means that the DBT individual therapist has primary responsibility for decision making related to the client's treatment plan. Although the DBT PE therapist may offer input, decisions that impact the client's treatment plan are left to the primary therapist.

2. *Who will provide between-session phone coaching?* This role typically falls to the primary therapist, which in most cases will be the DBT individual therapist. However, you may decide to split this responsibility between therapists. For example, clients may be instructed to contact the DBT PE therapist for coaching related to completing exposure tasks and to contact the DBT therapist for coaching related to all other issues.

3. *How will care be coordinated?* Consistent with DBT's consultation-to-the-client approach, the two therapists should strive not to discuss the client's treatment in detail when the client is not present or tell each other how to treat the client. During team meetings, each therapist can seek consultation about the client when needed but should limit the details they share to those that are relevant to the consultation issue. In general, it is recommended that clients be responsible for keeping each therapist updated about their progress in the other treatment, and when needed, both therapists and the client can meet together to share information and engage in collaborative treatment planning.

Structuring DBT Group Skills Training

In research trials, clients engaged in DBT PE also attended DBT group skills training (2–2.5 hours/week) as part of their comprehensive DBT treatment. The DBT skills group can be instrumental in helping clients to complete DBT PE successfully by providing regular opportunities to practice and improve their skills, as well as an important source of social support. In programs in which multiple clients are receiving DBT PE at once, the skills group often provides an opportunity for these clients to offer encouragement and reinforcement to one another for their hard work and progress while also serving as positive role models for other clients who may be considering receiving DBT PE. However, when implementing DBT PE in routine practice, some clients may no longer be participating in a DBT skills group at the time DBT PE is delivered. This may occur, for example, if clients continue in DBT individual therapy after graduating from their skills group. In such cases, it is up to you and the client to decide whether it would be useful for the client to reengage in a DBT skills group during DBT PE (e.g., for additional support or a refresher on the skills) or whether this is not needed (e.g., the client is knowledgeable about and continues to regularly use skills).

Structuring DBT Phone Coaching

Clients are also expected to have access to between-session phone coaching while they are engaged in DBT PE. Phone coaching is often used to help clients complete exposure homework effectively by offering support, troubleshooting problems (e.g., urges to avoid), and providing reinforcement. Coaching calls may also be scheduled in advance to occur either before or after exposure tasks as a way to increase motivation, particularly early in DBT PE when clients may be especially anxious about doing exposure on their own. Ideally, phone coaching will be provided by the DBT PE therapist, as they are likely to be in the best position to help clients navigate difficulties that may arise between sessions related to completing exposure exercises.

Structuring the DBT Therapist Consultation Team

In the standard model, DBT PE therapists are required to be members of a DBT consultation team, which means that teams need to consider how to provide therapists with consultation related to DBT PE. This may be more challenging when only some therapists on a DBT team are trained in DBT PE. My recommendation is to include DBT PE consultation issues as part of the agenda of regular DBT team meetings. From a theoretical perspective, the DBT team functions to build therapist motivation and capability to deliver DBT, which should include the delivery of protocols such as DBT PE that are integrated into DBT. From a clinical perspective, DBT PE can be an emotionally demanding treatment to deliver, and it is important that DBT PE therapists have an opportunity to receive "therapy for the therapist," which is a core function of a DBT team. Finally, from a practical perspective, it is often infeasible to schedule separate team meetings just for DBT PE therapists, although if there are enough DBT PE therapists and clients, this could certainly be considered.

Teams have a lot of flexibility in terms of how they structure their team meeting, and this is also true when considering how to include items related to DBT PE on the agenda. In general, the same principles that teams have used to prioritize agenda items should be applied to items related to DBT PE. In teams where priority is based on the DBT target hierarchy, therapists' needs related to DBT PE could fall into any tier depending on whether the therapist is struggling to manage life-threatening, therapy-interfering, or quality-of-life-interfering behaviors during DBT PE. If priority is determined by therapists' level of distress, then issues related to DBT PE could similarly fall anywhere on the priority list depending on how much they are impacting the therapist. Some teams may decide to create a standing item on the agenda to discuss therapists' delivery of DBT PE, which can be helpful when working to shape the team culture from focusing only on DBT to now considering both treatments. For example, at one point my team found it helpful to allot time every other week to check in on therapists' progress toward preparing clients to start DBT PE, which helped to make sure that this issue did not fall off the team's (or therapists') radar.

Another issue to consider is how much detail, if any, to share with your team about your clients' traumatic experiences when seeking consultation. In general, the focus of the DBT team should be on the therapist, not the client, and specifically on what the therapist needs to stay motivated and provide effective treatment. Therefore, my recommendation is that you share only as much information about a client's trauma as is required to get your needs met, and only when clients have been oriented to the fact that you may share information about them with your team. In most cases, therapists' needs can be met without disclosing detailed information about the client's trauma, as these details are often irrelevant to the problem and may even distract the team from providing the needed assistance.

Structuring Joint or Family Sessions

You and your client also need to decide whether and how to involve other people in the client's life (e.g., parents, spouse, partner) in DBT PE. For adult clients who elect to involve a support person in treatment, it is typical to have a single joint session at some point prior to starting imaginal exposure, and the exact timing of this session needs to be decided. For adolescent clients, parents or caregivers are generally more involved in treatment, although the frequency and type of involvement varies. Chapter 10 includes detailed information about how to conduct joint and family sessions to orient and elicit support from people in the client's life.

CLINICAL TIP

Can DBT PE Be Delivered via Telehealth?

Although no studies have evaluated the effectiveness of DBT or DBT PE delivered in a telehealth format, there is a sizable literature supporting the delivery of evidence-based PTSD treatments, including PE, via telehealth. These studies have shown that delivering PTSD treatments via videoconferencing is feasible and acceptable to clients and leads to improvements in PTSD that are comparable to those obtained in traditional face-to-face care (see Morland et al., 2020, for a review). Anecdotally, many therapists converted to delivering DBT PE via telehealth during the COVID-19 pandemic and similarly experienced this as an acceptable and effective method of treatment delivery. When delivering DBT PE via videoconferencing there are practical issues to consider, such as ensuring that clients have the necessary equipment and a private location to hold sessions, establishing methods for sharing and collecting treatment materials, and adhering to laws and insurance reimbursement policies related to delivering treatment via telehealth (and potentially across state lines). Clinically, it is also useful to consider the client's environment during DBT PE sessions (e.g., choosing locations with minimal distractions) and to ask clients to set up their cameras so that they are maximally visible (e.g., to better observe clients' behavior during exposure). Therapists may also ask clients to have relevant skills-related materials accessible to use during exposure as needed (e.g., an ice pack to manage dissociation) and/or to refrain from engaging in behaviors that may function as avoidance during exposure (e.g., being wrapped in a blanket or holding a pet). In general, clients should be asked to complete DBT PE via telehealth in a manner as similar as possible to how it would be done in a therapy office.

Ethical and Legal Considerations

Informed Consent

Consistent with professional ethical guidelines, it is important to ensure that informed consent to participate in DBT PE has been obtained and documented prior to beginning the treatment. For adults and adolescents able to provide their own consent, the process of obtaining informed consent to receive DBT PE typically occurs during Stage 1 as you work to obtain a commitment to engage in the treatment. You may choose to obtain written or verbal consent to participate in DBT PE, but in either case it is important to document that informed consent was obtained. For adolescents who are below the legal age to consent to mental health treatment, informed consent to receive DBT PE must be obtained from a parent or legal guardian. This is typically done in a family session that occurs in Stage 1 after the adolescent has decided they want to receive DBT PE. Parents should be provided with information about DBT PE (e.g., using *General Handout 4* [*What Is DBT PE?*] in Appendix A) and given an opportunity to ask questions. In addition, they should be informed about potential changes to the frequency and length of sessions and the fee implications of such changes. It may also be useful to review privacy guide-lines (e.g., reminding parents that they will not be privy to detailed information about what is happening in treatment), as well as mandatory reporting requirements (see below). The goal is to give parents enough information about DBT PE to provide informed consent without disclos-ing information that the adolescent prefers not to have shared. Once this is done, you should document that parents consented for their child to receive DBT PE.

Mandatory Reporting

During the course of DBT PE, therapists very often learn details about their clients' traumas that they did not previously know. Given this, you must be prepared for the possibility that your clients may disclose information about child abuse or neglect that you are legally mandated to report. In particular, it is critical that you make your clients aware in advance of the type of information that would obligate you to make a report so that they can make an informed deci-sion about what they choose to share during DBT PE. Although all clients should be oriented to mandatory reporting requirements prior to starting DBT, you may wish to review these requirements again before starting DBT PE and provide clients with an opportunity to ask questions about what would and would not necessitate a report. If clients then elect to share information that you are legally required to report, you can decide with the client how to do so. For example, you might make the report with the client present so that they can participate in or listen to the phone call, or they may prefer that you make the report on your own. If there is any uncertainty about whether a specific situation must be reported, you should seek consulta-tion about this from experts in this area.

The issue of mandatory reporting can pose a particular challenge in treatment with clients whose trauma history includes a reportable offense and who do not want a report to be made. There are many understandable reasons that clients may not wish to have their abuse reported to authorities. Very often shame, self-blame, minimization of the trauma, and/or fear of nega-tive consequences (e.g., retaliation, being disbelieved) lead clients to not want their abuse to be reported. In some cases, clients may be motivated by a desire to protect the perpetrator or others who might be negatively impacted by a legal investigation. These clients are faced with an incredibly difficult dilemma: to disclose their trauma to get effective PTSD treatment even though this may lead to an unwanted legal report or to not disclose their trauma and continue to suffer from PTSD.

For clients who are caught between these two opposing poles, you can help them think through the pros and cons of each course of action so that they can reach a wise-minded deci-sion about how they wish to proceed. In some cases, it may be possible to find a workable synthesis—for example, some clients may choose to leave out certain details (e.g., identifying information about perpetrators) when describing their traumas so that reports, if they are made, are unlikely to be acted on. If such an approach is considered, you need to weigh the potential benefits of being able to treat the client's PTSD against the potential downsides of doing so in a way that will reduce the need for or potential viability of a report. In some cases, therapists may understandably decide that such an approach would violate their own values or ethics even if it meets the letter of the law, perhaps particularly if there is reason to believe the perpetrator continues to pose a risk to children. It is also important to keep in mind that clients' concerns about having their abuse reported may decrease over the course of DBT PE as they stop holding themselves responsible for their own abuse, accept the reality of what happened to them, and no longer minimize its seriousness.

Logistical Issues

Recording Sessions

Each session of DBT PE is recorded for clients to listen to between sessions, typically as an audio recording but sometimes including video (e.g., if sessions are conducted via telehealth). This is done primarily to enable clients to complete imaginal exposure repeatedly throughout the week (i.e., by listening to the recording of their in-session imaginal exposure). In addition, clients are asked to listen to the entire session recording at least once per week (including the nonexposure session components) to aid in generalizing what is learned in session to the client's life out of session. Typically, clients are responsible for providing a recording device, and most choose to use their mobile phone or a digital voice recorder. In preparing to start DBT PE, you should therefore ensure that clients have a device to record sessions and help them to think through how they will secure the device to protect their own privacy (e.g., physical storage location, password protection, uploading of files to a shared cloud storage location).

Outcome Monitoring

Routine outcome monitoring is a core component of evidence-based practice. In DBT PE, therapists are expected to regularly assess clients' progress and to use these data to make adjustments to the treatment in a timely manner when progress is slow or insufficient. In preparing to start DBT PE, you must therefore select and obtain the measure(s) you will use for progress monitoring. Typically, PTSD symptom severity is assessed every other week using a self-report measure, such as the PTSD Checklist for DSM-5 (PCL-5; Weathers et al., 2013). On alternating weeks, you may choose to measure another outcome that is relevant to your client. I typically recommend measures that assess key mechanisms of action in reducing PTSD, such as the Post-traumatic Cognitions Inventory (PTCI; Foa, Ehlers, Clark, Tolin, & Orsillo, 1999), which can help to more precisely identify and target factors that may be maintaining clients' PTSD. Alternatively, you may choose to monitor another co-occurring problem that is particularly relevant to a client (e.g., dissociation, borderline personality symptoms). Appendix D includes a list of measures that may be useful.

DBT PE Case Formulation

On its surface, DBT PE may seem like a relatively straightforward treatment to deliver: It is a protocol with a clear structure that specifies which treatment strategies to deliver in each session, for approximately how long, and in what order. However, in the course of delivering this structured protocol, you will be required to make many clinical decisions about how to tailor the treatment strategies to fit the needs of your clients, as well as what to do when these strategies are not resulting in the desired changes. Given the severity and complexity of DBT PE's target population, these clinical decisions can be quite challenging to make as there is often no obvious "right" answer. Having a clear and theory-driven case formulation can function as a map that guides treatment, helping you to choose a route that is likely to be effective and to make timely course corrections when unexpected barriers are encountered along the way. For these reasons, it is recommended that you develop an initial case formulation in preparation for starting DBT PE.

In DBT, case formulation is typically done at the level of the case with the goal of developing a comprehensive description of a client's entire constellation of problems and the controlling variables that are hypothesized to be maintaining them. In contrast, the DBT PE case formulation focuses at the level of the disorder, specifically PTSD. This disorder-level case formulation is based on the theories of the development and maintenance of PTSD that underlie DBT PE and applies them to explain a specific client's PTSD. The initial DBT PE case formulation is typically based on knowledge you have acquired about the client's history and typical response patterns during Stage 1 DBT. Consistent with standard cognitive-behavioral case formulations (Persons, 2008), this information is condensed to create a concise summary of the problem (i.e., PTSD), the precipitants of the problem, the mechanisms hypothesized to be maintaining the problem, and the origins of the mechanisms (see the *DBT PE Case Formulation Worksheet— Therapist Form 1* in Appendix B).

Components of the Case Formulation

Defining the Problem

The primary problem targeted by DBT PE is PTSD. Therefore, this section should include a behavioral description of the type, intensity, and duration of the client's PTSD symptoms. Most often, this information is obtained via a standardized self-report measure of PTSD and the client's score on the measure, as well as the specific PTSD diagnostic criteria that they endorse, are briefly described.

Precipitants of the Problem

In contrast to many other problems and disorders, the precipitants of PTSD (i.e., the events that caused PTSD to develop) are typically clear and can be readily identified by the client. Accordingly, this section of the case formulation includes a list of the traumas that have caused the client's PTSD (including both Criterion A events and traumatic invalidation); the age(s) at which the traumas occurred; and, if applicable, the perpetrator(s) of the trauma. If known, the traumas can be rank-ordered by the severity of PTSD symptoms that they currently cause. Of note, potentially traumatic events that a client has experienced that have not caused PTSD do not need to be included on this list. When the client has experienced multiple traumas, it can be difficult to determine which are causing PTSD and which may not be. In these cases, you can list all of the traumas the client has experienced and make changes to the list later in treatment as the primary trauma(s) become clearer.

Mechanism Hypotheses

The cornerstone of the case formulation is the mechanism hypothesis—that is, a behavioral description of the factors believed to be maintaining the client's PTSD. In DBT PE, these hypotheses are based on an integrative framework that incorporates aspects of emotional processing theory, inhibitory learning theory, and DBT's biosocial theory. Figure 7.1 depicts a basic conceptual framework for understanding the factors that maintain PTSD, as well as the origins of these mechanisms. To develop an individualized mechanism hypothesis, you need to identify how this general model applies to your client so that it is clear what maintaining factors need to be targeted for their PTSD to improve.

As shown in Figure 7.1, PTSD is maintained by an interrelated set of emotional, cognitive, and behavioral responses to trauma cues. When a trauma cue (e.g., a person who resembles

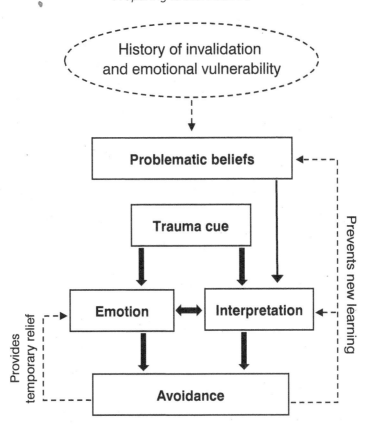

FIGURE 7.1. Model of the maintenance of PTSD.

an abuser) is encountered, it elicits a cascade of automatic reactions, including emotions and interpretations (expectancies) about the likelihood and severity of aversive outcomes. The person's interpretations (e.g., "She is going to laugh at me") stem from their underlying problematic beliefs (e.g., "People are likely to reject me") and may occur outside of conscious awareness. In contrast, the person is typically acutely aware of the cued emotions (e.g., fear, shame) and associated body sensations (e.g., racing heart, flushed cheeks), which can be intensely distressing in their own right and prompt additional interpretations (e.g., "I'm going to lose control"). To obtain relief from this emotional distress and increase a sense of safety, the person then engages in some type of avoidance (e.g., leaving the situation, self-injury). This avoidance provides short-term relief but maintains PTSD in the long run by preventing new learning about the accuracy of their interpretations and beliefs. As a result, their problematic beliefs are maintained and often strengthened over time. Each element of this model is included in the case formulation and described in more detail below.

TRAUMA CUES

Trauma cues can be internal experiences (e.g., thoughts, memories, sensations) as well as external situations (e.g., the smell of smoke, going to the doctor, asking someone for help) that have become paired with past trauma through a process of classical conditioning. Over the course of Stage 1, you are likely to become aware of a variety of your client's trauma cues. For example, trauma cues are often evident in the chain of events leading up to target behaviors or are uncovered when trying to understand why clients experience intense distress in certain seemingly neutral situations. More broadly, you are likely to be familiar with the types of activities, places, and people that your client regularly avoids that are contributing to impairment in their lives. These trauma cues can be included in the initial case formulation and expanded upon as treatment progresses.

PROBLEMATIC BELIEFS

Clients' problematic beliefs typically fall into three general categories, including (1) negative beliefs about the self (e.g., as bad, incompetent, and to blame for one's traumas), (2) negative beliefs about others and the world (e.g., as dangerous, untrustworthy, and rejecting), and (3) negative beliefs about emotions (e.g., as harmful, intolerable, and unacceptable). By the end of Stage 1, you are likely to be quite familiar with your client's typical problematic beliefs, such as self-invalidation, expectations of rejection, overestimations of danger, and distrust of others. These types of beliefs are often trauma related and can be included in the initial case formulation as hypotheses to be tested. Prior to starting DBT PE, you may be less aware of the beliefs clients hold about the specific traumas they have experienced (e.g., exactly why they think a trauma proves that they are bad) and these can be added to the case formulation as they become clear. Of note, the case formulation typically focuses on the client's broader problematic beliefs, whereas interpretations (expectancies) related to specific trauma cues are assessed and tracked in detail using *DBT PE Handout 8* (*Exposure Recording Form*; see Chapter 9).

EMOTIONS

Although PTSD has historically been viewed as a fear-based disorder, it is now well established that it is associated with a wide range of negative emotions that extend beyond fear. For many clients in DBT PE, trauma-related emotions, such as shame, guilt, and disgust, are often as or more intense than fear and play a significant role in maintaining PTSD. Frequently these emotions are fueled by a client's problematic beliefs and interpretations. You are likely to be well acquainted with clients' typical emotional responses by the end of Stage 1 and can make reasonable hypotheses about how these are linked to their problematic trauma-related beliefs.

AVOIDANCE

Avoidance includes any strategy the client uses to increase a sense of safety or reduce emotional distress when they encounter trauma cues. These avoidance strategies are highly individual and can include a wide variety of behaviors. Perhaps the most obvious type is when the client completely avoids entering certain situations or engaging in certain activities. However, avoidance is often more subtle and can be difficult to detect, such as when clients distract themselves with other thoughts, repetitively count, suppress emotional expression, or carry objects that make them feel safe (e.g., pepper spray). In addition, Stage 1 target behaviors often function as avoidance by providing relief from trauma-related emotions and thoughts. These avoidance behaviors are negatively reinforced through a process of operant conditioning and often become more frequent and pervasive over time. You should include the avoidance strategies your client relies on most often in the case formulation.

Origins of the Mechanisms

The final part of the case formulation focuses on how the hypothesized mechanisms were learned. Many factors may have contributed to clients' problematic beliefs and tendency to rely on avoidance to cope, such as the norms and values of their family, peer group, community, and culture. As shown in Figure 7.1, the biosocial theory is used as the primary framework for understanding how these maintaining factors developed. For example, many of the traumatic events clients experienced occurred within invalidating environments that blamed or judged them for these traumas, offered little or no emotional support, and punished their expression of distress. Consequently, clients' problematic beliefs and avoidant coping styles very often originated from past experiences of invalidation at both the interpersonal level (e.g., by family members, friends, and intimate partners) and cultural level (e.g., systemic exclusion and stigmatization of clients from marginalized groups).

Additionally, normal emotional reactions to trauma may have been exacerbated by a biology that predisposed them to have exceptionally strong emotional responses. For example, they may have experienced emotions in response to a wide range of trauma cues (emotional sensitivity) and these emotional responses may have been particularly intense (emotional reactivity) and long lasting (slow return to baseline). These overwhelming emotional responses may have increased the person's intrinsic motivation to avoid cues that elicit emotions and rely on avoidant coping strategies to manage emotions. When these biological vulnerabilities occurred within an invalidating environment that was intolerant of emotion, it is nearly inevitable that the person would have learned to respond to trauma cues and the intense emotions they elicit with avoidance and suppression no matter the cost.

Case Example: Maria's Case Formulation

The following example provides an illustration of how to create an initial DBT PE case formulation. The client, Maria, is described here and I continue to use her as a case example throughout the DBT PE protocol chapters. Maria is a 25-year-old single White woman who was referred to DBT after a serious suicide attempt via overdose on acetaminophen that resulted in psychiatric hospitalization. At intake, Maria reported her primary reason for seeking treatment was to "stop feeling miserable all the time and be able to have relationships." She met diagnostic criteria for borderline personality disorder (BPD), PTSD, major depression, bulimia nervosa, and social anxiety disorder. Maria also had a history of heavy alcohol and cannabis use but had been abstinent from both substances for the past 3 years. At the beginning of treatment, Maria had daily high urges to kill herself, was self-injuring via cutting one to two times per week, and binge eating and purging three to four times per week. She also dissociated frequently, and her self-injury often occurred while she was in a dissociated state. She had attempted suicide four times in her life, all via overdose, with the first attempt occurring at age 16. She had been psychiatrically hospitalized three times. She was unemployed, lived with her mother, and had no close friends other than a cousin who she sometimes spent time with.

During Stage 1 DBT, Maria reported having experienced several traumas, although these had not been discussed in detail. As a child, Maria had been repeatedly sexually and physically abused by her father. She also described her father as severely invalidating, including frequently criticizing and belittling her and holding her to strict standards of behavior that included total obedience to his frequent demands. She reported that she tried to be "the perfect child" all the time to not upset him, which included hiding her negative emotions and always trying to obey his orders without complaint. However, she stated that she was never good enough and always ended up "messing up" and being punished. Maria said that her mother had never abused her, but she also had not protected her from her father and had offered little emotional support. Her mother had also been physically abused by her father, including multiple episodes of domestic violence that Maria directly witnessed as a child.

In middle school, Maria became depressed, started self-injuring by cutting her arms and thighs, and regularly thought about killing herself to escape the abuse. At age 14, her father died in a car accident while driving under the influence. Maria began high school shortly after his death and became friends with a group of older kids with whom she began regularly drinking alcohol, smoking cannabis, and skipping school. She also began having sex frequently and impulsively with multiple partners. In her senior year of high school, Maria began seriously dating a man who was 10 years older than her who she met at a party and, after graduating, she moved in with him and worked as a waitress to support herself. Although their relationship was positive at first, over time her boyfriend became increasingly controlling and verbally abusive, and when she was 21, he violently raped her. She then left him, moved back in with her mother, and withdrew from her friends and social activities. She continued to work off and on in various jobs but was often fired due to poor attendance. Her most recent suicide attempt occurred near the anniversary of her father's death, which had prompted an increase in intrusive memories and flashbacks, self-loathing, and hopelessness.

Maria was very motivated to treat her PTSD as she viewed the traumas she had suffered as the main reason she was miserable and unable to have relationships. She worked hard in Stage 1 DBT and after 20 weeks of treatment she succeeded in meeting the readiness criteria for DBT PE. In the weeks leading up to starting DBT PE, her therapist created the initial case formulation shown in Figure 7.2.

CASE EXAMPLE DISCUSSION

The initial DBT PE case formulation for Maria includes information obtained from a variety of sources during Stage 1, including a standardized self-report measure of PTSD, the client's report of her developmental history, behavioral observation (e.g., of her tendency to inhibit emotional expression during therapy sessions), and chain analyses (e.g., indicating that making mistakes, self-critical thoughts, and shame often prompted Stage 1 targets). As is typical for early case formulations, several sections are relatively brief (i.e., the list of trauma cues) and others are noted as needing additional assessment (e.g., whether her father's death had been traumatic, the specific reasons she blamed herself for her abuse). This information will continue to be gathered during DBT PE and the case formulation will be updated accordingly.

A Case-Formulation-Driven Approach to Implementing DBT PE

The case formulation is used to guide all aspects of treatment during DBT PE. The information in the case formulation prepares you to deliver the rationales for treatment using examples specific to your client, which can be critical in helping them gain insight into the factors that are maintaining their PTSD. Additionally, the case formulation is used to guide treatment planning and help you select *in vivo* exposure tasks and traumas to target with imaginal exposure that will efficiently and effectively address these maintaining factors. These interventions are then

Client: _Maria_   Date completed: _January 28_

PTSD
Describe the type, severity, and duration of the client's PTSD symptoms.
PTSD Checklist–5 score = 61. In the past month, Maria reports extreme intrusive memories and emotional and physical reactions to trauma reminders. Nightmares and flashbacks each occur several times per week. She makes extreme efforts to avoid thinking about her trauma or being near things that remind her of it. She experiences strong negative emotions and endorsed extremely negative beliefs about herself, other people, the world, and blame. She feels extremely detached from other people, quite anhedonic and unable to experience positive emotions, and a little bit unable to remember important parts of her trauma. Hyperarousal symptoms range from quite a bit (e.g., hypervigilance, easily startled) to moderate (e.g., insomnia, trouble concentrating) to a little bit (irritability, risky behaviors). PTSD onset in early childhood and worsened after she was raped at age 21.

TRAUMA HISTORY
Briefly describe the client's history of trauma. For each trauma type, specify the client's age(s) at the time the trauma occurred and the perpetrator (if applicable). If known, rank-order the traumas by the severity of PTSD symptoms they currently cause.

Trauma type	Age(s)	Perpetrator (if any)
1. Sexual and physical abuse plus traumatic invalidation	Until age 14	Father
2. Witnessing domestic violence	Until age 14	Father to mother
3. Father's death in car accident (???)	14	n/a
4. Rape	21	Ex-boyfriend

TRAUMA CUES
Describe the primary internal and external trauma cues the client avoids.
1. Being near men
2. Going to social events/interacting with people she doesn't know well
3. Making mistakes
4. Trauma memories

MECHANISMS
A. **Problematic beliefs and emotions:** List the primary problematic beliefs and associated emotions that are hypothesized to be maintaining the client's PTSD.

Problematic beliefs: about the self, others, the world, and emotions	Emotions
1. People (especially men) are likely to harm me.	Fear
2. It's my fault that people have abused me. (*why? must assess)	Guilt
3. People won't like me and will reject me.	Shame, fear
4. I don't deserve love or care.	Shame, disgust
5. I always mess things up.	Shame
6. My emotions are unacceptable.	Shame
7. I will lose control if I allow myself to feel emotions.	Fear

(continued)

FIGURE 7.2. Initial DBT PE case formulation worksheet for Maria.

B. **Avoidance:** Describe the primary avoidance strategies the client uses to increase a sense of safety and/or reduce aversive emotions when confronted with trauma cues.

1. Isolation and social withdrawal
2. Trying to do things perfectly
3. Trying not to think about her trauma
4. Inhibiting or hiding emotions
5. Dissociation
6. Thinking about suicide or engaging in target behaviors (self-injury, bingeing/purging)

ORIGINS OF MECHANISMS

Briefly describe how the client learned or acquired the hypothesized mechanisms. Consider the role of the invalidating environment and biologically based emotional vulnerability.

Maria reports that she was a sensitive child who felt emotions intensely. As a young child, she learned to inhibit her emotions to avoid her father's anger and punishment. Her mother also modeled emotional suppression as a coping strategy and discouraged her from talking about things that were causing her distress. Maria's tendency to think negatively about herself stems from her father's severe invalidation and criticism of her as a young child and was reinforced by her ex-boyfriend's similarly invalidating behaviors.

FIGURE 7.2. *(continued)*

implemented according to the structure outlined in the protocol and outcomes are routinely monitored. If the interventions are not yielding the desired change in PTSD, adjustments are made to the case formulation to guide the selection of alternate interventions. In this way, case formulation is an ongoing and iterative process in which mechanism hypotheses are proposed, tested, and revised until PTSD is reduced. In the coming chapters, I describe in more detail how to implement DBT PE in a case formulation-driven manner that will help you to make effective clinical decisions about how to adjust and tailor the treatment to specific clients. Thus, you should rest assured that time spent creating a thorough initial DBT PE case formulation will yield a large return on investment as treatment progresses.

Concluding Comments

After working hard to prepare for DBT PE, it is understandable to feel more than a little anxious as Session 1 approaches. This can be an especially challenging time for clients who may have increasing urges to avoid DBT PE as the start date nears. In some cases, clients may have urges to engage in behaviors such as self-injury that would delay the start of DBT PE. It can be useful to remind clients that the decision to engage in DBT PE is entirely under their control and they need only tell you if at any point they no longer wish to continue. You can also predict and normalize that these types of second thoughts are likely to emerge and convey confidence that clients have the skills necessary to succeed. In the final days leading up to Session 1, you should encourage clients to focus on activities that will decrease emotional vulnerability and build resilience so that that they will begin DBT PE in as strong a state as possible. They have done everything that was needed to prepare for DBT PE and if they stay the course, there is every reason to believe they will achieve freedom from their trauma-related suffering.

PART III

THE DBT PE PROTOCOL

CHAPTER 8

Session 1

SESSION 1 COMPONENTS AND TIME ESTIMATES

	60-minute session	90-minute session
1. Review the DBT diary card and set the session agenda.	3 min.	3–5 min.
2. Orient to the treatment rationale and procedures.	10–15 min.	15–25 min.
3. Conduct the Trauma Interview and select the first target trauma.	25–30 min.	30–45 min.
4. Obtain and strengthen commitments.	3–5 min.	5–7 min.
5. Complete the Post-Exposure DBT skills plan.	5–10 min.	10–15 min.
6. Assign homework.	3 min.	3–5 min.

Reaching Session 1 of the DBT PE protocol is a dialectical experience if ever there was one. On the one hand, clients are likely to feel pride about having succeeded in obtaining the stability necessary to start this treatment, as well as hope about the relief it is likely to provide. On the other hand, clients are often filled with a sense of dread about what the treatment will entail and fear about their ability to tolerate the distress it will elicit. It is like a person who has prepared for months to climb a particularly steep mountain, including undergoing rigorous physical training, acquiring mountaineering skills and equipment, and hiring a guide to take them to the summit. The person then arrives at base camp, looks at the towering mountain above them, and thinks, "What in the hell have I gotten myself into?" Like climbing a mountain, completing DBT PE will require clients to keep moving forward one step at a time even when a nagging voice inside their head is urging them to turn back. Your job as their guide is to chart the path forward, help them keep their footing as they make their ascent, and maintain a stance of unyielding determination and optimism. The trek begins with Session 1 focused on orienting clients to the rationale for treatment and identifying the traumas that will be targeted via imaginal exposure. In this chapter, I describe each component of Session 1 in detail—a checklist for this session is included in Appendix C. All client handouts can be found in Appendix A and therapist forms are in Appendix B.

1. Review the DBT Diary Card and Set the Session Agenda

As in DBT, each session of DBT PE begins with reviewing the DBT diary card, which should be used to track suicide and self-injury urges and behaviors, as well as other target behaviors, particularly those that have the potential to interfere with DBT PE. However, in contrast to DBT sessions in which the diary card is reviewed in detail and used to determine the session agenda, in DBT PE sessions the diary card is reviewed briefly with the primary goal of determining whether any higher-priority behaviors have occurred that would require DBT PE to be paused. In other words, reviewing the DBT diary card allows the therapist to quickly make a "go/no-go" decision about whether to deliver DBT PE as planned versus revert to DBT. (Guidelines for determining when DBT PE should be paused are described in Chapter 14.)

Given that clients often experience anticipatory anxiety about starting DBT PE, it is not unusual to see higher than usual urges for suicide and self-injury in the days leading up to and at the start of Session 1. Typically, these increased urges are not a cause for alarm, as they often represent conditioned responses to increased distress rather than a true desire or intent to engage in those behaviors. Thus, if high but nonacute urges are evident on the diary card or at the start of the session, you can respond by normalizing this increase, reassuring clients that it is likely to be temporary, reinforcing their efforts to cope effectively with these urges, and continuing with the planned Session 1 components. In some cases, clients may report an increase in quality-of-life targets (e.g., binge eating, alcohol use) in the days leading up to Session 1. If this occurs, you can comment on this increase while reviewing the diary card but refrain from in-depth targeting of these behaviors until the DBT portion of the session or the separate DBT session (depending on your session structure).

After the diary card review is complete, a session agenda is briefly outlined. In general, the goal of setting an agenda is to make the treatment as clear and predictable as possible to the client by specifically outlining what they can expect to occur in the session. Given the heightened anxiety that clients often feel about DBT PE, providing this clear structure at the beginning of each session can be helpful in enhancing their sense of control and reducing the likelihood that they will be caught by surprise by any particular session component. In Session 1, the session agenda follows the list outlined at the beginning of this chapter.

2. Orient to the Treatment Rationale and Procedures

The first main task of Session 1 is to provide a clear and convincing description of the overall rationale for the treatment. This is not meant to be a didactic lecture but rather a collaborative discussion that will ideally increase clients' willingness to confront the things they are avoiding. By the time they reach Session 1, clients should already be reasonably familiar with the treatment rationale. Therefore, you can tailor your review of this information to best fit the needs and knowledge of your client while also ensuring that, by the end of this discussion, your client clearly understands the following: (1) why their PTSD is not getting better (and may be getting worse) and (2) how the core treatment procedures of DBT PE will help to reduce their PTSD.

Orientation to the Factors That Maintain PTSD

Helping clients understand what is maintaining their PTSD is critical to increasing buy-in for exposure. Indeed, the answer to why their PTSD is not getting better *is* the rationale for the treatment. The model of the maintenance of PTSD was described in detail in Chapter 7 and is illustrated in *DBT PE Handout 1 (How PTSD Is Maintained)*, which can be reviewed with clients in session and/or assigned as homework. Overall, the task in Session 1 is to present this information in a manner that is understandable and compelling to clients and help them see how it applies to their own experience. Table 8.1 includes the key points to be made when describing how PTSD is maintained.

Case Example: Orienting to the Treatment Rationale

The following example provides an illustration of how to orient clients to the factors that maintain PTSD using the case of Maria that was introduced in Chapter 7.

THERAPIST: The first thing I want to do today is make sure you understand what is keeping your PTSD going. Let's start by looking at DBT PE Handout 1. Do you see the oval at the top that says problematic beliefs?

MARIA: Yes.

THERAPIST: These are problematic things you learned as a result of trauma that influence how you think and feel about things in your life now. For example, what did your traumatic experiences teach you to believe about yourself?

MARIA: That I'm a bad person who always messes things up and makes people angry at me. If I hadn't been such a bad kid, my dad wouldn't have abused me. And the same thing happened with my boyfriend. I was always doing things wrong that made him mad and that's why he raped me. It makes me hate myself.

THERAPIST: Yes, people with PTSD often think they are bad or incompetent, and they usually blame themselves for the traumas they experienced. For the record, it makes me sad to hear you say these things about yourself. We are definitely going to have to work on changing how you think about yourself!

TABLE 8.1. Key Points in Orienting to the Factors That Maintain PTSD

1. PTSD is maintained by avoidance of trauma cues, including:
   a. Distressing thoughts, memories, and emotions about the trauma
   b. Situations, people, and things that prompt distressing thoughts and emotions associated with the trauma

2. PTSD is also maintained by problematic beliefs about:
   a. Others and the world (e.g., as untrustworthy, rejecting, and dangerous)
   b. Oneself (e.g., as bad, incompetent, and to blame for the trauma)
   c. Emotions (e.g., as harmful, intolerable, and unacceptable)

3. These problematic beliefs lead people with PTSD to interpret trauma cues in negative and inaccurate ways that set off intense emotions.

4. Avoidance provides temporary relief from this distress but keeps PTSD going in the long run by preventing new learning about the accuracy of problematic beliefs.

MARIA: OK.

THERAPIST: So, in addition to thinking negatively about yourself, trauma also teaches people to think negatively about other people and the world. For example, survivors of interpersonal trauma, like you, often believe that other people can't be trusted, and that people are likely to harm or reject them. In general, people with PTSD often believe they must be on guard all the time because dangerous things could happen at any moment.

MARIA: Yeah, that's me. That's why I avoid people, especially men. I just think they are going to do something to hurt me, or they won't like me. When I leave the house, I'm always looking all around to try to make sure I'm safe.

THERAPIST: That's really common. OK, the final type of problematic belief is related to how people think about their emotions. Often people believe that emotions are dangerous, they can't tolerate them, and they are likely to lose control or be rejected if they allow themselves to get emotional.

MARIA: You know that I don't like emotions! I feel like my emotions are so intense that I'll go crazy if I let myself feel them for too long.

THERAPIST: OK, you can clearly identify with these common types of problematic beliefs! So, what happens is that these beliefs influence your reactions to things you encounter in everyday life, particularly things that remind you of your traumas. Do you see the next box that says trauma cue?

MARIA: Yes.

THERAPIST: Trauma cues can be internal, like your own thoughts and memories about your trauma, or they can be external situations that remind you of your trauma. As an example, what reactions do you typically have when a memory of your dad abusing you comes into your mind?

MARIA: I get really anxious and ashamed, and I feel like I want to climb out of my skin.

THERAPIST: Right, so those trauma memories bring up uncomfortable emotions and sensations. What thoughts do you usually have either about the trauma memory or your emotional reactions to it?

MARIA: It makes me start thinking about how bad and disgusting I am.

THERAPIST: OK, so then what usually happens?

MARIA: I just feel like I can't tolerate it, so I try to distract myself and push the thoughts out of my head. In the past, when the memories got intense I would self-harm to try to make them stop.

THERAPIST: Yes, distraction is a very common strategy people use to avoid thoughts and emotions related to past trauma, and self-harm can be one way to distract yourself. So, what happens if a distressing trauma memory comes into your mind and then you distract yourself?

MARIA: I usually feel better, at least for a while. But the memories always come back eventually.

THERAPIST: Exactly. Avoidance provides temporary relief, but it doesn't keep the thoughts or emotions away in the long run. They always come back and often they get more frequent and intense the more you try to avoid them.

MARIA: I know, but it's still hard to stop myself from avoiding in the moment.

THERAPIST: Of course! Avoidance has become a habit that is hard to resist. So, if you always respond to trauma memories by pushing them out of your head, does that make you feel more or less confident in your ability to tolerate them?

MARIA: It makes me feel like I can't handle thinking about what happened, like I have to avoid it.

THERAPIST: Right. And what about those beliefs that you are bad and disgusting? Do those change if you avoid thinking about your abuse?

MARIA: No, I still think those are true.

THERAPIST: And that is the crux of the problem. If you avoid thinking about your trauma, then you can't learn anything new about it. That means you will continue to believe that you can't tolerate thinking about it, and that you are bad and disgusting because of what your dad did to you. As long as you are avoiding, those problematic beliefs that are fueling your PTSD are going to stay stuck. Does that make sense?

MARIA: Yes, I can see that.

THERAPIST: Good. Now, let's apply this model to an example of an external trauma cue. Can you think of a recent time that you encountered something in the world that reminded you of your trauma?

MARIA: I went grocery shopping yesterday and when I came out of the store there was a man standing near my car. You know that I hate being near men!

THERAPIST: Yes, which is understandable given that you have been harmed by multiple men in your life. So, seeing the man near your car was a trauma cue. Now use the handout to walk me through what happened.

MARIA: My interpretation was that he must be planning to attack me, and that I wasn't safe. I felt afraid and my heart was racing. I think I just immediately went into this fight-or-flight mode that happens when I feel threatened.

THERAPIST: It sounds like this was an intense trauma cue. Did you do anything to make yourself feel safer or less afraid?

MARIA: I put my keys in between my fingers so that I could use them to hurt him if he came near me. And then I walked to my car and threw my bags in as quickly as I could without making eye contact. As soon as I got in my car, I locked all the doors and drove away.

THERAPIST: So, you used a variety of avoidance behaviors, including holding your keys as a potential weapon, avoiding eye contact, locking your doors, and driving away as quickly as you could. Can you tell me how these kinds of avoidance behaviors keep your PTSD going?

MARIA: Well, they only give me temporary relief. If I saw another man today who was standing near my car, I would still be just as afraid.

THERAPIST: That's right. Avoidance only works to get short-term relief. The emotions are still going to be there in the long run. How did the avoidance prevent new learning?

MARIA: I guess by leaving the situation quickly, I didn't have a chance to find out if he was actually going to attack me.

THERAPIST: Exactly. It's entirely possible that he was just an innocent man who was going grocery shopping and had no ill intentions toward you. But avoidance made it impossible for you to learn if your interpretations were accurate.

MARIA: I can see that, but I still think that was a reasonable reaction to a strange man being near my car!

THERAPIST: I know you do, and that's because you haven't had enough experiences yet that disconfirm your belief that all men are dangerous. That is something we can work on during treatment. For now, do you feel like you understand how avoidance is maintaining those kinds of PTSD-related beliefs and emotions?

MARIA: Yes, I can see how avoidance is keeping me stuck.

THERAPIST: Do you have any questions about this?

MARIA: No, I think I get it.

CASE EXAMPLE DISCUSSION

This example illustrates how to have a collaborative conversation with clients about the factors that maintain PTSD. To help make this information both relevant and understandable, it is important to elicit examples from the client and then use these examples to illustrate key points. In the above case, the therapist asked Maria to provide examples of the three types of problematic beliefs, as well as internal and external trauma cues. These client-relevant examples were then used to explain how avoidance maintains PTSD by preventing new learning. Throughout this discussion, the therapist validated and normalized Maria's examples, thus modeling a nonjudgmental way of viewing her experiences. Of note, it can be tempting to begin trying to actively change problematic beliefs that arise during this discussion. For example, Maria voiced a number of self-invalidating beliefs, such as that she deserved to be abused by her father because she was bad. Given that the primary goal of this conversation is to orient clients to the treatment rationale, you should avoid getting derailed by significant efforts to modify cognitions. As was done in this example, you can simply highlight that these beliefs are problematic and will be addressed later in the treatment. Finally, it is important to assess the client's comprehension of the information. In this example, the therapist asked Maria to describe in her own words how the model in DBT PE Handout 1 applied to a recent experience of encountering a trauma cue. As was true for Maria, because clients have already received some orientation to the treatment rationale during Stage 1, they are often readily able to understand this information and may not have a lot of questions.

Orientation to the Treatment Procedures

Once the factors that maintain PTSD are described, this naturally segues into a discussion of how DBT PE will work to reduce PTSD by targeting these maintaining factors. Essentially, if avoidance of trauma cues is maintaining PTSD by making it impossible to correct problematic beliefs, then the solution is to stop avoidance. Thus, your task is to ensure that your client understands how the core procedures of DBT PE work to reduce PTSD by stopping avoidance so that new learning can occur and trauma-related emotions will decrease. In Session 1, the description of the core procedures should include an overview of each procedure and how it works. A more detailed rationale and description of the core procedures is provided in Session 2 (*in vivo* exposure) and Session 3 (imaginal exposure and processing). Table 8.2 describes the key points to cover when orienting clients to the core procedures of DBT PE—these are also included in *DBT PE Handout 2* (*How DBT PE Works to Reduce PTSD*).

TABLE 8.2. Key Points in Orienting to the Treatment Procedures

1. DBT PE works by helping clients approach rather than avoid trauma cues so that new learning can occur and distress will decrease.

2. *In vivo* exposure is used to approach safe but avoided situations, people, and things that bring up thoughts and emotions related to trauma.

3. Imaginal exposure is used to approach avoided trauma memories by repeatedly describing specific traumatic events out loud and in detail.

4. Processing is used to gain a new perspective on the meaning of the trauma and involves talking about and evaluating emotions and beliefs that are elicited by imaginal exposure.

Case Example: Orienting to the Treatment Procedures

Continuing with the case of Maria, the following transcript picks up where the last one left off to demonstrate how to orient clients to the core procedures of DBT PE.

THERAPIST: OK, so if avoidance is keeping your PTSD around, what do you think we need to do instead for your PTSD to get better?

MARIA: Not avoid.

THERAPIST: Exactly! For your PTSD to improve, we're going to have to stop the avoidance.

MARIA: I know that's true, but I still don't like it.

THERAPIST: I can understand why. So, the way we stop the avoidance is by doing exposure. Exposure is all about approaching instead of avoiding.

MARIA: Right.

THERAPIST: There are two types of exposure we will use. The first is *in vivo* exposure, which means exposure to things in real life that you are avoiding. These often include things like people, situations, objects, and smells that remind you of your trauma and bring up intense emotions.

MARIA: OK.

THERAPIST: In our next session, we'll start to figure out what types of things you will focus on for *in vivo* exposure, but based on what you've already told me, an example could be that we might have you do things that involve interacting with men.

MARIA: But what if that's dangerous?

THERAPIST: I would never ask you to do *in vivo* exposure to things that are objectively dangerous or that it would be wise to avoid. For example, I wouldn't ask you to approach a man on a deserted street late at night. Instead, we'll choose things for you to do that people do regularly without any danger, such as talking to men in public places. The goal is for you to learn that nothing terrible happens if you approach things you are avoiding so that these things will no longer be so distressing.

MARIA: OK.

THERAPIST: The other type of exposure is called imaginal exposure, which involves having you describe out loud to me exactly what happened during specific traumatic events you have experienced. We'll do that repeatedly in our sessions so that over time you will learn that your trauma memories aren't dangerous, and you can tolerate thinking about them.

MARIA: That is the part I am least looking forward to.

THERAPIST: Yes, it certainly isn't easy to think and talk about your traumas. And the more you do it, the less distressing it will get.

MARIA: I sure hope so.

THERAPIST: The last core procedure is called processing, which involves talking about and evaluating the emotions and beliefs that imaginal exposure brings up. The goal of processing is to help you get a new perspective on some of the beliefs that are keeping you stuck. For example, you said that you believe you deserved to be abused by your dad. During processing, we'll think through those kinds of beliefs and see if there are other ways to think about what happened that feel true to you now and will cause you less suffering.

MARIA: I would like that.

THERAPIST: Me too! So, that's the basic description of the treatment procedures and how they work. Do you have questions?

MARIA: What if I'm too ashamed to tell you what happened? I'm afraid you're going to think I'm disgusting.

THERAPIST: Most people I work with are afraid that I am going to think terrible things about them when I hear the details of their trauma. One really important thing this treatment will help you learn is that there are people, like me, who will not judge or reject you when they learn about your trauma. You're going to have to trust that I will respond to you with care and compassion, which I know feels hard to believe right now.

MARIA: It also makes me uncomfortable to tell you about sexual things that happened. I mean, who talks about that?

THERAPIST: You're right. We don't usually talk about our sexual experiences in detail with other people. The reason we're going to have you do that here is because it is critical to treating your PTSD. We need you to learn that you can talk and think about exactly what happened, including the most uncomfortable details, and nothing bad is going to happen.

MARIA: I'm really not looking forward to facing all these things that I don't want to face.

THERAPIST: Of course you're not! Nobody is excited to face things that make them afraid or ashamed, and it will be worth it in the long run.

CASE EXAMPLE DISCUSSION

In this example, the therapist provided a brief but clear description of the core procedures of DBT PE, including *in vivo* exposure, imaginal exposure, and processing. For each core procedure, the therapist described how it addresses the factors that maintain PTSD—that is, how it works to reduce avoidance, modify problematic beliefs, and reduce the intensity of trauma-related emotions. In addition, the therapist described the basics of how each procedure is implemented so that Maria would have at least a general understanding of what the treatment will entail. At the same time, the therapist did not provide detailed information about the rationale and instructions for each procedure, as these will be provided in subsequent sessions.

Throughout this discussion, the therapist used several examples that Maria had previously provided to help make the information more personally relevant. Maria also raised several common concerns about the treatment procedures, including that they would be hard, that *in vivo* exposure might be dangerous, and that it would be embarrassing to describe trauma details to her therapist. The therapist responded to each of these concerns with validation, providing information to address the concern, and cheerleading. In general, the therapist consistently conveyed confidence both in DBT PE's efficacy and in Maria's ability to do it while using "we" language to emphasize that they would work together as a team to get her through it.

3. Conduct the Trauma Interview and Select the First Target Trauma

The next task of Session 1 is to conduct the *Trauma Interview (Therapist Form 2)* to assess the client's lifetime trauma history, select the traumatic events that will be targeted via imaginal exposure, and gather more detailed information about the first target trauma. Given that most clients receiving DBT PE have a history of multiple and often chronic traumas, this can be quite a challenging task. Moreover, completing the Trauma Interview is essentially a small dose of imaginal exposure and is likely to cause your client some distress. While conducting the Trauma Interview, you will therefore need to balance being task oriented and emotion focused. On the one hand, you should follow the semistructured format of the interview, ask the questions in a matter-of-fact manner, and progress through the interview at a reasonable pace. On the other hand, it is important to pay attention to the client's affect, including highlighting and validating the emotions that arise, reinforcing efforts to allow emotions without avoiding, and providing coaching to regulate emotions as needed. Overall, the goal of the Trauma Interview is to prepare clients for imaginal exposure both by selecting the specific traumas they will address and getting some initial practice with talking about trauma details in session. In this process, you are likely to learn more about the client's trauma history and the mechanisms that are maintaining their PTSD, which can be added to the initial case formulation.

Section 1. Assessment of Trauma History (Item 1)

The Trauma Interview begins by gathering information about the client's lifetime history of trauma. Although this may seem daunting, particularly for clients with an extensive trauma history, this section is structured to make this as efficient as possible. As specified in the instructions, clients are not expected to provide a lot of detail about the traumas they have experienced and the only information that is needed at this point is (1) a brief description of each trauma, (2) the client's age(s) at the time of the trauma, and (3) the perpetrator (if any). The brief description of the trauma only needs to include the general type of trauma that occurred (e.g., sexual abuse, intimate partner violence) and specific, event-level details are not necessary. If clients provide more detail than is needed (e.g., describing exactly what happened during a traumatic event), you can reinforce their willingness to share more details, reassure them that these details are important and will be discussed as treatment progresses, and explain that the need to keep it brief is simply due to time management concerns.

To start, you will list any traumas that you already know about. This is done both to be efficient (i.e., the client will not have to repeat information that is already known) and to model the amount of detail that is expected. For example, you may say, "From what we have already discussed, I know that you were sexually abused by your father from the ages of 5 to 12. Did I get that right?" After you have finished listing the traumas of which you are aware, you should ask your client whether they have experienced any other traumatic events. Importantly, the client gets to decide which events they consider to be traumatic. Additional probe questions are provided that can be used as needed to help clients identify other potential traumas, including both Criterion A and traumatic invalidation events. Overall, the goal is to encourage your client to provide a complete list of the potentially traumatic events they have experienced without censoring themselves.

CLINICAL TIP

What If Clients Don't Want to Disclose Traumas?

Some clients may indicate that they have experienced traumas that they do not wish to disclose. When this occurs, you can validate the difficulty of disclosing trauma and emphasize that the client is in control of what they choose to share. You should also attempt to assess why the client does not wish to disclose a trauma. Common barriers include intense shame, fear of talking about the trauma, doubts about its validity, and/ or a desire to protect the perpetrator. In general, you should tailor your response to address the specific reason(s) the client wants to keep the trauma hidden and attempt to find a solution that would facilitate disclosure. To that end, specific points that may be useful to highlight include:

- Traumas that are particularly difficult to disclose are often the most distressing ones that are most in need of treatment.
- If they choose not to disclose the trauma, it won't be able to be treated and will likely continue to cause them distress.
- If they choose to disclose the trauma, they can decide how much detail to provide.
- Disclosing the trauma does not mean that they will have to target it in treatment. They will get to decide which traumas they will focus on.

Ultimately, the decision to disclose is up to the client and it is important that you do not try to pressure them into disclosing. If clients choose not to share certain traumas, you should remain nonjudgmental and validate this decision. Of note, it is not unusual for clients who are initially unwilling to discuss certain traumas in Session 1 to later change their minds and choose to disclose as treatment progresses.

Case Example

Continuing with the case of Maria, the therapist began by listing the traumas that were included in the initial DBT PE case formulation, including her father's sexual and physical abuse and traumatic invalidation, witnessing her father's domestic violence toward her mother, and the rape by her ex-boyfriend. Maria confirmed the accuracy of these trauma types and the ages at which they had occurred. Her therapist also asked whether she considered her father's death to have been traumatic. Maria said she mostly felt relieved when he died, and although she had some guilt about this, his death did not bother her significantly now. Her therapist validated this reaction and then asked whether there were any other events she had experienced that had been traumatic. Maria then disclosed several traumas that were new to the therapist. She said that she had gotten pregnant when she was 17, had decided to keep the baby, and then had a miscarriage that had been very distressing to her. Maria also said that a friend had died from a heroin overdose when she was 19. When asked whether there were any other traumas to add, Maria said there was something else but she wasn't sure if it counted as trauma. Her therapist encouraged her to share it and told her that what mattered was whether it had been traumatic to her. Maria then described being bullied by peers in high school for being sexually promiscuous. She said that a lot of boys boasted about having sex with her and in many cases this was not true, and that she was frequently taunted and called names by her peers. In addition, she said that boys would often make unwelcome sexual comments and advances toward her. She said these experiences occurred throughout high school and contributed to her first suicide attempt at age 16. Her therapist validated that these types of bullying experiences can be very damaging and traumatic, and thanked Maria for sharing this. Maria then confirmed that there were no more traumas to disclose—her final list of traumas is shown below in chronological order.

Brief description of the trauma	Age(s)	Perpetrator (if any)
Sexual and physical abuse plus traumatic invalidation	Until age 14	Father
Witnessing domestic violence	Until age 14	Father to mother
Bullying	15–18	Peers
Miscarriage	17	—
Friend died due to overdose	19	—
Rape	21	Ex-boyfriend

Section 2. Identification of Target Traumas

The most difficult task of the Trauma Interview is to narrow down the often long list of traumas identified in Section 1 to a limited number of specific traumatic events that will be targeted via imaginal exposure (i.e., target traumas). Overall, the goal is to select target traumas that will optimize both treatment efficiency and effectiveness—namely, we want to target the minimum number of traumatic events necessary to achieve the maximum amount of improvement. In my original studies, clients reported experiencing an average of 12 types of Criterion A traumas in their lifetime, many of which were chronic trauma types. However, it was typically necessary to target only two to three trauma memories via imaginal exposure to achieve the desired degree of improvement in PTSD. Given this, Section 2 requires you to work with your client to identify up to three target traumas.

Critically, the target traumas that are selected in Section 2 must be discrete traumatic events (i.e., single traumatic episodes). This is because imaginal exposure requires clients to describe a specific traumatic event as a detailed narrative, rather than talking generally about a type of chronic trauma they have experienced. When clients have experienced single-event traumas (e.g., a rape, accident, or sudden death of a loved one), these traumas are already at the level of a specific event and can be readily selected for targeting via imaginal exposure. However, when clients have experienced chronic traumas, the selection of specific traumatic events to target becomes more challenging. Chronic traumas include any type of trauma that occurred over and over again in a person's life, such as repeated child sexual abuse, traumatic invalidation, and intimate partner violence. To target a chronic trauma via imaginal exposure, you and your client need to identify one or more specific times that this type of trauma occurred that can be described as a detailed narrative.

Faced with a client who has experienced multiple types of trauma, often including a combination of single-event and chronic trauma types, how do you pick just three trauma memories to target? There are two main principles that influence the selection of these "top three" target traumas. *First, prioritize traumatic events that are causing the most current distress and impairment.* Although it may seem daunting to focus only on the most distressing traumatic events, this is likely to lead to the greatest improvement in the least amount of time. This approach is similar to that used in medicine: When a multiply injured person arrives at an emergency room after a serious car accident, their most severe and life-threatening injuries are treated first. In the case of psychological trauma, the same principle applies: Treat the traumas that are causing the most suffering before addressing less distressing events.

Second, prioritize traumatic events that are most likely to generalize to other traumatic events. In particular, the goal is to select specific traumatic events that, if targeted via imaginal exposure and processing, will be likely to reduce the distress associated with other related or similar traumatic events. Like the idiom about killing two birds with one stone, the intent is to solve multiple problems at one time with a single action. In this case, the hope is that conducting imaginal exposure to a single traumatic event will eliminate the need to directly target other associated traumatic events. The principle of generalization is particularly important to consider when selecting target traumas with clients who have experienced chronic trauma and/ or multiple single-event traumas of the same general type.

With these general understandings in place, let's now dive into the mechanics of how to actually identify the "top three" traumatic events. In Section 2 of the Trauma Interview, the first task is to identify up to three target traumas and rank-order them by level of distress (Item 2) before deciding the order in which they will be targeted via imaginal exposure (Item 3).

Identifying and Rank-Ordering Up to Three Target Traumas (Item 2)

For clients who have experienced fewer than three types of trauma and/or primarily single-event traumas, it may be quite straightforward to identify specific target traumas and rank-order them by level of distress. For example, if a client has experienced a rape and the suicide of a parent, then all that needs to be done is to order these two events by the level of distress they cause. However, most clients receiving DBT PE will have experienced more than three trauma types and/or one or more chronic traumas. For clients with more complex trauma histories, I recommend completing the task of identifying and rank-ordering the top three target traumas in the following steps.

STEP 1. RANK-ORDER LIFETIME TRAUMA TYPES BY LEVEL OF DISTRESS

To begin the process of narrowing down the list from Section 1 to three target traumas, I typically start by having the client rank-order these general traumas from most to least distressing. (For clients with a particularly long list of lifetime traumas, I may ask them to identify the three most distressing types of trauma they have experienced, rather than rank-ordering the entire list.) In this initial step, it is not necessary to narrow chronic traumas down to a specific traumatic event that will be targeted—this will happen in Step 3. Rather, the goal at this point is to determine which overall trauma types are causing the client the most distress or, alternatively, would provide the client with the most relief if they were resolved. When determining which trauma types are most distressing, both the client's subjective level of distress and current functional impairment should be considered.

Subjective Level of Distress. The most straightforward way to determine which traumas are most distressing is to ask the client. In general, it is important to keep in mind that distress is subjective—namely, what one client finds to be most distressing may not match what you or others would find to be most distressing. Thus, it is ultimately up to clients to decide what they find to be most distressing, and Item 2 includes several prompting questions that you can ask to help clients make this decision:

- Which traumas currently bother you the most?
- Which one(s) cause you the most distress?
- Which one(s) come up most often in your thoughts, nightmares, and flashbacks?
- Which one(s) upset you the most when you are reminded of them?
- Which one(s) make you feel the worst about yourself?

Functional Impairment. Another factor to consider is the degree to which specific traumatic events are linked to current functional impairment. For many clients, efforts to avoid situations that remind them of specific past traumas cause significant difficulties in functioning. For example, a client may be unable to work since being stalked by a former coworker. Or a client may not be receiving needed medical treatment because it reminds them of their mother's death. Or a client may avoid sexual intimacy with their partner because it triggers flashbacks of child sexual abuse. Often you will already be familiar with the ways in which trauma-related avoidance is causing significant problems in your client's life and can use this knowledge to help identify traumas that are most closely linked to disabling avoidance. You can also assess this with questions such as:

- Which traumas cause the most problems or interfere in your life the most?
- Which one(s) make it hardest for you to do things that are important to you?
- Which one(s), if resolved, would most improve your ability to function?

When significant functional impairment is evident, it may be useful to prioritize targeting the traumas that are fueling those problems in order to improve functioning most rapidly.

CLINICAL TIP
But All of My Traumas Are Distressing!

Although most clients can identify the traumas that are most distressing to them without too much difficulty, some really struggle to make this decision. This indecision is often due to feeling as if all of their traumas are equally distressing and, in some cases, not wanting to minimize the seriousness of any trauma they have experienced. If this occurs, it can be helpful to validate the importance of all the client's traumatic experiences and reassure them that selecting specific events to target via imaginal exposure will not negate or invalidate the others. Furthermore, traumas that are not selected for targeting via imaginal exposure may still be discussed in treatment. For example, it is common to discuss other traumas during processing in order to generalize learning from a target trauma to other similar or related traumas. For clients struggling to decide which traumas are more versus less distressing, it may also be helpful to focus on more objective indicators of distress. For example, the specific traumas that intrude most often in the form of unwanted thoughts, nightmares, and flashbacks and/or that cause avoidance that makes it most difficult to achieve important life-worth-living goals are typically good candidates for imaginal exposure.

Case Example

In this first step, the therapist asked Maria to rank-order the six trauma types she had identified in Section 1 from most to least distressing. Maria had some difficulty deciding whether the child abuse by her father or the rape by her ex-boyfriend was more distressing, as both traumas were associated with severe PTSD symptoms and impairment. Her therapist suggested she consider which one had had a more damaging effect on the way she thinks and feels about herself. Maria said that her father's abuse and invalidation was the reason she began to view herself as bad, unlovable, and a burden, and that these beliefs had continued to plague her throughout her life. In addition, she said that her father's abuse was linked to the onset of most of her mental health problems, including PTSD and self-injury. For these reasons, she decided to rank the child abuse and invalidation by her father as the most distressing type of trauma, followed by the rape. After that, she picked the bullying she experienced in high school as the third most distressing type of trauma because it had made her self-loathing even worse and had prompted her first suicide attempt. She then decided that witnessing her father physically assault her mother was the fourth most distressing trauma type, as this had contributed significantly to her chaotic home environment and the pervasive sense of threat she felt while growing up. Maria then quickly ranked the remaining traumas in terms of the amount of distress they caused at the time they happened but noted that neither of them bothered her very much now. Thus, Maria's list of trauma types from Section 1 was reordered from most to least distressing as follows:

1. Sexual and physical abuse and traumatic invalidation by father (until age 14)
2. Rape (age 21)
3. Bullying by peers (ages 15–18)
4. Witnessing domestic violence (until age 14)
5. Miscarriage (age 17)
6. Friend's death by overdose (age 19)

STEP 2. LOOK FOR EVENTS THAT COMBINE MULTIPLE TRAUMA TYPES

Unfortunately, many of our clients have experienced traumatic events in which they were exposed to multiple types of trauma and/or perpetrators of trauma in a single event. For these clients, it may be possible to increase the efficiency of the treatment by identifying target traumas that span multiple categories. For example, a client may have been repeatedly physically abused by her father and severely invalidated by her mother. In such a case, it may be possible to identify a single event in which both the mother and father engaged in these behaviors. This may also occur when a single perpetrator engaged in multiple types of abusive behavior. For example, if a client was both sexually and physically abused by her brother, it may be possible to identify an event in which both types of abuse occurred. For clients who did not experience intersecting trauma types or perpetrators, then this step can be skipped.

Case Example

Given that Maria had experienced multiple types of abuse from her father and had witnessed him physically abuse her mother, her therapist asked whether she had experienced any events in which her father had engaged in all of these abusive behaviors at one time. Her therapist provided a brief rationale for this, saying that it can speed up the treatment if more than one type of trauma can be addressed in a single event. After taking a minute to think about this, Maria said that she could remember several times when she had witnessed her father hit her mother right before he then physically and sexually abused her. Maria agreed that it would make sense to choose one of those episodes for targeting since this would allow her to address her top four types of trauma in three events. Thus, her rank-ordered list of traumas was condensed to:

1. Sexual and physical abuse and traumatic invalidation by father and witnessing domestic violence (until age 14)
2. Rape (age 21)
3. Bullying by peers (ages 15–18)
4. Miscarriage (age 17)
5. Friend's death by overdose (age 19)

STEP 3. IDENTIFY A SINGLE TARGET TRAUMA FOR EACH CHRONIC TRAUMA TYPE

If any of the top three most distressing trauma types are chronic traumas, then this final step requires you to help the client identify one specific time that the chronic trauma occurred that can be targeted via imaginal exposure. When picking one episode, the goal is to maximize generalization by selecting a specific traumatic event that, if targeted via imaginal exposure and processing, will be likely to reduce the distress associated with other events from the same chronic trauma type. To that end, there are four main factors to take into consideration.

Level of Distress. Consistent with the selection of target traumas more generally, the traumatic events that cause the most distress are typically prioritized over those that are less distressing. In the case of chronic trauma, the level of distress often varies across episodes such that there are some events that stand out to clients as being particularly distressing. For example, there may be some events that were especially terrifying or humiliating at the time they occurred and/or that resulted in unusually negative consequences for the client. As described above, both the client's subjective level of distress and current trauma-related functional impairment can be taken into account when determining which events from a chronic trauma are causing the most distress.

Representativeness. To maximize generalizability, it is also useful to select a traumatic event that is reasonably representative of the way in which the chronic trauma typically occurred. It can be helpful to consider the perpetrator's typical behavior, the client's typical reaction, the usual context in which the trauma occurred, and the environment's characteristic response. For example, if a client experienced chronic sexual abuse by her brother for over 10 years, the goal would be to select a single time the sexual abuse occurred that exemplifies the way in which her brother typically abused her (e.g., vaginal intercourse), the location where the abuse typically occurred (e.g., when they were home alone together), and the way in which the client typically responded (e.g., going along with it, feeling fear and disgust, not telling anyone).

At times, an event may be selected that includes representative elements of the chronic trauma, as well as distinctive elements that make the event particularly distressing. For example, it is not unusual for clients to choose an event in which the perpetrator engaged in their typical behavior, but the client did not (e.g., they initially fought back when they were typically compliant). Or, conversely, the client engaged in their typical behavior, but the perpetrator did not (e.g., they were more physically violent than usual). Alternatively, both the perpetrator and client may have engaged in their typical behaviors, but the environment responded in an unusual way (e.g., a parent discovered the abuse and punished the client for it). Overall, you should strive to find an event that is both highly distressing and reasonably representative of the chronic trauma.

CLINICAL TIP

Should More Than One Target Trauma Be Selected from a Chronic Trauma?

In most cases, targeting a single traumatic event that is distressing and representative of a chronic trauma will be sufficient to reduce distress associated with all episodes of the chronic trauma. When this generalization occurs, it is not necessary to directly target other events from the same chronic trauma type via imaginal exposure. Given this, it is typical during the Trauma Interview to identify only one target trauma per chronic trauma type. There are two main exceptions to this approach:

1. *The client has experienced fewer than three types of trauma overall.* In these cases, the client's top three most distressing events may include more than one event from the same chronic trauma because there are no other types of trauma that require targeting.

2. *There are important variations in how a chronic trauma occurred.* In some cases, more than one event may be selected if there were distinct and meaningful differences in how the chronic trauma occurred. For example, many survivors of chronic child sexual abuse experienced episodes in which the perpetrator initiated the sexual behavior, as well as episodes in which they, as a result of past learning, initiated the sexual behavior. These two types of abusive experiences are likely to elicit different trauma-related beliefs and emotions, and it may be necessary to target both variations of the abuse to achieve maximum improvement.

Of note, the decision to target more than one event from a chronic trauma is often made later in treatment rather than during the Trauma Interview. In particular, after the first target trauma is treated via imaginal exposure, if other events from the same chronic trauma remain highly distressing, then a second event may be selected for targeting at that time. This is discussed in more detail in Chapter 12.

Link to Beliefs. Another factor to consider when selecting a specific event is its link to the primary problematic beliefs that clients have about the chronic trauma they experienced. This can be particularly helpful when targeting traumatic invalidation that was the cumulative effect of many day-to-day criticisms and slights rather than the result of any particularly extreme episodes of invalidation. In these cases, events can be prioritized based on the degree to which they contribute to clients' problematic beliefs about themselves and others rather than by the distress any one episode may cause. For example, if the client's primary problematic beliefs are "I am not important" and "People don't care about my suffering," then you can help them identify an event that taught them to think this way about themselves and/or that they view as providing the strongest evidence that those beliefs are true. The goal here is to identify an event that, once processed, will help to decrease the believability of the global negative beliefs that arose from a chronic trauma.

Memory Quality. A final factor to consider is how clearly the client remembers the event. Typically, the clarity of a client's memories varies, with some episodes being quite foggy or vague and some being quite clear and well remembered. All things being equal, it is preferable to select an event that is clearly remembered over an event that is fragmented or blurry. Thus, if there are multiple events that seem like good candidates for imaginal exposure, select the memory that has the most detailed narrative.

Case Example

Maria's top three most distressing trauma types included one single-event trauma (the rape) and two chronic traumas (her father's abuse and the bullying by peers). Thus, she and her therapist set out to select a specific event for each of the two chronic traumas. Her therapist started by asking whether there was one time that her father had abused both her and her mother that stood out to her as particularly distressing. Maria said there was one event when she was about 7 years old that was particularly upsetting to her because she had done something that caused her father to hit her mother and then abuse her. She became tearful as she said that she had made her father angry by accidentally knocking over his beer while he was watching TV. She said he had then physically assaulted her mother for not keeping Maria away from him and demanded that she go out and buy him more beer. As soon as her mother left the house, she said her father physically and sexually abused her as punishment for her misbehavior. Maria began crying and her therapist responded by praising her for sharing these painful details and for allowing herself to cry. The therapist then asked Maria if this type of abusive behavior was typical of what her father would do to her and her mother, and Maria said it was. The therapist then asked her how well she remembered this event and whether she thought she could describe it as a story with a beginning, middle, and end. Maria said she couldn't remember much about what was happening before she spilled his beer, but that she clearly remembered knocking it over and most of what had happened afterward. They both agreed that this seemed like a good episode to select for targeting.

Next, they turned their attention to Maria's third most distressing type of trauma: the bullying by peers in high school. When asked whether there was any event that was particularly distressing to her from this chronic trauma, Maria said that it happened so frequently, often multiple times per day, that it was hard to pick just one event. Since Maria had previously said that this harassment had contributed significantly to her self-hatred, her therapist suggested that they pick an event that made her feel particularly intense self-hatred and perhaps even prompted her suicide attempt. Maria said there was one especially humiliating event that had occurred a few days before she tried to kill herself, and then she covered her face with her hands and slumped over in her chair. After a brief period of silence, Maria quietly said that she had gotten drunk at a party and performed oral sex on a boy that she did not know well. She said that the next week he and several of his friends approached her in the hall at school and began calling her a "whore" and asking her if she would give them all blow jobs. She said they offered to pay her $20, which she found extremely humiliating, particularly because this event was witnessed by a lot of other students.

Her therapist reinforced her for disclosing these details and said she was doing a great job. Maria then added that this event really made her hate herself because her "slutty" behavior had caused it and she had deserved to be treated "like a prostitute." Her therapist again thanked her for sharing this information and encouraged her to look at her so she could take in her response. Maria then peered out from behind her hands and the therapist smiled at her warmly and said that Maria was doing exactly what was needed to make this treatment work and she was proud of her. Her therapist also told her that she was very sorry this had happened to her and that she did not agree that Maria had deserved to be treated in this way. Maria then uncovered her face, sat up straight, and thanked her therapist for not judging her. Her therapist then wrote Maria's top three target traumas from most to least distressing in Item 2 as follows:

1. Father got angry when she spilled his beer, hit her mother, and then physically and sexually abused her (age 7)
2. Rape (age 21)
3. Bullying episode of boys calling her a "whore" and offering to pay for sexual favors (age 16)

Ordering of Target Traumas for Imaginal Exposure (Item 3)

The final item of Section 2 involves determining the order in which the top three target traumas will be addressed via imaginal exposure. It is important to emphasize that this is entirely up to the client: Your role is to function as a consultant to the client during the decision-making process. In general, it is typically recommended that clients start imaginal exposure with the most distressing target trauma so that they obtain the greatest relief most quickly. In addition, the effects of targeting the most distressing trauma may be more likely to generalize to other lesser distressing traumas, perhaps reducing the overall number of traumas that require targeting. On the other side, starting with a less distressing target trauma will allow for a more gradual approach, which may be useful for clients who wish to gain experience and confidence with imaginal exposure before targeting the most distressing event. However, this approach may take longer, as clients who start with a less distressing trauma will typically need to subsequently target the most distressing trauma, whereas the opposite may not be true. To help clients make this decision, you can help them think through the pros and cons of starting with the most distressing versus a lesser distressing target trauma.

Case Example

When asked which trauma she wanted to focus on first, Maria said she wasn't sure what to do. Her therapist responded by telling her that it was ultimately her decision to make, and then shared her perspective on the potential pros and cons of starting with the most versus a lesser distressing memory. Maria then decided that she would target her traumas in order from most to least distressing, starting with her father's abuse. She said, "I've already decided to do this so I might as well do it all the way." Her therapist reinforced her for making this choice and told her that she had faith in her ability to take on the hardest trauma first.

CLINICAL TIP
What If We Don't Choose the "Right" Target Traumas?

A common concern among therapists (and sometimes clients) is that if you don't choose the "right" target traumas during the Trauma Interview, the entire treatment will be doomed to fail. Never fear! The target traumas that are selected in Session 1 are not set in stone. As treatment progresses, you may discover that some traumas that you initially thought would be important to target become less distressing and don't need to be addressed. Conversely, some traumas that were not originally in the top three may become more salient and therefore need to rise higher on the list. Sometimes clients may change their minds about which single events to focus on from a chronic trauma. In general, the exact memories that are targeted and the order in which this occurs can change during treatment in response to the client's progress and changing levels of distress. Therefore, the target traumas identified in Session 1 can be viewed as your and the client's best guess about how treatment will progress, while also acknowledging that this may change if a more effective path forward becomes clear.

Section 3. Trauma Narrative and Prior Disclosure

Once the first target trauma is selected, the remainder of the Trauma Interview is much more straightforward for the therapist, although it is still likely to be emotionally challenging for the client. Section 3 focuses on identifying start and end points for the imaginal exposure narrative and assessing the client's prior disclosure experiences.

Identifying Start and End Points (Items 4 and 5)

Imaginal exposure involves telling the story of exactly how a specific traumatic event unfolded. As with any story, the narrator, who in this case is the client, will need to decide where to start the story and where to end it. For the purposes of imaginal exposure, we want the narrative to include all of the central and most difficult elements of the traumatic experience while ideally also being brief enough to allow for multiple repetitions to be completed within the 20–45 minutes typically allotted for imaginal exposure. With this goal in mind, the first question asks clients to estimate how long the entire traumatic event lasted. Answers may range from only a few minutes (e.g., a mugging in which a person was hit once and the assailant immediately ran away) to days or weeks (e.g., an abduction in which a person was held captive and repeatedly assaulted before they eventually escaped).

It almost always takes less time to tell the story of an event than it took for the event to occur. This means that traumatic events that lasted 3 hours may only take the client 10 minutes to narrate. On the other hand, some clients will describe events in such rich detail that a 3-hour event may take 45 minutes to narrate. Although it is impossible in Session 1 to know for certain how long an imaginal exposure narrative will be, it is generally recommended that the start and end points be no more than a few hours apart in real time. When traumatic events were particularly long in duration, it may be necessary to select only one part to focus on to shorten the narrative and allow for a detailed description. For example, if a combat veteran was involved in an 8-hour firefight, the imaginal exposure narrative may focus only on the most distressing part (e.g., the moments leading up to and immediately following his friend being killed). For events that took place across several hours where it is not clear if the narrative may end up being longer than ideal, it is also reasonable to select the entire event now with the plan of shortening it later in treatment if needed.

START POINT

Ideally, the start point for the imaginal exposure narrative will be a few minutes before anything bad or scary started to happen to allow the client to have at least a brief lead-in to the exposure that does not include anything intensely distressing. Given that many of the traumas our clients have experienced are interpersonal in nature, the start point often involves a description of what the client was doing right before the perpetrator entered the scene or began to threaten them. For example, they may have been alone in their bedroom, watching TV, or arriving home from school. For other types of trauma, the start point may be what they were doing right before they realized they were in danger. For example, a person who was in a car accident may start by describing where they were driving in the minutes before their car was hit. Given that many clients have fragmented memories of their traumatic experiences, it is not always possible to select a start point that occurs before the acute trauma began. For example, a person who was raped may not remember what they were doing beforehand and their memory may start in the middle of the rape. For these types of fragmented memories, the start point will be whatever the first thing is that the client can remember about the traumatic event.

END POINT

The end point for the imaginal exposure narrative will ideally be the point at which the person was out of immediate danger or experienced some relief even if it was only temporary. The goal is to allow the client to end the narrative at a point that is not the most intensely distressing moments of the trauma. The end point can be particularly tricky to identify for clients who were repeatedly traumatized by the same person, which means they were often never truly out of danger. In these cases, it can be helpful to validate the reality of the chronic danger they were in and clarify that the end point may have only been a temporary break from imminent danger. Again, given the interpersonal nature of much of our clients' trauma, the end point is often after the perpetrator and/or the client had left the situation. For example, the perpetrator left the client's bedroom or the client left the perpetrator's house. If clients cannot remember how the event ended (e.g., because they dissociated during the event), then the end point will be whatever the last thing is that they remember.

Case Example

Maria reported that she thought the entire abusive episode with her father had lasted about 2 hours. Given this time frame, her therapist suggested that they plan to have Maria describe the entire event for imaginal exposure. Her therapist then oriented Maria to the goal of starting the narrative right before anything scary happened and asked her what she thought a good start point would be. Maria suggested starting when she was sitting on the living room floor playing with her toys and mistakenly bumped into the coffee table and spilled her father's beer. Her therapist then asked her where she thought the narrative should end and said that ideally the end point would be after Maria felt as if she was out of imminent danger. Maria said that after her father finished punishing her, he told her to go to her room and leave him alone. She then hid in her closet because she was afraid he might come in and hurt her again. She said that she didn't really feel safe until she heard her mother come home about 30 minutes later. Maria began to cry as she thought about this, and her therapist responded by validating how scary this must have been. Given that Maria had stayed in the closet for more than 30 minutes and her father had never entered her room, her therapist suggested that they end the narrative closer to when the abuse was over and she first went into her bedroom. Maria then suggested that she could describe the first few minutes of hiding in the closet and then stop, and her therapist agreed this sounded like a good plan.

CLINICAL TIP
What about the Middle of the Trauma Narrative?

As you have likely noticed, the Trauma Interview does not include any questions to assess what happened between the start and end points of the trauma narrative. Although this may feel odd, this is because it is not necessary to know the details of the trauma itself in order to prepare clients to tell the story of what happened. Moreover, asking clients to provide these details now would be likely to turn the Trauma Interview into full-fledged imaginal exposure rather than assessment. Additionally, there is not usually enough time for clients to discuss the details of the trauma in depth. This means that you typically have very little if any information about the details of the actual traumatic event before the client's first imaginal exposure session. This may feel like you're being asked to walk into a booby-trapped room wearing a blindfold. However, there will be plenty of time to learn about and process the details of the trauma during the exposure sessions, and for the sake of time, you are encouraged to steer away from asking clients to provide these details in the Trauma Interview.

Assessing Prior Disclosure Experiences (Items 6 and 7)

For some clients, imaginal exposure may be the first time they have ever talked about the trauma with another person. For other clients, they may have told the story of their trauma many times to friends, family members, partners, prior therapists, or the police. In some cases, other people may have shared information about the client's trauma with others—for example, a parent may have told other family members about the client's allegations that her grandfather had sexually abused her. If other people know about the target trauma, it is useful to know whether the decision to disclose was under the client's control. It is not unusual for disclosures to have been made without the client's permission, and in some cases, the way in which traumas were disclosed may have been equally or even more distressing than the traumatic event itself. For example, a client's traumatic experience may have been widely publicized on social media or they may have been forced by their parents to file a police report, which may have added another layer of trauma to their experience.

If other people know about the trauma, it is also useful to know how those people responded. In all too many cases, clients report that they have been blamed, criticized, disbelieved, humiliated, ignored, rejected, or even punished when others learned about their trauma. Very often these negative disclosure experiences shaped the client's social support-seeking behavior, leading them to stop talking to or trying to get support from other people and instead setting them on a path of avoidance, isolation, secrecy, and shame. Alternatively, some clients may shift to the end of overdisclosing by frequently talking about their traumatic experiences to people with whom this is not appropriate or effective. Not surprisingly, research has shown that negative social reactions after a trauma are strongly correlated with the development of PTSD (e.g., Ullman, 2007). Some clients will have had one or more people who responded in positive ways, such as by expressing compassion or providing support. However, even in these cases it is common that clients also experienced negative responses to their trauma disclosures, which may have outweighed the potential buffering effect of the more positive reactions.

As the therapist, it is helpful to know about these prior disclosure experiences for two main reasons. First, this information can help to inform how you respond to the client after you hear the details of the target trauma in the first imaginal exposure session (and beyond). If it will be the client's first time ever telling someone about the trauma, you may choose to respond to this first disclosure with particular care, reinforcement, and praise. Alternatively, if clients have had negative disclosure experiences in the past, they will often expect you to respond in similarly hurtful and invalidating ways. In such cases, knowing how others have responded will help you to choose responses that will be most likely to disconfirm the client's expectancies. For example, if a client has previously been accused of lying about being raped, an effective response at the end of the first imaginal exposure may be to say, "I believe you."

Second, information about prior disclosure experiences can be useful from a case formulation perspective, as it often offers important insights into the origins of clients' problematic beliefs that are maintaining PTSD. If clients were blamed by others for the trauma, they will very often blame themselves in similar ways. If others appeared indifferent or unaffected when they learned about the trauma, clients will often believe that what happened to them was not a big deal. If clients were told they were damaged, dirty, or disgusting because of what was done to them, they will often hate themselves for these same reasons. Knowing that clients' problematic beliefs may have stemmed from others' negative responses can provide you with useful information about how best to tailor treatment to change these beliefs. Overall, it may help to shape the goal of treatment as being about helping clients to get a new perspective on their trauma that reflects their own wise mind and not the invalidating views of other people.

Case Example

Maria said that her mother was the only person who knew about her father's abuse. She said that her mother had witnessed his physically abusive behavior many times during her childhood but had never been present when he sexually abused her. Maria first told her mother about the sexual abuse after her father died when she was 14. Her mother was very distressed to learn this had occurred and had said Maria should have told her sooner because there was nothing she could do about it now. Her mother also told her to try to forget about it and move on as she herself was doing. As a result of this disclosure experience, Maria said that she had felt like she had done something wrong by not telling her mother sooner. She also said that she felt like she was supposed to act like it hadn't happened and didn't bother her, so she had never talked to her mother or anyone else about it again.

Section 4. Beliefs, Emotions, and Radical Acceptance (Items 8–10)

The final section of the Trauma Interview focuses on assessing the specific trauma-related beliefs and emotions that are likely maintaining the client's PTSD related to the first target trauma. As in the earlier rationale, when clients express clearly maladaptive beliefs during this portion of the interview, it is best to avoid the temptation of moving into in-depth cognitive modification strategies. There will be plenty of time to address these beliefs later in treatment: for now, the goal is to begin to more clearly understand what they are. If new information is obtained during this portion of the interview, the initial case formulation should be updated to enable more precise targeting of mechanisms as treatment progresses.

Item 8 assesses who, if anyone, the client blames for the occurrence of the traumatic event. Clients are asked to assign blame for the event (totaling to 100%) across multiple potential people, the environment, organizations, or the broader culture. Given that self-blame is a robust risk factor for developing PTSD, self-blaming beliefs are among the most common and intense maladaptive beliefs that clients express. For example, at the beginning of treatment a typical survivor of rape may blame herself 90%, the perpetrator 5%, and the culture 5%. For each domain to which the client assigns blame, they are then asked how that person or entity is responsible. For example, the client may say that the rape was her fault because she made poor decisions and put herself in danger, the perpetrator took advantage of her, and the broader sexist culture promoted violence against women.

Item 9 assesses the emotions clients currently have when they think about the target trauma. Clients are asked to rate the intensity of each emotion from 0 to 100 and to briefly describe what it is about the traumatic event that makes them feel that emotion. At the beginning of treatment, the typical pattern is that unjustified emotions are high (e.g., fear, guilt, shame, and self-directed disgust), whereas justified emotions are low (e.g., sadness and anger). (As a reminder, the term *justified* in DBT refers to whether emotions fit the facts of the present situation, which is different from whether they are understandable.) When asked why they have the emotions they have, clients will again begin to articulate more specific beliefs about the trauma and its impact. For example, a client might say that they feel shame at 100 because they believe the trauma is proof that they are a terrible person, or disgust at 85 because they believe the trauma has made them permanently dirty and contaminated. The goal here is to get a quick read on the client's emotions and the beliefs that may be driving them without getting too bogged down in a detailed discussion of the trauma and its aftermath.

The final question, Item 10, asks clients to rate from 0 to 100 how much they radically accept that this traumatic event happened. On the surface, it might seem that clients should have high ratings of radical acceptance—if they are seeking treatment to address the event, then surely they must recognize that it happened. However, clients often acknowledge the facts of a traumatic event and still do not wholly and completely accept that it occurred, which is required for radical acceptance. Nonacceptance of trauma may mean that clients are questioning reality ("Maybe I'm making it up"), distrusting their perceptions ("I'm probably overreacting"), harboring bitterness about what happened ("It shouldn't be this way"), or fearing the sadness acceptance will bring ("I will be overwhelmed by despair"). In addition, a common barrier to radical acceptance of past trauma is the belief that acceptance means they approve of the horrific things that have happened to them. This is absolutely not the case. Radical acceptance means only that they fully and completely accept that this painful event happened exactly the way that it did. Alternatively, if clients are unable to remember significant portions of the trauma, radical acceptance may instead focus on accepting the uncertainty of not knowing exactly what happened. Both of these realities are incredibly hard to accept, and nearly all clients begin treatment with a low level of radical acceptance.

Case Example

For Item 8, Maria said that she blamed herself 85% for her father's abuse, her father 10%, and her mother 5%. She said it was almost entirely her fault because she was constantly doing things that made him angry. She said if she had been a better-behaved child, that he wouldn't have had to punish her so much. The little blame she assigned to her father was because she thought he was sometimes excessively harsh, particularly when he used sexual behavior to punish her. Finally, she said that she thought her mother was at least a little responsible because mothers are supposed to protect their children from harm and her mother had not done that for her, even though she understood why she had not. Her therapist responded by saying it was common for child abuse survivors to blame themselves for their abuse, and that this was something that they would talk a lot more about during treatment.

Maria's ratings of the intensity and reasons for her current emotions about the abuse by her father are shown below.

Emotions	Intensity (0–100)	What is it about this event that makes you feel [*insert emotion*]?
a. Fear	95	Reminds her of how scared she was of him
b. Sadness	40	Sad that she and her mom had to go through this, also that she could never seem to do things right
c. Anger	20	Anger that her father hit her mother
d. Guilt	100	Thinks it was her fault for spilling his beer, she made him so angry that he hit her mother, she should have been more careful
e. Shame	100	Feels like she is bad and deserved his punishment
f. Disgust	100	Feels disgusted by her body, particularly the sexual parts

Finally, Maria rated her radical acceptance of this episode of her father's abuse as a 40. She said, "I mean, I know that it happened, I'm not making it up. I just think it shouldn't have happened. I just wish I could go back and change myself to be a better kid so that none of this would have happened." Her therapist normalized this, saying it is hard for most people to accept the painful reality of their traumas. She also told Maria that although acceptance may be painful in the short run, it reduces suffering in the long run and that this was something they would work on during treatment. Her therapist then congratulated her for finishing the Trauma Interview and said she had done a great job answering the questions and allowing herself to experience the emotions that the discussion had elicited. The therapist finished this portion of the session by saying, "This is a really good sign that you're ready for this treatment. I can't wait to see what a difference this is going to make for you!"

CLINICAL TIP

An Opportunity for Behavioral Observation

Although the primary function of the Trauma Interview is to assess the client's trauma history and prepare for imaginal exposure, it also provides you with an important opportunity to observe the client's ability to talk about their trauma and tolerate the distress this evokes. Some examples of the kinds of behaviors that may be useful to pay attention to include:

- What avoidance behaviors, if any, are evident (e.g., dissociation, hiding, distracting, unwillingness to disclose, avoiding certain words)?
- How much detail does the client provide about the trauma? Do they have difficulty saying much or do they provide the amount of detail needed without much hesitation?
- What emotions are present? Is the client either highly distressed or very numb or flat? What strategies are they using to regulate or tolerate emotions?
- Does the client self-initiate skills use when needed or do you have to provide significant coaching? If so, how responsive are they to coaching?
- What seems to be an effective validation-to-change ratio? Is frequent validation needed to keep the client engaged and moving forward, or are they able to stay task focused without a lot of validation?

In general, carefully observing the client's behavior during the Trauma Interview can help you to be better prepared for imaginal exposure, including being able to anticipate challenges that may be likely to occur and begin to identify potential solutions.

---

4. Obtain and Strengthen Commitments

At this point in treatment, clients should be well aware of the contingencies that were established during Stage 1 in order to demonstrate readiness to start DBT PE. In Session 1, it is important to ensure that clients are similarly aware of the contingencies that will be applied during DBT PE, as well as the general expectation that they will not revert to severe behavioral dyscontrol. Using DBT's standard strategies for obtaining and strengthening commitments, clients are asked to commit to three goals that align with the Stage 1 DBT target hierarchy:

1. Not engaging in suicidal or self-injurious behaviors.
2. Actively participating in DBT PE, including both in-session tasks and homework.
3. Not engaging in escape-related quality-of-life behaviors immediately before, during, or after sessions, or when completing exposure homework.

The first commitment is simply an extension of what clients have already agreed to during Stage 1, and it is therefore typically a straightforward and quick task to confirm that clients remain committed to not killing themselves or self-injuring during DBT PE. It is also important to ensure that clients are aware that there will be zero tolerance for these behaviors during DBT PE—namely, if they attempt suicide or self-injure, then DBT PE will be paused. Like the requirement of abstinence from these behaviors to start DBT PE, this contingency is used primarily as a strategy for increasing clients' motivation to prevent these behaviors from occurring in the first place. Thus, it is critical that clients are informed of this contingency at the beginning of DBT PE. You might also remind clients that the treatment is under their control, and if they decide at any point that they don't want to continue, they should just tell you rather than potentially engaging in self-injurious behavior to get DBT PE to stop. (The decision about how long to pause DBT PE if these behaviors recur is discussed in detail in Chapter 14.)

The second and third commitments are intended to optimize outcomes by reducing the likelihood that therapy-interfering and quality-of-life behaviors will decrease the effectiveness of DBT PE. Clients are asked to either refrain from or sufficiently control behaviors that may prevent them from receiving an adequate dose of the treatment (e.g., nonattendance, homework noncompliance) and/or interfere with the mechanisms of exposure (e.g., in-session dissociation). These commitments should be personalized to reflect the behaviors most relevant to a given client. When quality-of-life behaviors are still active (e.g., substance use, disordered eating, impulsive sex, gambling), and particularly when these behaviors function to escape from emotions, clients are asked to commit to not engaging in these behaviors before, during, or for 2 hours after any exposure task. There are no specific rules about the frequency or intensity of these behaviors that may cause DBT PE to be paused, but clients should be oriented to the general principle that significant therapy-interfering or quality-of-life behaviors may result in a temporary suspension of DBT PE (for more details on this decision-making process see Chapter 14).

5. Complete the Post-Exposure DBT Skills Plan

The next task of this session is to identify DBT skills that clients can use after exposure to help them effectively manage intense emotions without engaging in problem behaviors. These are written on *DBT PE Handout 3* (*Post-Exposure Skills Plan*) and should include a balance of acceptance and change skills. Typically, these plans include skills designed to reduce the intensity of aversive emotions (e.g., distraction, self-soothing, TIP), as well as skills to experience emotions at their natural intensity (e.g., mindfulness of current emotion, radical acceptance, willing hands). As is true for DBT skills more broadly, clients need to know which skills to apply in which contexts—for example, the TIP skills may be used when clients have reached a skills breakdown point and are at high risk of acting on problematic urges, whereas mindful experiencing of emotion may be used in noncrisis situations. It is also important to ensure that clients include skills that can be used anywhere at any time (e.g., paced breathing, imagery), as well as those that may be situation specific (e.g., spending time with a friend, going to a movie). The Post-Exposure Skills Plan also includes space to list behaviors to be avoided after exposure. Often these will overlap with the behaviors that clients were asked to commit to controlling but may also include other types of behaviors that may be ineffective (e.g., isolating, sleeping) or unwise (e.g., making important life decisions, spending a large amount of money).

At this time, it is also helpful to start working with clients to figure out a plan for what they will do after their first imaginal exposure session, which is typically still a few weeks away. In outpatient settings, it may be preferable to ask clients to make a plan that involves spending time with a support person after their first imaginal exposure session. Because this may take some time to arrange, it is useful to have clients start thinking about this now. If clients do not have a person with whom they either can or want to spend time after their first exposure session, then it will be important to have them start thinking about what they will do on their own.

6. Assign Homework

At the end of Session 1, clients are asked to complete the following homework assignments. As is standard in DBT, you should obtain a commitment to complete the homework and troubleshoot factors that might interfere before ending the session.

SESSION 1 HOMEWORK ASSIGNMENTS

1. Review the rationale for treatment (DBT PE Handouts 1 and 2).*

2. Practice skills from the Post-Exposure Skills Plan daily and add more skills if needed (DBT PE Handout 3).*

3. Listen to the entire session recording once.

4. Make a plan for after the first imaginal exposure session.

*Clients may choose to share these with support person(s) when appropriate.

CHAPTER 9

Session 2

SESSION 2 COMPONENTS AND TIME ESTIMATES

	60-minute session	90-minute session
1. Review the DBT diary card and set the session agenda	3 min.	3–5 min.
2. Review homework	3–5 min.	5–7 min.
3. Discuss dialectical reactions to trauma	15–20 min.	25–30 min.
4. Orient to the rationale for *in vivo* exposure	7–10 min.	10–15 min.
5. Construct the *in vivo* exposure hierarchy	15–25 min.	30–40 min.
6. Assign homework	3–5 min.	5–10 min.

The primary tasks of Session 2 are to provide psychoeducation about common dialectical reactions to trauma and prepare clients to begin the *in vivo* exposure portion of the treatment. Clients are likely to be experiencing increased anxiety as the time to start exposure nears, and you should strive to attend to these underlying tensions while also remaining laser focused—Session 2 is packed with treatment tasks and you will need to manage time effectively to complete them all. A checklist for Session 2 is included in Appendix C and can be used in session to guide you through each of these tasks. All client handouts are in Appendix A.

1. Review the DBT Diary Card and Set the Session Agenda

To start, the DBT diary card is briefly reviewed to confirm that no life-threatening or other higher-priority behaviors have occurred that might require DBT PE to be paused (see Chapter 14 for details). As in Session 1, it is not unusual for clients to exhibit a pattern of elevated urges to engage in a variety of target behaviors in the weeks leading up to starting exposure. Typically, you can respond by reinforcing clients for not acting on these urges and then proceed with the planned DBT PE session tasks. When needed, increased urges or target behaviors can be more fully addressed during the DBT session (or portion of the session). Once the diary card has been reviewed, present the session agenda by outlining the components listed at the beginning of this chapter.

2. Review Homework

Homework is a critical component of DBT PE and adherence to homework assignments is likely to improve outcomes. Therefore, it is important to set the expectation that homework will be reviewed—and homework noncompletion will be addressed—at the start of every session. In Session 2, homework review involves confirming that clients read *DBT PE Handout 1* (*How PTSD Is Maintained*) and *Handout 2* (*How DBT PE Works to Reduce PTSD*) and addressing any questions, reviewing any changes to *Handout 3* (*Post-Exposure Skills Plan*), and discussing clients' practice of skills from the plan. Clients are also asked whether they have finalized plans for after the first imaginal exposure session and any barriers to making this plan are problem-solved. Finally, clients are asked whether they listened to the recording of Session 1, which is typically the assignment that clients have the most difficulty completing. Given that listening to recordings of in-session imaginal exposure is a critical component of DBT PE, it is essential that problems related to reviewing session recordings are assessed and problem-solved immediately. This is usually done via a brief missing links analysis followed by commitment and troubleshooting. (See Chapter 14 for details on conducting missing links analysis.) If homework noncompliance becomes a repeated or significant problem, more in-depth targeting may become necessary in subsequent sessions—however, in Session 2 the goal is primarily to establish effective contingencies related to homework completion.

3. Discuss Dialectical Reactions to Trauma

The first major task of the session is to engage the client in a discussion about common reactions to trauma. As shown in *DBT PE Handout 4* (*Dialectical Reactions to Trauma*), these trauma reactions are organized as a set of three dialectical dilemmas related to emotions, behaviors, and relationships that each include a pole of extreme undercontrol and overcontrol. Clients may shift rapidly from one pole to the other with movement in one direction quickly reversed by countermovement in the other direction. Alternatively, the shift between poles may be more gradual and long lasting. For example, clients may have been undercontrolled throughout their adolescence and young adulthood before becoming overcontrolled as adults. This movement between poles can be both confusing and overwhelming for clients, and conceptualizing trauma reactions within a dialectical framework can help them to better understand their own extreme and seemingly opposite behaviors. Importantly, not all clients will experience all poles of these dialectical dilemmas. Regardless, awareness of these dialectical reactions can help clients to identify balanced goals that represent a synthesis between these extremes. Of note, these dialectical reactions to trauma are intended to be transdiagnostic and to provide a comprehensive picture of the types of trauma-related problems common among people with a recent history of Stage 1 level of disorder, including PTSD symptoms as well as behaviors characteristic of other disorders (e.g., BPD, depression, substance use disorders, obsessive–compulsive disorder [OCD]). These dialectical reactions to trauma are not intended to replace the original dialectical dilemmas in DBT (e.g., emotional vulnerability vs. self-invalidation), but rather to augment them with a set of dialectical dilemmas that are particularly relevant for clients with a history of trauma and PTSD.

Extremes in Emotions

Emotional Flooding

Emotional flooding refers to uncontrollable experiences of intense and aversive trauma-related emotions, such as fear, shame, guilt, sadness, disgust, and anger. These emotions are often prompted by intrusive reexperiencing of trauma via flashbacks, nightmares, and recurrent memories, as well as exposure to external trauma reminders. Once triggered, these powerful trauma-related emotions are a full-system response that includes biological changes (e.g., increased heart rate, rapid breathing), physical sensations (e.g., dizziness, nausea), urges (e.g., to escape or hide), body language (e.g., looking down, clenching fists), and actions (e.g., sobbing, verbally attacking). The rapid onset, intensity, and unpredictability of these overwhelming trauma-related emotions often leave the person feeling depleted and out of control. In addition, many people with PTSD experience chronically high levels of negative emotions. For example, they may feel ashamed, sad, or angry most of the time and these emotions may spike even higher when they encounter a trauma cue. Thus, clients typically view emotions as intolerable, dangerous, and potentially even traumatizing, and will go to great and at times highly destructive lengths to avoid them.

Emotional Numbness

At the other end of this dialectic is emotional numbness, a less outwardly dramatic but equally impairing type of extreme emotional experiencing. Clients often describe emotional numbness as feeling as if they are hollow or dead inside and unable to feel anything. At times, emotional numbness may be intentionally induced to obtain relief from intense emotions. At other times, emotional numbness may occur unintentionally and be experienced as beyond the person's control. Emotional numbness may involve a general inability to access any emotion or it may be restricted to only certain emotions (e.g., positive emotions, such as happiness, love, and joy). In some cases, emotional numbness is a chronic state—for example, numbness may be due to long-standing depression, which can lead to a general feeling of flatness and difficulty finding pleasure in life. For many clients, numbing can also take the form of dissociation, including feeling disconnected from themselves or the world around them. Dissociation may occur briefly and intermittently, such as in times of high stress, or it may be a more frequent state lasting many hours. Often clients view temporary emotional numbness to be preferable to emotional flooding, whereas prolonged or chronic emotional numbing is often an excruciating state that clients work to avoid.

The Dialectical Dilemma

The central dilemma for the client is how to experience emotions without being completely flooded or becoming totally numb. Should emotions be experienced even though they are likely to rapidly become overwhelming? Or should emotions be suppressed even though this may result in an unbearable state of chronic numbness? Since neither extreme is a viable solution in the long term, the client often vacillates between the two. Emotions may be present for a period of time until the person becomes flooded and reverts to emotional numbness as an escape.

Conversely, efforts to suppress and numb emotions often result in a paradoxical effect in which emotions subsequently rebound and become more intense. Clients are at high risk of engaging in problematic behaviors at both ends of the emotional spectrum. When left to choose between falling into a pool of emotional despair or grabbing for a life preserver that is full of holes but will float temporarily, clients will often choose the short-term, maladaptive way of obtaining emotional relief. On the other end, clients will also go to great lengths to alleviate excruciating numbness, resorting to behaviors likely to generate feelings and induce sensations even if painful or damaging. The goal is to achieve nonanguished emotional experiencing, a dialectical synthesis of these two extremes in which clients are able to experience the full range of emotions without suppressing and use adaptive strategies to modulate emotional intensity when needed.

Extremes in Behavior

Reckless Dyscontrol

At this extreme, people engage in reckless, impulsive, and damaging behaviors without restraint. These behaviors often occur suddenly and without forethought: An impulse arises and it is quickly acted on with little to no consideration of the negative outcomes of these behaviors. Instead, the focus is on short-term goals, such as obtaining relief from intense emotions, escaping a painful situation, or experiencing a rush through behaviors, such as suicidal and nonsuicidal self-injury, substance use, and binge eating. When in a disinhibited state, poor risk assessment is common and clients may engage in risky behaviors, such as reckless driving, stealing, physical aggression, and unsafe sex. Impulsive decision making is also common, such as deciding to quit a job with little thought and purchasing things on a whim that can't be afforded. Impulsivity is often accompanied by other problems, such as restlessness, hyperactivity, and inattention. Overall, the person's experience is one of danger and loss of control.

Rigid Control

At the other extreme, people are constantly on guard and perceive danger lurking around every corner. They live their lives in a state of high alert, actively scanning the environment for potential threats and being prepared to act to protect themselves or others. They often follow rigid rules that they believe are necessary to keep themselves and others safe—for example, they may check the locks repeatedly before going to bed, not allow their children out of their sight, or always sit close to an exit. This hypervigilance is often accompanied by other types of physiological arousal and reactivity, such as irritability, difficulty sleeping, an exaggerated startle response, and poor concentration. In addition, many clients are rigid and overcontrolled in their behavior more broadly. They may be extremely clean and orderly, excessively prepare and plan before taking action, inhibit spontaneity, and adhere to perfectionistic standards. These behaviors often serve a similar function of increasing their sense of safety and predictability in a world that feels dangerous and out of control.

The Dialectical Dilemma

The juxtaposition of reckless dyscontrol and rigid control can be particularly disorienting both to clients and those around them. On the one hand, clients grossly underestimate danger: They directly harm themselves via suicidal and self-injurious behaviors, put themselves in objectively dangerous situations, and take excessive risks. On the other hand, clients completely overestimate danger: They rigidly control their behavior to reduce their risk of harm or rejection, perceive danger in objectively safe situations, and take excessive precautions. These contradictory perceptions of risk can feel as if one has entered a parallel universe in which safety and danger have been reversed. However, what is constant at both ends is the client's experience of being in danger and out of control. Whether the danger is from themselves or the world, they are engaged in a constant and exhausting battle for survival. Clients often shift between these poles with periods of dangerous behavioral dyscontrol leading to fervent efforts to rigidly control their behavior in perfectionistic ways that are doomed to fail. At times both poles are present simultaneously—for example, disinhibited behaviors may occur while the client is engaged in activities in the outside world and be counterbalanced by extreme rigidity and overcontrol in their home environment. Ultimately, the goal is to find a dialectical synthesis in which the person can accurately assess danger and modulate their behavior to reduce their risk of harm without overly restricting their lives.

Extremes in Relationships

Desperate Connection

The defining characteristic of this extreme is the person's sense of desperation for close connections with others to escape the intolerable pain of aloneness. They often depend on other people to make them feel whole, complete, and as if they matter, and they feel unsafe and insecure without close relationships. This strong emotional need for connection may lead them to behave in ways that others experience as clingy, demanding, or needy, which can have the undesirable effect of pushing people away. Alternatively, in an effort to be as likable as possible, many people will regularly prioritize others' needs above their own, rarely say no to requests, and make few demands on others. Often people endure destructive relationships in which they are repeatedly mistreated because it feels preferable to being alone. If a relationship does end, they may quickly rush to find a new relationship to replace it. When building new relationships, they often become quickly attached, are overly trusting, and share personal information too quickly. In general, they may behave in overly familiar ways with people they do not know well, acting as though they are in a stable, reciprocal relationship when in fact they are merely acquaintances. When close relationships are hard to find, they may seek out sex with people they do not know well, which may help them to feel connected and less alone even if only temporarily. Ultimately, this pattern of desperately pursuing closeness with others increases clients' vulnerability to being victimized by others.

Detached Independence

At the other end of this dialectic, people seek isolation, are uncomfortable with emotional closeness, and strive to be independent and self-sufficient. They often deny needing close relationships and feel alienated and detached from others. These problems stem from a pervasive distrust of people and an expectation that others will cause them harm, particularly if they allow themselves to become attached. To prevent themselves from getting hurt, they will actively work to emotionally distance themselves from people and may even behave in off-putting ways so that people will leave them alone. In addition, they often work to appear strong and invulnerable, sending a clear message that they do not want or need anyone's help. When another person offers support or expresses care, they often question the person's intentions, do not reciprocate, and may even disavow the relationship. In the relationships they do have, they may feign close-ness, seeming to be connected to a person while at the same time not allowing themselves to become emotionally attached. If they do become attached to another person, this leaves them feeling weak, exposed, and vulnerable, resulting in high ambivalence about and difficulty main-taining the relationship.

The Dialectical Dilemma

There is validity both in the need for closeness and the need for autonomy, and the dilemma for the client lies in how to achieve both simultaneously and in a balanced way. When clients are unbalanced in the direction of desperately seeking closeness, they feel as if their existence is dependent on being connected to others and they tend to overestimate others' trustworthiness. In contrast, the detached independent person feels as if their survival is dependent on being free from the control or influence of others and they regularly underestimate others' trustwor-thiness. In both cases, clients are seeking safety either by being in relationships (even when they are unsafe) or by shunning relationships (even when they are safe). However, both extremes are likely to be dangerous in the long run. The desperate search for connection often leads to relationships with people who cause them harm, whereas the resolute pursuit of disconnection often leads to a painful lack of belonging that increases the risk of suicide and other problem behaviors. The dialectical synthesis of these extremes lies in the ability to be connected to and dependent on others while also being able to tolerate being alone and independent, at least at times. Moreover, the goal is to be able to flexibly move between connecting and detaching based on one's own needs, as well as accurate assessment of the needs and trustworthiness of others.

Discussing the Dialectical Reactions to Trauma with Clients

In Session 2, your task is to review these dialectical reactions to trauma with clients in an inter-active manner while helping them apply this information to their own experiences. To facilitate this discussion, DBT PE Handout 4 is used to orient clients to this dialectical framework for conceptualizing trauma reactions and to provide a brief overview of each extreme reaction. *DBT PE Handout 5* (*Understanding Your Reactions to Trauma*) provides a more detailed description of each dialectical dilemma, gives examples of common reactions that map onto each extreme, and asks clients to check off the reactions they have personally experienced.

Case Example: Maria's Dialectical Reactions to Trauma

THERAPIST: I want to talk with you about common reactions to trauma. My goal is to help you better understand how the traumas you have experienced have affected you, and to help you see that your reactions are very typical for trauma survivors. Let's start by looking at Handout 4.

MARIA: OK.

THERAPIST: As you can see, this handout describes trauma reactions as dialectics. Do you remember what a dialectic is?

MARIA: Doesn't it mean that two things that are opposite can both be true at the same time?

THERAPIST: Yes, and when these types of opposite or extreme reactions are present, the goal is to find a balanced middle ground that honors the truth in both sides.

MARIA: Right.

THERAPIST: The reason we think about trauma reactions as dialectics is because it is very common for people to have multiple and sometimes opposite reactions to trauma. If you look at this handout, you can see that all the reactions above the dotted line are ways in which trauma can lead people to become out of control, whereas all the reactions below the dotted line are ways in which trauma can cause people to become overly controlled. Do you see that?

MARIA: Yes.

THERAPIST: There are three dialectics that refer to different ways that trauma can impact people's emotions, behaviors, and relationships. So, on the one hand, people may feel as if their emotions, behaviors, and relationships are out of control, and on the other hand, they may feel as if they are too controlled. In general, would you say you have responded to your traumas in a way that feels more out of control, more overly controlled, or both?

MARIA: I think both. Sometimes I feel totally out of control and sometimes I try too hard to control things.

THERAPIST: I agree—I can see both sides fitting for you. So, let's start by focusing on the dialectic about emotions. It is really common for trauma survivors to experience both ends of this one. On the out-of-control side, people experience emotional flooding. This is when they have intense and painful emotions and feel totally overwhelmed by them. Often these emotions come on quickly and can last a long time.

MARIA: That happens to me.

THERAPIST: Yes, and that's totally normal. Often these intense emotions can be triggered by things that remind you of your trauma. For example, you might have a memory about your father's abuse come into your mind and then all of a sudden you're feeling intensely ashamed. Or you may come across something in the world that reminds you of the rape and become very afraid.

MARIA: Just last night I was watching a movie and there was a scene in it that reminded me of my rape where this drunk guy was hitting on a woman and wouldn't listen to her when she told him to leave her alone. It made me really anxious and my heart started racing. And all I was trying to do was relax and watch a movie!

THERAPIST: I know. These intense emotions and physical sensations can sneak up on you when you don't expect them and suddenly you're totally overwhelmed.

MARIA: Yeah, I ended up turning off the movie because I didn't want to risk that happening again.

THERAPIST: Well, that's a good example of how people often move from the end of emotional flooding to the other end of emotional numbing. Very often people will try to shut off or suppress their emotions, particularly after they've just experienced an intense one. They might do this by avoiding things that are likely to cause emotions, like your example of shutting off the movie, or they might dissociate so that they can feel numb.

MARIA: Yeah, I sometimes just let myself zone out so that I don't have to feel anything.

THERAPIST: Right, and sometimes people may want to have emotions and not be able to. For example, people may feel empty or hollow inside and like they can't feel anything. For some people, that emotional flatness can be related to depression.

MARIA: There are times when I just feel dead inside. Like I have no emotions at all.

THERAPIST: Exactly—that's also a very common reaction to trauma. One of our goals in doing DBT PE is to help you find a balance between these two extremes. Ideally, we want you to be able to experience emotions without getting totally flooded or totally numb. And to be able to effectively increase or decrease the intensity of your emotions when needed.

MARIA: I would like to be able to do that. Right now, it feels like it's all-or-nothing, like I either have emotions on full blast or they are totally shut off.

THERAPIST: Well, DBT PE is going to help you find a midpoint on your emotional dial. Let's look at Handout 5. Read that first section on emotional reactions and check off any that fit for you. [*Maria then reads and checks off reactions on both sides of the emotional experiencing dialectic, and she and her therapist have a brief discussion about them.*]

OK, let's look back at Handout 4 at the dialectic about behaviors. You see reckless dyscontrol is at the top on the undercontrolled side. This is when your behaviors are out of control and you are engaging in a lot of impulsive, damaging behaviors without really thinking about the consequences.

MARIA: I've done that a lot in my life with self-harm and attempting suicide. I also used to drink and smoke pot a lot. I still binge sometimes, but my behavior is less out of control than it was.

THERAPIST: Yes, you have worked hard to get control over those kinds of self-damaging behaviors. Another thing that falls into this category is generally being impulsive, which happens for a lot of trauma survivors. For example, you might make decisions quickly and without really thinking things through.

MARIA: I do that sometimes. I have quit a lot of jobs impulsively. In my last job, I just got really stressed out one day by a customer and told my boss I quit.

THERAPIST: That's a good example. OK, so let's think about the other end, which is called rigid control. On that end people tend to be on guard and perceive lots of situations as dangerous. You told me in our last session that you often feel on guard, right?

MARIA: All the time. I'm constantly looking over my shoulder and expecting bad things to happen.

THERAPIST: That's very common, and hypervigilance is one of the symptoms of PTSD. Often people with PTSD will try to keep tight control over their behavior to make themselves feel safer. They may take a lot of precautions to avoid things they think could be dangerous, or may have strict rules about things they can and can't do in order to stay safe. Do you have any examples of that?

MARIA: I try never to be around people who are drinking alcohol. It's too risky.

THERAPIST: That's a good example. Sometimes people also try to be in control more generally by doing things like being excessively clean or orderly, or doing a lot of planning.

MARIA: I keep my room really clean. I always make my bed as soon as I get up and I put my clothes away as soon as they come out of the laundry. You should see my closet, it is totally organized! I can't stand when things are messy, it just makes me really anxious. My mom has always called me a neat freak. I guess I've been this way since I was a little kid.

THERAPIST: Well, having things be orderly and predictable can help people feel safer in a home like yours that was often unsafe and chaotic.

MARIA: I can see that.

THERAPIST: Our goal is to help you find a middle path where you can be both controlled and flexible in your behavior and make effective decisions about what is and is not likely to be dangerous for you.

MARIA: OK.

THERAPIST: Now go ahead and read the next section on Handout 5 about behavioral reactions and check off the ones that fit for you. [*Maria and her therapist then briefly review and discuss the behavioral reactions she identified as relevant to her.*] You can see on Handout 4 that the final dialectic is about relationships. On the undercontrolled end is desperate connection. Many people respond to trauma by trying hard to be in relationships or stay connected to people. This is often because they are afraid of being alone and they depend on other people to feel safe in the world. Does that fit for you?

MARIA: I think that used to be true for me, but it's not now. In high school, I had sex with a lot of guys just because I wanted to feel cared about by someone, even if they only cared about me for sex. That caused a lot of the bullying I experienced, but I kept doing it anyway because it was better than feeling totally alone and unloved.

THERAPIST: That makes a lot of sense, and many sexual abuse survivors engage in frequent or impulsive sexual behavior. You are certainly not alone in that.

MARIA: Really? I always thought I was just a slut. It's one of the things I hate the most about myself.

THERAPIST: Well, that is definitely one of the beliefs we have to work on changing as we do DBT PE. For now, just know that your behavior in high school is normal for someone with a history of sexual abuse.

MARIA: OK, that's helpful.

THERAPIST: There is another piece of the desperate connection pole that I thought might fit for you. Specifically, people who have experienced trauma often ignore their own needs and instead prioritize the needs of other people. They often have difficulty standing up for themselves and may end up in relationships with people who don't treat them well. Does that apply to you?

MARIA: My relationship with my ex-boyfriend wasn't good for me. He didn't seem to care about my needs very much, and I always just did what he wanted to do. I put up with it because I thought that was normal, like that's how men are.

THERAPIST: It makes sense you would think that given that you grew up with an abusive father.

MARIA: Yeah, I was just used to men being jerks who don't treat me or other women well. And then my boyfriend ended up raping me, which I should have known was going to happen. So now I just stay away from men completely.

THERAPIST: And that is the other end of this dialectic, which is called detached independence. On that end, people try to avoid connection, including physical and sexual intimacy, and feel as if they are better off alone. They don't trust people and try not to get close to anyone in order to keep themselves from getting hurt.

MARIA: That is definitely true for me. Since the bullying in high school, I have always been a loner and haven't had close friends. And now I don't trust men at all. I think they're all going to hurt me. I haven't dated anyone since I was raped, and I have no desire to. I'd rather be alone than risk getting hurt again.

THERAPIST: I agree that detached independence fits for you now. Ideally, we want you to find a more balanced approach to relationships, where you are not avoiding them completely and you are not staying in relationships with people who don't treat you well.

MARIA: I don't know about that one. I don't trust myself to pick men who are not going to hurt me.

THERAPIST: We'll keep thinking and talking about that as we do DBT PE. For now, let's have you take a look at the last section on Handout 5 about interpersonal reactions and check off any boxes that fit for you. [*Maria and her therapist then review and discuss her interpersonal reactions. Her therapist ends this portion of the session by generating hope that DBT PE will help to improve many of the trauma reactions Maria has experienced.*]

CASE EXAMPLE DISCUSSION

This example illustrates how to engage clients in an interactive discussion about the dialectical reactions to trauma. The therapist briefly described each of the reactions, elicited examples from Maria, and normalized her experiences. As is typical, Maria endorsed a variety of reactions on both sides of these dialectics. Some of these polar opposite reactions were present in her current life (emotional flooding and numbing), whereas others had primarily been present earlier in her life (reckless dyscontrol, desperate connection) and been replaced by the other extreme in her current life (rigid control, detached independence). In addition, some of these reactions appeared to primarily be in response to her childhood trauma (e.g., self-harm, substance use, impulsive sexual behavior), whereas other reactions had occurred since the rape (e.g., avoiding relationships, being constantly on guard). Throughout this conversation, the therapist worked to build hope that DBT PE would help Maria to find a more balanced middle ground and to no longer lead a life characterized by extreme reactions to trauma.

It is also useful to note that the approach used in this example, which included having the client go back and forth between Handouts 4 and 5 during the session, is only one option of how to use these materials. You may instead review all six dialectical poles using Handout 4 before having the client read and complete all of Handout 5. Alternatively, you may choose to refer only to Handout 4 during the session and ask clients to review Handout 5 on their own for homework. Overall, the goal is to end this part of the session with the client having a reasonable understanding of their emotional, behavioral, and interpersonal reactions to trauma, as well as how their reactions may shift from one extreme to another over time. Ideally, this conversation will also serve a validating function for clients, helping them begin to see that their own reactions are normal rather than a sign that they are bad, incompetent, or crazy.

4. Orient to the Rationale for *In Vivo* Exposure

The next task of Session 2 is to orient clients to the rationale for *in vivo* exposure (see Table 9.1). This discussion builds on the general rationale for DBT PE that was provided in Session 1 by providing the client with more detailed information about *in vivo* exposure and how it works. When delivering this rationale, it is important to provide examples of important concepts and

---

TABLE 9.1. Key Points in Orienting to the Rationale for *In Vivo* Exposure

1. Behavioral avoidance (e.g., of people, places, and things) works temporarily to reduce distress, but maintains PTSD in the long run by preventing new learning.

2. *In vivo* exposure works to reduce PTSD by:
   a. Breaking the habit of reducing distress by avoidance or escape
   b. Disconfirming beliefs about the expected outcome of exposure to avoided situations
   c. Increasing the ability to tolerate intense emotions
   d. Reducing the intensity of distress over time (habituation)
   e. Building mastery and confidence
   f. Improving quality of life and increasing joy

---

personalize the information to the client. Overall, the goal is for clients to understand (1) the role of behavioral avoidance in maintaining PTSD, and (2) how *in vivo* exposure will help to reduce PTSD.

Case Example: Orienting Maria to the Rationale for In Vivo Exposure

THERAPIST: Now I want to talk with you about *in vivo* exposure and how it works. First, do you remember the main thing that maintains PTSD over time?

MARIA: Do you mean avoidance?

THERAPIST: Yes. Today I want to focus specifically on behavioral avoidance, which refers to avoiding people, places, and things in the world that remind you of your trauma or that bring up distressing emotions related to your trauma.

MARIA: OK.

THERAPIST: You mentioned an example of behavioral avoidance earlier when you said you shut off the movie you were watching last night because it had a scene in it that reminded you of your rape.

MARIA: Uh huh.

THERAPIST: How did you feel when you turned off the movie?

MARIA: I felt less anxious.

THERAPIST: Right, avoidance works in the short run to make us feel better. But what do you think would happen if you watched that movie again today?

MARIA: I would still get anxious. I'd probably be even more anxious because I would know that the scene was coming.

THERAPIST: The problem with avoidance is that it doesn't solve the problem in the long run and it can even make distress more intense over time. So, the way we address behavioral avoidance is by doing *in vivo* exposure. *In vivo* means "in life" and this type of exposure involves repeatedly approaching safe situations in your life that you typically avoid so that you can learn that you don't need to be so afraid of them.

MARIA: OK.

THERAPIST: I'm curious, is there something that you used to be afraid of that you're not afraid of anymore?

MARIA: When I was a little kid, I used to be afraid to go anywhere without my mom. I was basically always with her. When I first started school, I remember being really scared and crying every day when she would drop me off.

THERAPIST: So how did you get less afraid of being away from your mom?

MARIA: I just had to keep doing it. I mean, I had to go to school. So eventually it just stopped bothering me.

THERAPIST: Well, I have good news for you! You have already done *in vivo* exposure and it clearly works for you!

MARIA: I see what you mean. I guess we can do exposure without even realizing it.

THERAPIST: That's right. And we are often encouraged to do exposure-like things. Have you ever heard the saying about what you're supposed to do if you fall off a horse?

MARIA: Get back on.

THERAPIST: Right—that is *in vivo* exposure, because it means you should face things that feel scary rather than avoid them. We often do that in our lives without really thinking about it as exposure.

MARIA: I guess that's true.

THERAPIST: So, let me explain how *in vivo* exposure works, because there are several reasons why it is so effective at reducing PTSD.

MARIA: OK.

THERAPIST: One of the reasons it works is that it helps you to break the habit of using avoidance to reduce painful emotions. For a long time, avoidance has been one of the main ways you have regulated your emotions, and although it can help in the short term, it has had some negative long-term consequences for you, including chronic PTSD. *In vivo* exposure will help you to break that habit by having you repeatedly approach rather than avoid things that cause difficult emotions. Ideally, we want to make approaching hard things your new habit, rather than avoiding. Does that make sense?

MARIA: Yes, I think so, but it sounds scary.

THERAPIST: I get that. The thing is, by approaching the things you are avoiding you will be able to learn some important lessons. One is that bad things are unlikely to happen if you approach these situations. For example, you mentioned in our last session that you avoid men. What are you afraid will happen if you were to be near men?

MARIA: I'm afraid they would rape me or try to hurt me in some way.

THERAPIST: So, *in vivo* exposure will help you to learn that those kinds of negative outcomes are unlikely to happen. For example, if you were to interact with men in a variety of everyday places, you would learn that being around men is generally safe and they are not going to hurt you.

MARIA: I just don't know if that is true.

THERAPIST: Right—that's exactly why we need to do *in vivo* exposure. Beliefs are like hypotheses and we can't think ourselves out of believing they are true. The way to change them is to conduct experiments to test them out and learn what actually happens.

MARIA. OK, I see your point.

THERAPIST: Good. Another benefit of *in vivo* exposure is that it is going to make you even more skillful at being able to experience and tolerate intense emotions. Right now, you live a lot of your life as if emotions are dangerous and should be avoided as much as possible, right?

MARIA: Yeah, I do not like emotions.

THERAPIST: Well, *in vivo* exposure will help you learn that you can tolerate uncomfortable emotions and they don't have to stop you from doing things that are important to you.

MARIA: That would be good.

THERAPIST: And the more you approach difficult things without avoiding, over time those emotions will become less intense. For example, the more you interact with men, the less distressing it will be—just like your experience of getting used to being away from your mom as a kid.

MARIA: OK. It just sounds really hard.

THERAPIST: It will be hard, and it would be hard for anyone. In fact, that's another reason we do it. How do you usually feel after you do something really hard?

MARIA: I guess I feel proud of myself.

THERAPIST: Well, you and I are both going to feel proud when you do *in vivo* exposure! Do you remember the skill of building mastery from DBT?

MARIA: Yes.

THERAPIST: *In vivo* exposure is a way to build mastery. It will help you to feel like a strong and competent person who is able to do hard things.

MARIA: I would like that because I usually feel the opposite about myself.

THERAPIST: Well, you're going to feel much more competent after this! The final thing that *in vivo* exposure will do is help you reach your life-worth-living goals. Do you remember when you started treatment you said that one of your main goals was to have more relationships?

MARIA: Yes.

THERAPIST: Well, *in vivo* exposure will help you to engage in activities that are meaningful to you, including finding ways to meet new people and have more joy in your life.

MARIA: I definitely want that.

CASE EXAMPLE DISCUSSION

In this example, the therapist covered the key points in Table 9.1 about how and why *in vivo* exposure works in a conversational manner that engaged the client. Multiple examples from Maria's life were used to illustrate these concepts and make the information as personally relevant as possible. During this conversation, the therapist utilized a variety of DBT strategies to balance change (e.g., orienting, clarifying contingencies) and acceptance (e.g., validation, warm engagement) to keep Maria engaged and moving forward despite her anxiety about doing *in vivo* exposure. In this process, the therapist conveyed unwavering confidence both in the benefits of *in vivo* exposure and in Maria's ability to do it despite its difficulty.

5. Construct the *In Vivo* Exposure Hierarchy

The final major component of Session 2 is to construct an *in vivo* exposure hierarchy. The hierarchy includes approximately 15 *in vivo* exposure tasks that are rated using the Subjective Units of Distress Scale (SUDS; see below) and written on *DBT PE Handout 7* (In Vivo *Exposure Hierarchy*). The hierarchy should include tasks that are expected to elicit a range of distress levels (SUDS = 40–100) and are designed to test and disconfirm clients' primary problematic beliefs. Depending on time constraints, it may not be possible to complete the entire hierarchy in the session, but you should aim to identify at least five well-defined *in vivo* exposure tasks, including at least two in the moderately distressing range (SUDS = 40–60). In this section, I review common types of *in vivo* exposure tasks and the principles underlying the selection of specific tasks to include on the *in vivo* exposure hierarchy.

> **CLINICAL TIP**
> **Using the Subjective Units of Distress Scale (SUDS)**
>
> When building the *in vivo* hierarchy, clients are asked to provide a SUDS rating to indicate how much distress they expect each task will elicit. Often clients are already familiar with SUDS because it has been used for other purposes during Stage 1 DBT. If not, you should provide a brief orientation to SUDS by explaining that you will ask the client to use this scale to rate their overall level of emotional distress, using numbers ranging from 0 (*no distress at all*) to 100 (*the most distress they have ever felt*). It can be helpful to reassure clients that these ratings do not have to be exact, but rather are intended to provide a quick and dirty method of estimating how much distress they expect different tasks will elicit. If clients struggle to provide SUDS ratings, it can be helpful to have them identify personal examples of past experiences that illustrate what a 0, 50, and 100 SUDS rating feels like for them, but this is not required. If this is done, the 0 should be a time they felt reasonably calm, the 50 should be a time they felt moderately distressed, and the 100 is often how they felt during a traumatic event. These anchor points can be used to help clients estimate SUDS by linking the abstract numbers to their own concrete past experiences.

Types of *In Vivo* Exposure Tasks

The *in vivo* exposure hierarchy is a list of real-life situations that clients are currently avoiding and want or need to be able to approach. There are four main types of *in vivo* exposure tasks that may be included on the hierarchy, including three types that are derived from standard PE and one that was added to DBT PE to target unjustified shame. *DBT PE Handout 6* (*Common Avoided Situations*) includes examples in each of these four categories and can be used with clients to help generate ideas for the hierarchy.

1. Situations Perceived as Dangerous

People with PTSD routinely overestimate the likelihood of danger and avoid many things that they believe will be risky or harmful to themselves or others. These avoided situations are generally things that people regularly do with little to no risk of harm but that clients view as dangerous, such as going to locations similar to where a trauma occurred, being in crowds, walking outside at night, or riding public transportation. Very often these situations elicit fears of being retraumatized—for example, a person who was raped will avoid situations in which they believe there is a high probability of being raped again. At other times, the perceived danger may involve other types of physical injury, illness, threat, or emotional discomfort.

Example Questions to Ask
- "Are there situations you avoid because you think they are dangerous, but that other people generally think are safe?"
- "Are there things you either do or don't do that help you to feel safer and less at risk of being harmed?"

2. Situations That Are Reminders of the Trauma

People with PTSD also typically avoid many things that remind them of their trauma. These reminders often include situations or activities that are directly related to the trauma, such as driving a car for someone who was in a motor vehicle accident, or sexual intimacy for someone who was sexually abused. Trauma reminders may also include things that have become paired with traumatic experiences through a process of classical conditioning. For example, objects, sounds, smells, or physical sensations that were present at the time of a trauma are often avoided because they are associated with the traumatic event. Clients also frequently avoid things that depict traumas similar to their own experiences, such as movies about war for a combat veteran, or news reports about sexual assault for a rape survivor.

Example Questions to Ask
- "Are there activities, situations, or people you avoid because they remind you of your trauma?"
- "Are there certain smells, sounds, physical sensations, or objects that are associated with your trauma that you currently avoid?"

3. Activities the Client Lost Interest in Due to Depression

This type of *in vivo* exposure is similar to behavioral activation for depression (Martell, Dimidjian, & Herman-Dunn, 2013) and can be used with clients for whom depression is a significant co-occurring problem. These tasks typically involve engaging in pleasurable or mastery-building activities that clients lost interest in due to depression-related fatigue and anhedonia, rather than activities they may be avoiding because of PTSD-related distress and arousal. This may include things such as engaging in hobbies, exercising, socializing with friends, and completing household tasks. These types of behavioral activation tasks have often already been addressed during Stage 1 DBT but can also be done during DBT PE if needed.

Example Questions to Ask
- "Are there activities you used to enjoy that you have lost interest in since the trauma?"
- "Are there things you want or need to do but that you find hard to do because of depression or fatigue?"

4. Situations That Elicit Unjustified Shame

Given that shame is a particularly pervasive and impairing emotion in this client population, DBT PE includes *in vivo* exposure tasks that are explicitly designed to target unjustified shame. Shame is considered unjustified when the thing about which a person feels ashamed will not lead people they care about to reject or criticize them if it is revealed. Therefore, the goal of *in vivo* exposure for unjustified shame is to disconfirm clients' expectations of rejection by others. As described in DBT PE Handout 6, there are six common types of situations that cause clients to experience unjustified shame, including being genuine (e.g., sharing personal information), being deserving (e.g., asking for what you want), being imperfect (e.g., making a mistake), being competent (e.g., talking about your strengths), being vulnerable (e.g., showing emotions that feel weak), and being seen (e.g., doing things that call attention to yourself). Importantly, it is possible for shame to be justified in some contexts and not others—for example, a client's family may respond critically to something that their close friends support. Therefore, you and your client will need to work together to identify contexts in which they will be unlikely to be rejected for engaging in the shame-eliciting behavior. At times, it may also be useful to do *in vivo* exposure to situations in which shame is justified (i.e., rejection is likely to occur) when being rejected is unlikely to have serious consequences (e.g., the client may be stared at by strangers). This can be helpful when clients believe they cannot tolerate any form of rejection and efforts to avoid nonserious forms of rejection are causing significant impairment.

Example Questions to Ask
- "Are there things that you avoid doing because you believe people will reject or criticize you, but that are things other people routinely do?"
- "Are there important things about yourself that you keep hidden because of shame?"

CLINICAL TIP
But I'm Not Avoiding Anything!

Some clients have difficulty identifying situations they are avoiding that could be targeted via *in vivo* exposure. However, if a person meets criteria for PTSD, it is rare that they are not engaging in at least some behavioral avoidance. In my experience, there are three main factors that can interfere with identifying *in vivo* exposure tasks:

1. *Avoidance.* For some clients, not identifying potential *in vivo* exposure tasks is itself avoidance. Clients may find it difficult to acknowledge the things they are avoiding because even saying the words out loud causes distress. Sometimes clients are ashamed of the things they are avoiding and want to keep them hidden. Some clients may withhold information because they are afraid you will force them to do *in vivo* exposure to any situation they identify. When avoidance is the problem, you can address this with validation, cheerleading, reorienting to the rationale, and enhancing the client's sense of control over the hierarchy construction process.

2. *Recognizing safety behaviors as avoidance.* Clients may not be aware that they are avoiding when they rely on safety behaviors to help them get through certain situations. For example, a client may regularly walk outside at night, but always bring her dog, cell phone, and a can of pepper spray. This client may genuinely say that she doesn't avoid walking outside at night and not recognize her safety behaviors as

avoidance. You can address this by asking clients if there are things they will only do under certain circumstances—for example, at certain times of day, with other people, or while carrying certain objects. These rules of living can also be framed as "have tos" (e.g., "I have to do X to be safe") and "only ifs" (e.g., "I can only do X if I'm not alone").

3. *Difficulty distinguishing preferences and avoidance.* In some cases, behavioral avoidance may be so ingrained and long-standing that it can seem more like a personal preference or one's identity than intentional or active avoidance. For example, a client may say, "I don't avoid interacting with people, I just prefer to be alone" or "I have never been a person who likes to go to crowded places." This is particularly likely to occur for clients with early-onset trauma who have never known another way of being in the world. When this occurs, it can be helpful to frame *in vivo* exposure as a way to experiment with new behaviors and activities to find out whether they may be enjoyable or otherwise improve their quality of life. In this way, the goal may be less about reducing avoidance and more about finding new ways of engaging with the world that are more fulfilling and empowering.

Selecting *In Vivo* Exposure Tasks for the Hierarchy

Often there are many avoided situations that could be targeted with *in vivo* exposure and you and the client will need to decide which ones to focus on during treatment. Table 9.2 summarizes the guidelines that are used to select tasks that are likely to be most effective in maximizing the impact of *in vivo* exposure and improving the client's quality of life.

Choose Tasks That Will Improve Quality of Life

In vivo exposure is intended not only to reduce distress but also to improve quality of life. Often people with PTSD lead very restricted lives in which behavioral avoidance causes them to miss out on many potentially enjoyable and meaningful activities. For clients in DBT PE, this limited engagement in the world and the isolation and lack of belongingness it causes, is often a primary reason they wish to be dead. *In vivo* exposure is a very effective strategy for helping clients achieve the ultimate goal of DBT: to build a life they experience as worth living. With this in mind, *in vivo* exposure tasks that are likely to significantly improve a person's quality of life should be prioritized over those that will have less of an impact.

TABLE 9.2. Guidelines for Selecting *In Vivo* Exposure Tasks

Choose *in vivo* exposure tasks that:

1. Most improve quality of life
2. Maximally violate expectancies
3. Vary stimuli and distress levels
4. Involve acceptable risks
5. Occur in multiple contexts
6. Are particularly challenging

Clients nearly always avoid things that are not causing impairment or that they do not want or need to have in their lives. For example, a client whose friend died in a motorcycle accident may avoid riding motorcycles. However, if riding motorcycles is not a valued or necessary activity, then there is no need to target this type of avoidance. Instead, time would be better spent on reducing avoidance of things that are causing impairment or decreasing the client's potential for joy. For example, I once treated a woman who loved football and was a passionate Seattle Seahawks fan. Although she religiously watched football games on TV, she had never been to a live game because she was terrified of crowds and being around men she did not know, particularly if they were drinking alcohol. We set out to design *in vivo* exposure tasks that would enable her to eventually attend a Seahawks game, which she succeeded in doing. It makes me smile now to think about how that first live football game and being part of the massive crowd of zealous fans brought her so much joy.

Example Questions to Ask
- "Are there things that you would like to be able to do in your life that you currently don't do at all, or that you only do with intense distress?"
- "Which activities would bring you the most joy if you were able to do them?"
- "Are there activities or situations that you avoid that are making it difficult or impossible to complete important tasks or function in your life in ways that matter to you?"

Choose Tasks That Maximally Violate Expectancies

A key reason that exposure works to reduce PTSD is that it provides clients with information that disconfirms their inaccurate beliefs about themselves, others, and emotions. To maximize this new learning, *in vivo* exposure tasks should be designed so that the actual outcomes of approaching an avoided situation are as different as possible from the client's predicted outcomes. The larger the mismatch between the client's expectancies and reality, the more likely it is that beliefs will change and be readily retrieved in the future (Craske, Treanor, Conway, Zbozinek, & Vervliet, 2014). Given this, *in vivo* exposure tasks that maximally violate expectancies should be prioritized over tasks that minimally violate expectancies.

To determine this, you need to understand exactly what your client expects will happen if they approach the avoided situation. This may include a variety of feared outcomes, such as being rejected, threatened, or harmed; feeling intense emotions; and engaging in problem behaviors. Once the specific feared outcomes are identified, *in vivo* exposure tasks should be selected that will be most likely to help clients learn that these outcomes are unlikely to occur or are not as bad as they thought they would be. For example, for clients who believe that asking for things they want will result in people refusing to fulfill their requests, *in vivo* exposure tasks that involve making extreme requests will more fully violate their expectancies than tasks that require them to make small requests. For example, you might have a client go to a shoe store and ask a sales associate to bring them 10 pairs of shoes to try on, rather than only asking to try on one pair of shoes.

Example Questions to Ask
- "What is the worst outcome that could happen in this situation?"
- "Why do you avoid this situation?"
- "What exactly are you afraid will happen if you approach this situation?"

Choose Tasks That Maximize Variability

Conducting exposure to varying stimuli at varying levels of arousal has been found to enhance the retention and retrieval of newly learned information (Craske et al., 2014). To maximize stimulus variability, it is important to include items on the hierarchy that elicit a wide range of distress levels (e.g., SUDS from 40 to 100). If clients have identified primarily low or high distress tasks, there are a number of stimulus characteristics that can be adjusted to achieve greater variability (see Table 9.3). Stimulus variability may also involve selecting multiple stimuli that elicit the same fear—for example, a fear of being rejected by others may be triggered by exposure to sharing personal information, saying "no" to requests, and initiating social contacts. In addition, stimulus variability can involve having items on the hierarchy that target distinct fears—for example, exposure to smells present during a trauma may elicit fears of having a flashback, whereas exposure to being in a crowd may elicit fears of being assaulted.

Choose Tasks That Involve Acceptable Risks

Very often clients are afraid that *in vivo* exposure tasks will be dangerous and will result in them being harmed in some serious way. In most cases, these fears reflect erroneous beliefs about the likelihood of danger and the effective course of action is to proceed with selecting *in vivo* exposure tasks that will disconfirm these inaccurate beliefs. However, in some cases, the situations that clients are avoiding may be objectively dangerous or at least involve some reasonable possibility of serious negative outcomes. In addition to it clearly being unethical to ask clients to do dangerous things, it is also likely to be ineffective as it would reinforce rather than disprove clients' beliefs. (Of note, there is some evidence emerging that occasional reinforced exposure may enhance learning, particularly when the feared outcome is not excessively severe, such as social rejection or having a flashback; Craske et al., 2014.)

In most cases, differentiating between low-risk and high-risk situations is reasonably straightforward. A helpful guideline is to choose situations that people similar to the client regularly find themselves in either purposefully or by accident without any severe consequences. For example, is the situation something that the client's friends and family or other people in the client's environment regularly do or would do? If so, it is likely to be low risk. For example, people routinely drive cars, ride in elevators, go to crowded places, and talk to strangers. These types of everyday situations are therefore reasonable activities to ask clients to expose themselves to.

TABLE 9.3. Identifying Tasks That Elicit Variable Levels of Distress

Consider varying the following to achieve a wide range of SUDS values:

1. *Distance to the stimulus:* for example, looking at versus touching; standing close versus far away
2. *Stimulus intensity:* for example, a photo versus real life; one versus multiple stimuli present
3. *Length of time:* for example, 15 versus 30 minutes in contact with the stimulus
4. *Contexts:* for example, day versus night; at home versus in public
5. *Use of safety behaviors:* for example, alone versus with others; with versus without a phone

---

CLINICAL TIP
But It Could Be Risky!

As some clients will argue, risk can occur even in situations that are generally safe. On the one hand, it can be useful to acknowledge the kernel of truth in this concern. Car accidents do occur, elevators do break, crowds do become violent, and people are attacked by strangers. Given this, we should never promise clients that a situation will absolutely be safe. On the other hand, it is important to highlight that people with PTSD tend to greatly overestimate the likelihood that these negative outcomes will occur and their attempts to avoid these low-probability events often increase suffering and reduce the quality of their lives. The important question therefore becomes "Is it worth it to take reasonable risks if this will help you to create a fuller and more meaningful life?" Ultimately, *in vivo* exposure requires clients to engage in activities that involve acceptable or "everyday" risks and to tolerate the reality that risk can never be fully eliminated.

In some cases, it may be unclear whether an avoided situation may be excessively risky and further assessment may be needed. For example, clients from marginalized populations (e.g., racial and sexual minorities) may believe there is a high likelihood they will be rejected, harassed, discriminated against, or physically attacked, and in some contexts, these beliefs are likely to be accurate. If you do not share your client's identity, it may be difficult to estimate the potential risks for people of the client's group. In such cases, assessment may be needed to figure out whether continued avoidance may be wise minded versus excessively cautious. To make this determination, it can be helpful to have clients ask family members, friends, or others with similar identities whether they ever engage in the proposed exposure task or if they think it is likely to be safe. You may also be able to obtain objective information about risk levels (e.g., crime rates) to help inform this decision. When working with adolescent clients, it may also be important to consider whether the activity is normative in their family and peer group (e.g., watching R-rated movies with sexual scenes) and to consult with their parents about whether certain tasks are considered to be acceptable and/or age appropriate.

CLINICAL TIP
But Nobody Would Do That on Purpose!

At times, *in vivo* exposure tasks may involve doing things that people typically do not do intentionally, but that they may do inadvertently or by accident. For example, many *in vivo* exposure tasks for unjustified shame involve intentionally engaging in behaviors designed to elicit embarrassment, such as making errors. In addition, some *in vivo* exposure tasks may involve doing things that most people try to avoid, such as leaving important items (e.g., phones, wallets) at home. When these types of *in vivo* tasks are suggested, clients may protest that they are unreasonable because they are not things that other people normally do. While there is validity in this argument, these types of tasks can nonetheless be very helpful when clients' efforts to avoid these behaviors are causing significant impairment. To help in deciding whether these types of tasks are appropriate, it is important to ask, "Do people inadvertently perform this exposure without serious negative consequences?" If the answer is "yes," then these tasks are likely to be reasonable when there is a clear rationale for how they will help to disprove important beliefs that are maintaining the client's PTSD.

Example Questions to Ask
- "From your own wise mind, do you believe that this task is objectively dangerous?"
- "Do people ever do this exposure even if it is not done on purpose?"
- "Would your friends or family members agree that this task is dangerous?"

Choose Tasks That Occur in Multiple Contexts

At times, relapse (i.e., a return of emotional distress about a previously extinguished stimulus) can occur when the stimulus is encountered in a context that is different from the one in which exposure was conducted. For example, if a person who is afraid of riding buses repeatedly completes exposure to riding the same bus from his home to his place of work at approximately the same time each weekday, then he is quite likely to become less afraid of riding the bus. However, his fear may be likely to return if he were to ride a different bus, get on or off at a different stop, or travel at a different time of day. To reduce the likelihood of relapse, *in vivo* exposure to an avoided stimulus should therefore be conducted in as many contexts as possible. These contexts may be external (e.g., location, time of day, day of the week, presence of others), as well as internal (e.g., mood, level of hunger, medication status).

Example Questions to Ask
- "Where do you typically encounter [the stimulus] in your current life?"
- "Are there other places you would like to be able to go where [the stimulus] is likely to be present?"
- "Are there certain times or days that you are more or less likely to come across [the stimulus]?"

Choose Tasks That Are Particularly Challenging

Another strategy for reducing the likelihood of relapse is to conduct *in vivo* exposure to situations that are more difficult than those that are likely to be routinely encountered in the person's life. This concept of "pushing the envelope" is done so that daily life will seem relatively easy in comparison to the more challenging situations the person approached for exposure. For example, if a client is afraid of seeing her own menstrual blood because it reminds her of vaginal bleeding caused by a rape, then routine activities she would need to be able to complete would include being able to use feminine hygiene products when menstruating. However, pushing the envelope might involve having her touch her own menstrual blood, look at the blood for 20 minutes, or put blood on her underwear. Relatedly, it is important to always include the client's worst fear on the hierarchy. For example, if a client is afraid of driving, you should identify the worst-case driving scenario that the client can imagine. This might involve having to drive alone on an interstate in the middle lane during rush hour. Whatever this worst fear is, it is important that clients confront it. Otherwise, they are likely to continue to believe that some element of their fear is justified, which may increase their vulnerability to later relapse.

Example Questions to Ask
- "In what ways do you typically come into contact with [the stimulus]? What would be even harder than that?"
- "What would be the most challenging way you could imagine doing exposure to [the stimulus]?"
- "What are you most afraid of when it comes to [the stimulus]?"

> ### CLINICAL TIP
> ### Should We Make More Than One Hierarchy?
>
> Given that most clients in DBT PE have experienced multiple types of trauma, they often avoid multiple types of situations that are quite distinct from one another. For example, situations that are avoided because of past sexual abuse are likely to be quite different from situations that are avoided due to a motor vehicle accident. In such cases, it can be useful to create one *in vivo* hierarchy for each trauma that will be targeted via imaginal exposure so that both types of exposure are addressing the same trauma. Once the first trauma has been sufficiently treated, then a new hierarchy can be created that includes avoided situations related to the second trauma and so forth. When using this approach, it may be useful to restrict the assessment in Session 2 to situations related to the first target trauma.

Case Example: Building Maria's In Vivo Hierarchy

THERAPIST: What I'd like to do next is work on building your *in vivo* exposure hierarchy. This is a list of real-life things that you are currently avoiding related to your trauma.

MARIA: OK, but I avoid a lot of things. It could be a really long list!

THERAPIST: That's true for most people. So how about if we start by identifying things that you think would improve your life the most. What are the things that you most wish you could do that you currently either avoid completely or can only do with a lot of distress?

MARIA: Probably the biggest thing is just being around people and being able to have relationships. I hardly interact with anyone except my mom and my cousin.

THERAPIST: I think that would be a great thing to work on. So, what are you afraid of that makes you avoid interacting with people?

MARIA: I'm afraid of being hurt by people. With men, I'm afraid they will actually physically hurt me. But I'm also afraid that people will be mean to me or won't like me, so I just stay away from everyone.

THERAPIST: OK, so it sounds like there are two main beliefs we need to try to disprove with *in vivo* exposure. The first is that men are dangerous and likely to physically hurt you, right?

MARIA: Yes.

THERAPIST: All right, so what kinds of situations are you avoiding related to men?

MARIA: I avoid talking to or being near men basically all the time.

THERAPIST: Are there specific situations you avoid because you are likely to have to interact with men?

MARIA: It can really happen anywhere. Like at the grocery store, I try never to get in a checkout line with a male cashier. Or on the bus, I won't sit next to a man. If I'm walking down the street and pass a man, I'll always look the other way.

THERAPIST: OK, so using the SUDS scale from 0 to 100, let's get ratings for each of those. How distressing would it be to interact with a male employee in a store?

MARIA: Maybe a 65.

THERAPIST: How about sitting next to a man on the bus?

MARIA: I'd say 70.

THERAPIST: And what about making eye contact with a man as you pass on the street?

MARIA: That's not as hard, maybe a 40.

THERAPIST: What would be the most difficult situation for you to have to interact with men?

MARIA: Anything related to dating or sex.

THERAPIST: Do you want to include things on the hierarchy about dating or having sex?

MARIA: I don't think so. I want to date eventually, but I don't feel ready for that now.

THERAPIST: I can understand wanting to wait and I'm worried this may be avoidance that is not helpful. Do you think it's wise mind to wait or should we try to tackle dating during DBT PE?

MARIA: It is avoidance, but I think it's wise. I don't think a relationship would work while I'm still struggling so much with PTSD. I'd rather get my PTSD under control and then try to date when I'm feeling stronger.

THERAPIST: OK, that sounds reasonable. How would you feel if we start working on things now that would help you feel more able to date later, but we'll wait to work on dating until after you finish DBT PE?

MARIA: That sounds good to me.

THERAPIST: OK, so besides getting more comfortable interacting with men, are there other things that would need to be different for you to feel more able to date?

MARIA: I would need to feel more comfortable with my body. That's part of why I can't imagine dating or having sex. I can't even stand to look at myself in a mirror or shower with the lights on or wear anything that exposes my body—like shorts—so how could I possibly be naked around another person?

THERAPIST: That makes sense. Let's get some concrete examples. What would your SUDS be if you were to look just at your face in a mirror?

MARIA: About a 55.

THERAPIST: And what about looking at your entire body in a full-length mirror?

MARIA: If I was wearing clothes, maybe a 70.

THERAPIST: What if you were naked?

MARIA: That would be the worst, 100.

THERAPIST: And what about taking a shower with the lights on?

MARIA: Maybe a little less, like a 99, just because I wouldn't be directly staring at myself.

THERAPIST: OK. And the other thing you mentioned was wearing shorts. How distressing would it be to wear shorts in public?

MARIA: Maybe an 80. It makes me really uncomfortable to be so exposed.

THERAPIST: Yes, that is true for a lot of people. Are there other things related to your body that you avoid?

MARIA: I don't like being touched.

THERAPIST: OK, so what if we were to have you do things that would cause people to touch you, like get a pedicure or a massage?

MARIA: That would be hard!

THERAPIST: I'm sure it would be, but would it make sense to do?

MARIA: I've never been interested in massages, and they would be expensive. But maybe a pedicure or manicure.

THERAPIST: OK, so what would your SUDS be for getting a pedicure or manicure?

MARIA: They would both be about a 75.

THERAPIST: Are there other things you are avoiding because of shame or disgust about your body that you would like to be able to do?

MARIA: This is partly why I isolate and avoid being around people. Like, I avoid going to the gym even though I'd like to. I'm just afraid people will stare at me or be critical.

THERAPIST: OK. What would your SUDS be if you went to the gym?

MARIA: About an 80.

THERAPIST: Are there other activities that you'd like to be able to do that would help you be less isolated?

MARIA: I've thought about joining a support group for women who have been raped or sexually abused. I've seen those advertised, but I've been too afraid to go.

THERAPIST: I love that idea! What would your SUDS be if you were to join a group like that?

MARIA: I assume I'd have to talk about my own traumas, which would be hard. So probably an 85.

THERAPIST: OK, so we've got lots of things related to getting more comfortable around people and with your body. Since we're going to start by focusing on your dad's abuse, I'm wondering if there are any negative beliefs you developed because of his abuse that make you avoid things now?

MARIA: I think the biggest thing with my dad is that he made me feel like I'm bad and always mess everything up. So now I try to be perfect all the time.

THERAPIST: What are you afraid will happen if you make a mistake or do something less than perfectly?

MARIA: I know it's not logical, but it makes me afraid that someone will hit me or sexually abuse me, since that's what he would do when I did something wrong.

THERAPIST: That makes complete sense to me.

MARIA: It also just makes me hate myself and feel like I am not good enough and never will be if I don't do everything perfectly.

THERAPIST: Well, that's an impossible standard to live up to! It sounds like it would be useful to get you comfortable with being imperfect. What are some examples of things you try to do perfectly?

MARIA: I am always on time to everything. I can't stand being late. I usually get here an hour early and wait in the lobby just to be sure I will be on time. And since I'm not working and my mom is currently supporting me, it's my job to do all the household chores. I make a list each day of all the things I need to get done and I can't relax until they are all complete.

THERAPIST: Those are great examples. So, let's got SUDS ratings. How distressing would it be to show up late to something?

MARIA: My dad used to get so angry at me if I ever made us late anywhere, so being late makes me really anxious. I'd give it a 90.

THERAPIST: How about if you didn't complete everything on your chore list or didn't do some chores perfectly?

MARIA: That would be hard because my dad used to punish me for that. Things that only affect me would be a little easier. So not making my bed or leaving dirty clothes on my bedroom floor would be like a 45. But things that would affect my mother, like leaving dirty dishes in the sink or not sweeping the kitchen floor, would be really hard, like a 90.

THERAPIST: And how about if you were to relax and take a break before you finish your chores for the day?

MARIA: It's really hard for me to take a break when there are things I should be doing. Maybe 75?

THERAPIST: OK, well that gives us a good list to start with and we can always add more things later if needed.

Maria's *In Vivo* Exposure Hierarchy	
Exposure task	SUDS (Session 2)
1. Looking at body naked in a full-length mirror	100
2. Taking a shower with the lights on	99
3. Leaving chores undone that affect mom (e.g., dirty dishes in sink, not sweeping kitchen floor)	90
4. Being late	90
5. Going to a women's sexual trauma support group	85
6. Wearing shorts in public	80
7. Going to the gym	80
8. Taking a break before chores are done	75
9. Getting a pedicure or manicure	75
10. Looking at body while clothed in full-length mirror	70
11. Sitting next to a man on the bus	70
12. Talking to a male employee in a store	65
13. Looking at face in mirror	55
14. Leaving chores undone that don't affect mom (e.g., not making bed, leaving dirty clothes on bedroom floor)	45
15. Making eye contact with men in public	40

CASE EXAMPLE DISCUSSION

In this example, the therapist focused on identifying avoided situations that would most improve Maria's quality of life and that would disprove specific trauma-related beliefs. Although several of the items on the hierarchy are specific to beliefs related to her father's abuse (e.g., about needing to be perfect), most of the exposure tasks represent more general beliefs (e.g., of being harmed by men, of being ashamed of her body) that are likely to generalize across Maria's multiple traumas. In addition, the hierarchy includes different types of exposure tasks, including situations that are direct reminders of her father's abuse (e.g., being late), situations that are perceived as dangerous (e.g., interacting with men), and situations that elicit unjustified shame (e.g., looking at her body).

The therapist also followed the recommended guidelines for selecting *in vivo* exposure tasks to put on Maria's hierarchy. To ensure that the tasks would be likely to improve Maria's quality of life, the therapist confirmed that the avoided situations were things she wanted or needed to be able to do. Potential tasks that Maria indicated were not important to her (e.g., getting massages) or were longer-term goals (e.g., dating and having sex) were not included, whereas those she reported wanting to be able to do (e.g., go to the gym, join a women's support group) were included. To ensure that the tasks would violate Maria's expectancies, the therapist assessed the specific feared outcomes of each potential task and selected tasks that would be likely to disconfirm them. To maximize variability, tasks were included that elicited varying levels of distress (i.e., SUDS ranged from 40 to 100) and targeted multiple fears (e.g., of being harmed, making mistakes, and feeling body-related shame). In addition, multiple tasks were included to target the same fear (e.g., several ways of doing exposure to her body). To include tasks that would occur in multiple contexts, the therapist also assessed the typical situations in which Maria would be likely to encounter a feared stimulus (e.g., interacting with men in stores, on the bus, and on the street). Finally, Maria's most challenging situation was included on the hierarchy: looking at herself naked in the mirror.

It is also important to acknowledge that there are almost certainly other things that Maria is avoiding that are not included on the hierarchy. The hierarchy is rarely an exhaustive list of all the situations that a client is avoiding, but rather is a selective and representative list of tasks that are most likely to target key fears and improve the client's life. The selection of tasks should be informed by the case formulation, particularly the primary beliefs that are believed to be maintaining the client's PTSD. Importantly, the hierarchy that is created in Session 2 is not set in stone. If additional avoided situations that would be important to target become apparent as treatment progresses, they can always be added to the hierarchy. In addition, some items may be revised as treatment progresses to more specifically target the client's fears and expectancies. Similarly, if situations that were originally included on the hierarchy become less important, they can be removed. Finally, the initial hierarchy that is created in Session 2 often includes items that remain somewhat general (e.g., "being late" on Maria's hierarchy) that will need to be more specifically operationalized at the time they are assigned for practice (e.g., being 10 minutes late to DBT skills group).

Select *In Vivo* Exposure Homework Tasks and Give Instructions

Once an initial hierarchy has been constructed, the next step is to select the specific tasks the client will complete for their first *in vivo* exposure homework, instruct the client on how to do *in vivo* exposure, and orient to *DBT PE Handout 8/8A* (*Exposure Recording Form*).

Select *In Vivo* Exposure Tasks for Homework

Typically, two tasks are selected from the hierarchy and clients are asked to complete at least one of these *in vivo* exposure tasks every day. The primary goal of these first *in vivo* exposure practices is for clients to be successful in completing them. Importantly, *success is defined as completing the tasks as instructed and not by whether clients experience a reduction in distress during the task*. Therefore, you should aim to select initial *in vivo* exposure tasks that clients believe with near certainty they will be able to complete before the next session. One way to increase the "doability" of these initial *in vivo* exposure assignments is to start with tasks that are challenging but not unmanageable. Therefore, it is typical to select initial *in vivo* exposure tasks that are expected to elicit a moderate degree of distress (e.g., SUDS of 40–60). Although more distressing tasks could be assigned, using a gradual approach is likely to increase home-work compliance.

In addition, you should consider whether there may be practical barriers that will make it difficult for clients to complete these initial exposure tasks. For example, do clients have access to the materials they will need to do the exposure (e.g., objects, sounds, photos, articles), or will they need to find or purchase them? If the exposure involves going to certain places (e.g., parks, malls, hospitals), do they have transportation to and from those locations? If they are doing exposure to a specific type of activity (e.g., eating at a restaurant) or event (e.g., a concert), will this be possible and affordable to do before the next session? If the exposure task involves other people (e.g., sharing personal information), is there someone available to do these activi-ties with? If clients think that they will be unlikely to complete a specific *in vivo* exposure task, then make changes to the task to make it more doable or select a different task that they feel confident they will be able to complete.

Instruct on How to Do *In Vivo* Exposure

Because clients complete *in vivo* exposure entirely on their own outside of sessions, it is essen-tial that they understand how to do *in vivo* exposure effectively. *DBT PE Handout 9* (*How to Do Exposure Homework*) provides detailed instructions on how to complete exposure homework and can be reviewed in session. There are four main things clients should be instructed to do during exposure tasks to make them as effective as possible. The first involves fully focusing their attention on the exposure task. Consistent with the DBT skill of one-mindfulness, this means that when they are doing exposure, that is all they should be doing (i.e., no multitask-ing). In addition, they should select a time and place to do exposure when they are unlikely to be interrupted. Second, for exposure to work it is important that they allow themselves to fully experience the emotions that arise without trying to block them. Third, clients should avoid avoidance during exposure. Avoidance can be broadly defined as anything that functions to arti-ficially reduce distress or increase their sense of safety, including using DBT skills (e.g., distress tolerance) during exposure. It is often helpful to identify in advance how the client is likely to avoid during exposure and troubleshoot what they will do to prevent this.

Finally, clients should be instructed to continue the exposure task until they have achieved their goals. For each exposure task that is assigned, you should work with the client to set clear goals about the specific behaviors to engage in (or not) and where, when, how often, and for how long to do them. For example, the goal may be for a client to continue with an exposure task for a specific length of time (e.g., 30 minutes) or until a specific behavior is emitted (e.g., sending back food in a restaurant after telling the server that they did not like it). In addition, a goal should be set for the number of times the client will repeat the exposure task before the next session. Setting these types of behaviorally specific goals will make it possible for clients to objectively evaluate whether they have successfully completed exposure tasks.

Orient to the Exposure Recording Form

You will also need to orient clients to the Exposure Recording Form, which should be filled out before and after every exposure task they complete. There are two versions of the Exposure Recording Form that can be used: a full-page form (DBT PE Handout 8) and a condensed diary card format (DBT PE Handout 8A). Instructions for completing the form are in DBT PE Handout 9 and can be reviewed with clients in session. The first section of the Exposure Recording Form asks clients to rate the probability and cost of up to three feared outcomes of the exposure as well as whether these outcomes actually occurred. This is intended to consolidate learning by highlighting discrepancies between expected and actual outcomes, as well as to monitor progress in changing problematic beliefs that are maintaining PTSD. The second section includes ratings of overall distress (SUDS) to track habituation, as well as potential problems that may arise during exposure (e.g., suicide and self-harm urges, dissociation) that may require intervention. The third section assesses the intensity of seven specific emotions, as well as radical acceptance of the trauma—these ratings are used to monitor progress in changing these potential

---

Why Does the Exposure Recording Form Track Specific Emotions Instead of Just SUDS?

In many exposure treatments, clients are only asked to rate their pre-, peak, and post-SUDS, and improvement is signaled by decreases in peak SUDS across exposure trials ("between-session habituation"). When I began developing DBT PE, I had three main concerns about relying only on SUDS to monitor clients' experiences and progress:

1. *SUDS ratings are nonspecific.* SUDS ratings assess overall distress as opposed to specific emotions. Although SUDS are often assumed to reflect fear or anxiety, in most cases these ratings reflect a combination of different emotions that clients are experiencing. Thus, obtaining only a SUDS rating obscures important differences in the types and intensities of the emotions that clients experience.

2. *Not all emotions are created equal.* The use of SUDS to monitor progress assumes that it is desirable for all emotions that may be captured by the rating to decrease over time. However, some emotions reliably increase over the course of treatment (anger and sadness), and when these emotions are justified and effective, there is no need to decrease them. Indeed, the goal may instead be to increase emotions that are ineffectively low and decrease other emotions that are excessively intense, which requires more specific emotion ratings to tease apart.

3. *Labeling emotions is an emotion regulation strategy.* In DBT, clients are taught to label the specific emotions they are experiencing using primary emotion names rather than general terms like "distress." Indeed, this is the first emotion regulation skill taught in DBT because knowing the specific emotion is necessary to identify the regulation strategies that will be most effective in changing it. Of note, asking clients to label their emotions during exposure has also been shown to improve outcomes (Craske et al., 2014).

For these reasons, DBT PE includes a much more granular focus on specific emotions to monitor progress over the course of treatment and tailor interventions to the specific emotions that clients are experiencing.

PTSD-maintaining factors. Finally, there is space for clients to describe what they learned as a result of completing the exposure, which is intended to further consolidate new learning. Although the amount of information collected in this form can seem overwhelming, it typically only takes clients a minute or two to complete once they are familiar with it.

Case Example: Maria's In Vivo Exposure Homework

Maria and her therapist decided that Maria would start with the two least distressing *in vivo* exposure tasks on her hierarchy: making eye contact with men in public (SUDS = 40) and leaving chores undone that would not affect her mother (SUDS = 45). Maria's therapist gave her instructions about how to complete *in vivo* exposure effectively and they set specific goals for each of her initial tasks. For the first one, they decided that Maria would make eye contact with at least three men while in public places and would do this four times in the next week. Maria identified the specific locations where she would do this, including her local grocery store, the bus, the public library, and while walking down the street in her neighborhood. For the second task, she agreed that she would leave her bed unmade on 3 days in the next week and would leave her bedroom door open on those days.

6. Assign Homework

At the end of Session 2, clients are asked to complete the homework assignments listed below. An optional phone check-in can be scheduled to occur after the client completes their first *in vivo* exposure task so you can provide immediate reinforcement and troubleshoot any problems that may have interfered with completing the task. If clients have not yet finalized their plan for after the first imaginal exposure session, this can be added as homework.

SESSION 2 HOMEWORK ASSIGNMENTS

1. Review the dialectical reactions to trauma (DBT PE Handouts 4 and 5).*

2. Review the common avoided situations (DBT PE Handout 6)* and add items to the *In Vivo* Exposure Hierarchy (DBT PE Handout 7)* if needed.

3. Read the instructions for doing exposure homework (DBT PE Handout 9).

4. Complete the assigned *in vivo* exposure tasks (at least one per day) and fill out an Exposure Recording Form (DBT PE Handout 8 or 8A) before and after each practice.

5. Practice skills from the Post-Exposure Skills Plan (DBT PE Handout 3) as needed.

6. Listen to the session recording once.

*Clients may choose to share these with support person(s) when appropriate.

CHAPTER 10

Joint and Family Sessions

A client's family members, spouse, partner, and friends can be important allies during DBT PE, offering encouragement and support in ways that help to facilitate the client's effective engagement in treatment. They can also, often unwittingly, be a hindrance to treatment, interfering with or slowing the client's progress. For these reasons, DBT PE includes the option of having one or more joint or family sessions with the client and their primary support person(s) to provide them with information about DBT PE and discuss how they can be helpful during treatment. With adult clients, this typically occurs once sometime between Sessions 1 and 3 so that the support person is involved before the client starts imaginal exposure. With adolescent clients, family sessions with parents or caregivers typically occur prior to starting DBT PE and as needed during treatment.

Although the focus of these joint or family sessions is on topics relevant to DBT PE, they are delivered in accord with the principles and strategies of DBT. The main function of these sessions is to structure the client's environment in ways that will promote exposure and skillful coping with the emotions it elicits, discourage avoidance, and ideally, disconfirm rather than reinforce trauma-related beliefs. When it is available, this type of environmental support can make a tremendous difference in helping our high-risk clients effectively navigate the challenges of DBT PE. In this chapter, I discuss how to elicit that support in the context of a joint or family session. Some clients may elect to talk with their support person(s) on their own, and if so, information in this chapter may be useful in helping them prepare for these discussions. Alternatively, some clients may choose not to discuss their treatment with others or do not have supportive people in their lives, in which case you can skip this optional session.

General Guidelines

When conducting a joint or family session during DBT PE, there are three general guidelines to follow.

Enhance the Client's Control

First, it is important to empower the client to make decisions about if and how to involve friends and family members in their treatment. For adult clients, the decision about who, if anyone, they might want to involve in their treatment and in what ways is completely under their control. For adolescent clients, parents or caregivers are generally involved in the consent process and are given some feedback about how treatment is progressing, but the degree to which parents are involved and the specific information that is shared with them is under the adolescent's control. When making decisions about involving others in DBT PE, clients should consider who in their life is likely to be willing to provide support in ways that would be helpful, as well as who might become an obstacle to treatment if they are not informed about what the client is doing and why. Your role is to function primarily as a consultant in this decision-making process by helping clients to think through the pros and cons of involving or not involving certain people in treatment.

Use a Consultation-to-the-Client Approach

Consistent with DBT's approach to managing the client's environment, you should adhere to consultation-to-the-client strategies as much as possible when interacting with people in the client's life. This means that your primary role is to help the client communicate effectively with their support person(s) and not to speak on their behalf. For this reason, sessions with family members and friends should not occur without the client present, and clients are encouraged to take an active role in leading these sessions. Frequently, clients will both provide some description of DBT PE to their support person and make direct requests about what they would like the person to do (and not do) to be helpful. During these interactions, you can provide coaching and support to the client, clarify or expand on information the client has shared, and reinforce and validate the client's requests. However, you usually do not take the lead in this discussion. Environmental intervention (e.g., making a direct request on the client's behalf) is typically used only when the client's efforts to shape the environment are not working and the other person is seriously interfering in treatment.

Maintain Confidentiality and Privacy

You should always be careful to maintain the client's confidentiality and privacy during joint and family sessions. This is particularly important when it comes to discussing trauma, as it is essential that clients be in control of if and how much they share about their trauma history with their support person(s). In some cases, this may be tricky to navigate—for example, if parents were not previously aware that their child had experienced trauma, they may understandably want to know what happened. In such cases, you can validate the parents' desire to know details about the trauma while explaining that private details of therapy (other than life-threatening or seriously high-risk behaviors) will not be discussed with them without the client's permission. Therefore, if a client does not want their support person(s) to know about the trauma they have experienced, you should not disclose this information to them. Instead, you can help the client think through the pros and cons of keeping this information secret, as well as whether there may be any amount of detail that would be beneficial to share.

CLINICAL TIP

Including Trauma Disclosure on the *In Vivo* Hierarchy

Disclosing trauma to supportive friends, family members, and others in the client's life is often a task that is included on the *in vivo* exposure hierarchy. Typically, this is done to reduce unjustified shame by disconfirming beliefs that others will judge and reject them if they know about their trauma. At times, disclosing trauma may be done for other reasons, such as to improve a relationship with a parent or partner who has expressed a desire to know what happened. If clients have a goal of eventually telling the support person(s) about their trauma, but they are unwilling to do so at the beginning of DBT PE, it may be useful to orient the support person(s) to this goal during the initial joint or family session.

Preparing for Joint or Family Sessions

It is important that you and the client spend time preparing in advance for any joint or family session. This will ensure that the goals of the session are clear and provide an opportunity to strategize about how best to reach these goals. When preparing for a joint or family session as part of DBT PE, the following issues should be considered:

What Does the Client Want the Person to Know (or Not Know) about Their Treatment?

While a key goal of this session is to provide information about DBT PE to the support person, the amount of detail that is provided varies widely. For example, the client may choose to share only a general description of what the treatment entails (e.g., talking about their trauma and approaching feared situations), or they may provide detailed information about the specific types of imaginal and *in vivo* exposure tasks they will be completing. If there is information the client does not want to share with the support person, they should communicate this in advance to you. It may also be useful to have a plan for how the client will manage a situation in which the support person pushes for or demands information that the client is not ready to share.

What Does the Client Want the Person to Do (or Not Do) to Be Helpful during Treatment?

Clients should think in advance about what the support person could do that would help to increase their motivation and ability to complete exposure tasks effectively, as well as what the support person might do that would make it harder to engage in the treatment. *DBT PE Handout 10* (*Asking for Support during DBT PE*) in Appendix A can be given to clients to help them decide what they want to ask the person to do and not to do to be helpful. Once they are clear about their request, they should be encouraged to prepare a script (using the DEAR MAN and GIVE skills) and practice it on their own or with you in advance of the joint or family session.

What Skills Can the Client Use to Cope with Stressful Interactions That May Occur?

Joint and family sessions are often stressful for both the client and the support person. It can be uncomfortable to meet together with a therapist, the topics that are being discussed are often particularly personal and emotional, and the likelihood that one or both people may behave in less than optimal ways in some moments is high. Therefore, clients should prepare in advance for how they will manage their own emotions during the session to try to prevent unskillful interpersonal behavior, as well as how they will respond effectively to their support person's potentially stressful behaviors. For example, if they plan to share information about their trauma with the person, how do they anticipate the person will respond and how will they manage this? What will they do if the person is unwilling to fulfill some of their requests for support? What would they like you to do to provide support and help them remain skillful? In preparation for the session, clients can be encouraged to create and rehearse a cope ahead plan with specific skills they will use as needed.

What Role Will You and the Client Each Play in the Session?

A final issue to consider is how the tasks of the session will be divided between you and the client. Consistent with the consultation-to-the-client approach, the client will ideally take primary responsibility for leading the conversation and you will largely be there to offer coaching and support. In addition, although clients are often quite capable of describing DBT PE to their support person, it is reasonable for you to act as the expert on the treatment, offering additional information and/or correcting any inaccuracies as needed. In general, however, the client should be encouraged to lead the session as much as possible, and it should be clear in advance what each of your roles in the session will be.

Conducting the Orientation Session

Next, I outline a general structure for the orientation session that occurs prior to starting imaginal exposure and suggest potential topics that can be discussed. The specific content of this session should be tailored to fit the needs of your client and their support person(s).

Setting an Agenda

As with any session, it is useful to start joint and family sessions by creating an agenda so that everyone is clear from the outset about the goals of the session. The agenda is mostly predetermined by the goals that you and the client have planned for the session, but the support person can also request to add items to the agenda. A typical agenda for the orientation session includes:

1. Sharing information about DBT PE with the support person.
2. Discussing how the person can support the client during DBT PE.
3. Discussing other issues raised by the support person (if any).

Providing Information about DBT PE

The session typically starts by providing information about DBT PE to the support person and answering questions they may have. If the support person is not familiar with PTSD, it may be helpful to start with psychoeducation about PTSD—*General Handout 1* (*What Is Posttraumatic Stress Disorder?*) can be used to facilitate this discussion. It is also important that the support person understand the general rationale for treatment, particularly the role of avoidance in maintaining PTSD and how exposure works to reduce PTSD. If helpful, the support person can be provided with a copy of *General Handout 4* (*What Is DBT PE?*), which explains the treatment rationale and procedures. The support person should have at least a basic understanding of what the client will be expected to do during the treatment. This may include providing a brief description of *in vivo* and imaginal exposure, and highlighting that clients will be asked to regularly complete both types of exposure outside of therapy sessions. It may also be helpful to provide estimates of how much time exposure homework will require.

Finally, it can also be useful to talk about how the client is likely to react during the treatment. Clients may wish to emphasize that this will be an emotionally challenging treatment and that there will be times when they are likely to become quite distressed while doing exposure. I often tell the support person that the client may look worse before they look better—that is, it is common to experience an increase in emotional distress at the beginning of the exposure portion of the treatment as the client begins to confront trauma cues that have previously been avoided. I encourage the support person to view this as progress and a sign that the client is doing exactly what is needed to get better, rather than thinking it means that the treatment isn't working. The support person should be reassured that an increase in distress, if it does occur, is typically temporary and can be expected to decrease as the client continues with the treatment.

CLINICAL TIP

Identifying Acceptable In Vivo Exposure Tasks

When working with adolescent clients, it may be necessary to involve parents or caregivers in identifying *in vivo* exposure tasks that they will allow the teen to engage in. For example, parents may have concerns about their child engaging in certain types of *in vivo* exposure, such as going to parties, driving alone, leaving the house without a cell phone, or watching an R-rated movie. In such cases, you and the client may need to explain the rationale for these types of tasks to the parent and work together to craft a reasonable list of *in vivo* exposures that they will allow the client to complete. In addition, if there are questions about the potential riskiness of certain *in vivo* exposure tasks (e.g., walking around the neighborhood alone at night), it may be helpful to consult with the support person(s) about whether the task may pose an unacceptable level of risk.

Asking for Support

Friends and family members often want to know "How can I help?" The answer to this question depends both on what the client would find helpful and on what the support person is willing and able to do. There are multiple roles that friends and family members could play in supporting the client to complete DBT PE, including being a cheerleader, confidant, coach, and/or assistant (see DBT PE Handout 10). As a cheerleader, the support person's main task is to keep the client's morale high and inspire them to keep going. This often means that the person helps by encouraging the client to complete exposure tasks rather than avoid. This can be hard to do when they see their loved one experiencing distress and they may have urges to say things like "Don't do it" or "Listen to the recording tomorrow instead." Maintaining the stance that the client has the ability to do what is needed—without invalidating the difficulty of the task—is essential. Clients can suggest specific things the person can say that would be helpful, such as "I know this is hard and I believe you can do it" or "Keep going and it will get easier." As a cheerleader, the support person can also praise the client's efforts, look for evidence of improvement, and celebrate successes.

Support people may also serve as a confidant with whom private matters can be discussed and painful emotions can be shared. This might include listening to the client talk about their struggles in treatment and providing a shoulder to cry on after a particularly challenging exposure task. Ideally, the support person will both encourage the client to express their emotions and validate them when they do arise. Although clients are typically discouraged from sharing their imaginal exposure recordings with others, they may want to talk about their trauma with someone other than you. If so, having a support person who is open to hearing about the client's trauma and responding with care and compassion can be incredibly helpful. Whatever the client does choose to share, it is essential that the support person keep this information private and refrain from discussing it with others without the client's permission.

Many support people, perhaps particularly parents and caregivers, naturally gravitate toward the role of the coach. A coach helps to strategize about the most effective course of action and stays steady and levelheaded in stressful situations. As a coach, the support person may assist the client in completing exposure tasks when asked. This may include going with the client to complete certain *in vivo* exposure tasks or being nearby while the client listens to their imaginal exposure recording. In some cases, the support person may be the exposure cue (e.g., when the client is working on *in vivo* exposure to sexual intimacy with a spouse). If the support person is asked to participate in exposure tasks, it is important to provide them with instructions about what to do to be helpful during exposure. For example, they can offer praise, encouragement, and validation, but should not provide excessive reassurance (e.g., repeatedly telling the client that they are safe) or reinforce avoidance (e.g., encouraging the client to stop prematurely). In addition, they should be careful not to do things that may make the exposure task easier (unless this is preplanned/strategic), such as speaking for the client in social interactions, or holding the client's hand throughout the task. During exposures, the support person should strive to appear calm and confident, and refrain from showing intense emotions, such as fear, horror, or disgust. They may also help by assessing the client's SUDS throughout the task. The support person can also function as a coach in helping the client to implement their Post-Exposure Skills Plan when needed. Although support people may initially function as a coach during exposures, it is important to ensure that the client does not become overly reliant on the person as a safety cue. Therefore, clients should be asked to eventually complete the exposure on their own without the support person present.

The perhaps least glamorous but no less essential role is the assistant. For adults, this role is often fulfilled by spouses or partners and involves relieving the client from the stress of daily life tasks—such as running errands, paying bills, and caring for children—so that the client will have more time and energy to devote to treatment. For teens, parents might relieve them of selected chores or provide help with homework to allow more time for treatment. The support person can be involved in scheduling times for the client to do exposure homework when they will be available to provide logistical support. This may involve keeping other people (e.g., children, siblings) away from the client and taking over household tasks (e.g., cooking dinner) so that the client can focus on doing exposure assignments. The support person may also offer other types of logistical support, such as driving the client to and from therapy sessions or helping to locate objects (e.g., photos, music, movies) that are needed to complete *in vivo* exposure tasks.

An important part of asking for support is also to ask the person to refrain from behaviors that would be unhelpful. Often these requests are informed by the client's history with the person and their predictions about how the person is likely to respond. Common responses that are likely to be unhelpful are included in DBT PE Handout 10. Some of these are ways in which a support person might respond negatively to the challenges of doing exposure, such as invalidating, judging, or making fun of the client's distress or urges to avoid. In some cases, there may be concern that the support person may become overinvolved in treatment by, for example, excessively pressuring the client to complete exposure tasks or not respecting their privacy. Clients may worry that some support people may become intensely distressed themselves, including potentially expressing high levels of anxiety or worry about the client and frequently checking on the client's well-being. Other unhelpful responses are things that would reduce the effectiveness of exposure, such as distracting, excessively reassuring, or encouraging avoidance during exposure tasks.

There are clearly many potential ways in which support people could be helpful and unhelpful during DBT PE, and it is up to clients to decide what exactly they want to ask for. In making this decision, clients should consider what they would find most helpful in keeping them motivated and able to do the treatment effectively. For example, some clients find cheerleading to be aversive, whereas others may strongly dislike it when their support person offers skills coaching. Just as critically, however, clients must consider whether the support person is likely to be capable of and willing to provide the desired support. This may influence what the client asks for in the first place and should also be assessed with the support person during the session. What is feasible for the support person to do given other demands in their life? What are they willing to do assuming it is possible for them to do it? What concerns do they have about their ability to provide the requested support or to refrain from the behaviors that would be unhelpful? As with any request, the needs and preferences of both parties should be taken into account before any support plan is finalized.

Addressing Other Issues

The last portion of the session typically includes discussing any other topics the support person may have placed on the agenda. For example, the support person may want to talk about how the client's PTSD impacts them, share things they have noticed that the client avoids, or highlight problems that they would like to see the client work on during treatment. It may also be helpful to discuss whether and how the friend or family member may want to seek their own support if they are having difficulty managing their own emotional reactions or otherwise struggling to provide the support the client has requested.

Case Example: Maria's Joint Session

Returning to the case of Maria, her therapist raised the topic of potentially having a joint session with a support person in the weeks leading up to starting DBT PE and provided her with DBT PE Handout 10 to help her decide whether she would like to do this. Given Maria's social isolation, the only person she thought might be reasonable to ask was her mother, particularly because her mother already knew about her trauma. However, she had concerns that her mother might be critical of the treatment given her avoidant approach to coping with her own trauma and her tendency to discourage Maria from expressing negative emotions. At the same time, her mother had generally been supportive of her in the aftermath of her rape and Maria believed she might be able to offer some support that would be helpful during DBT PE. Given that they were living together, she also thought it would be important for her mother to have some understanding of what she was working on in treatment so that she might be less likely to inadvertently do things that would be unhelpful, such as encourage Maria to avoid doing her exposure homework. After weighing these pros and cons, Maria decided that she would ask her mother to attend a joint session, and she and her therapist planned for this to occur between Sessions 2 and 3.

Maria spent time thinking about what she would like her mother to know about her treatment and what types of support she would ask her to provide. Given that her mother generally discouraged her from talking about emotionally distressing topics and had never been open to talking with her about her father's abuse, Maria did not think it would be wise to share information about the details of the traumas she had suffered or the specific exposure practices she would be completing. Instead, she decided that she would provide her mother with general information about DBT PE but would not provide specific examples of what she would be doing during treatment or ask her to serve in the role of confidant. She also did not think her mother would be effective as a coach during exposure given her own tendency to avoid emotions, but that she might be helpful after she had completed exposure in implementing certain skills. She also did not anticipate needing any logistical support from her. Therefore, Maria decided to focus her request for support on asking her mother to function as a cheerleader by encouraging her efforts to do DBT PE even if she seemed more distressed. She also wanted to ask her mother whether she would be willing to spend time with her after exposure doing activities like watching TV or going for a walk at times when Maria might need help distracting. To accomplish these goals, Maria prepared a DEAR MAN with GIVE and practiced it several times with her therapist. They also planned how Maria would respond if her mother suggested that she would be better off not thinking or talking about her trauma or otherwise discouraged her from doing DBT PE.

The session started with Maria providing her mother with a general description of the rationale for DBT PE, including the role of avoidance in maintaining PTSD. She then told her that she would be working on processing traumas she had experienced by talking about them in therapy and confronting things that reminded her of them outside of therapy. Her therapist reinforced what Maria had said and provided additional information about the research supporting DBT PE's safety and effectiveness. Maria's mother responded by saying that she could not personally imagine doing the treatment, but that she could see how it could be helpful. Maria then asked her mother to support her efforts to do exposure even though it might go against her typical ways of coping. Her mother said that she was fully supportive of her daughter's desire to treat her PTSD and she would do her best to provide encouragement to stick with it. Maria gave her some examples of things she might say that would be encouraging, such as "I'm proud of you for working so hard" and "I believe you can do this." Her mother also readily agreed to spend time with Maria when it would be helpful, including at times when she might be struggling with intense emotions. Maria thanked her mother for her support, and they agreed to check in with each other periodically as the treatment progressed.

Conducting Ongoing Joint or Family Sessions

In some cases, particularly with adolescent clients, it may be useful to continue having joint or family sessions during DBT PE. These sessions may focus on topics such as reinforcing what is going well in terms of providing support, addressing things that are not going well and asking for changes, and providing updates on progress. In addition, the support person can be asked to share observations about the client's progress in treatment, ask questions, and communicate any concerns they may have. These ongoing sessions should adhere to the same general principles for the joint/family sessions described above and can be conducted on an as-needed basis or according to a previously established schedule for family sessions.

Concluding Comments

Having a support person from the client's life involved in DBT PE can be an effective way to reduce obstacles and improve outcomes. Of course, a support person would need to be nearly superhuman to fulfill all the potential roles described in this chapter. Instead, friends and family members should be asked to provide assistance in targeted ways that will both augment the support you provide and capitalize on the support person's strengths. In some cases, the most effective plan may be to limit the role that certain friends and family members play in treatment or not involve them at all. In other cases, clients may not have anyone in their life that they could ask to be involved. Importantly, clients should be assured that they and you together have what it takes to make DBT PE successful. Involving other people in treatment can be helpful, but it is not necessary to make the treatment work.

CHAPTER 11

Session 3

SESSION 3 COMPONENTS AND TIME ESTIMATES

	60-minute session	90-minute session
Review the DBT diary card and set the session agenda	3 min.	3–5 min.
Review homework	5–10 min.	10–15 min.
Orient to the rationale for imaginal exposure and processing	5–10 min.	10–15 min.
Give instructions on how to do imaginal exposure	3 min.	3–5 min.
Conduct imaginal exposure	20–30 min.	30–45 min.
Conduct processing of the imaginal exposure	15–25 min.	20–30 min.
Assign homework	3–5 min.	5–10 min.

Session 3 is the point at which clients' anxiety typically peaks as they prepare to do their first imaginal exposure. This highly anticipated moment has been the focal point of the entire treatment plan for months and it is now finally here: The proverbial rubber is about to meet the road. Clients often arrive at this session jittery and agitated with their stomach in knots. No matter how much they have prepared or how motivated they are, they are likely to be scared and having worry thoughts: What if they aren't able to tolerate this? What if this ends up making them worse? What if you think badly of them once you find out what happened? From the first moments of the session, you should assume a stance of unwavering centeredness that conveys belief in the client's ability to do imaginal exposure, in your own ability to guide them through it, and in the effectiveness of the treatment itself. You must be the calm in the middle of the client's storm, providing a clear-eyed vision of the gains they stand to make in the long run and not balking in the face of their mounting distress in the short run.

Although clients may be focused on the upcoming imaginal exposure, there are several other treatment tasks that must be completed first, including reviewing their homework and presenting the rationale and instructions for imaginal exposure. It can be challenging to get through these initial tasks in a timely manner because clients' anticipatory anxiety can make it difficult for them to engage in a productive discussion. In addition, you and/or your client may have urges to avoid starting the imaginal exposure and thus be vulnerable to spending longer than is necessary on these initial session tasks. Therefore, it is important to find a balance between giving these initial tasks the time they require and keeping the session moving forward to ensure that there will be sufficient time to do imaginal exposure and processing. A checklist for Session 3 is included in Appendix C to guide you through each session component and handouts are found in Appendix A.

1. Review the DBT Diary Card and Set the Session Agenda

As in every DBT PE session, Session 3 begins with a quick review of the DBT diary card to make a "go/no-go" decision about whether to continue with the planned DBT PE session. (Behaviors that may cause DBT PE to be paused are described in Chapter 14.) Given the high anticipatory anxiety leading up to Session 3, the diary card frequently reveals higher than usual urges to quit therapy, as well as to engage in target behaviors that have historically functioned to provide relief from distress. These increased urges, if present, should be normalized and clients can be reassured that they are typically temporary and will decrease as the treatment progresses. Clients should also be commended for coming to this pivotal session despite having urges to quit, and reinforced for effectively using skills to manage urges without acting on them. Following this brief diary card review, the session agenda is presented according to the session outline shown above.

2. Review Homework

In Session 3, homework review typically begins by checking in with clients about the *Dialectical Reactions to Trauma* (DBT PE Handout 4) and *Understanding Your Reactions to Trauma* (Handout 5) to see whether any questions or important insights came up as they read through these materials. In addition, new *in vivo* exposure tasks that clients may have identified from *Common Avoided Situations* (DBT PE Handout 6) are briefly discussed and added to the hierarchy. Clients are asked whether they listened to the recording of Session 2 and any obstacles to doing so are addressed. Most of the homework review time is then spent discussing the client's *in vivo* exposure homework. To start, you should reinforce clients for having successfully completed their first *in vivo* exposures. If clients completed all of the assigned practices, then wholehearted reinforcement is called for using whatever strategies the client finds to be motivating. If clients completed some but not all of the *in vivo* exposure assignments, you can apply the principles of shaping by reinforcing whatever tasks they did complete and conveying approval of small steps toward their goals.

For clients who completed *in vivo* exposure homework, you then review the tasks that they completed to identify signs of progress as well as potential problems. Table 11.1 includes steps for reviewing exposure homework. Ideally clients will have filled out an *Exposure Recording Form* (DBT PE Handout 8 or 8A) for each *in vivo* exposure task they completed, which means that there may be a lot of information to review. It often takes practice to feel facile in reviewing these forms in a way that doesn't skim over important information while also not getting bogged down in all of the details. Key ratings and patterns of change to look for when reviewing the

TABLE 11.1. How to Review Exposure Homework

1. Review one exposure task at a time, including each repetition of the task.
2. Start with open-ended questions, such as "What did you learn by doing this task?"
   - Reinforce and strengthen corrective learning that may have occurred.
3. Look for patterns of change (or lack thereof) in key mechanisms across repetitions.
   - Are SUDS and emotions decreasing across multiple practices?
   - Are problematic probability and cost estimates getting corrected?
4. If change is occurring, reinforce the client's progress.
5. If change is not yet occurring, emphasize mastery and emotional tolerance.
   - Encourage clients to keep going and express faith that it will eventually get easier.
   - Provide coaching as needed on how to complete the exposure task more effectively.
6. Look for potential increases in state dissociation and urges to engage in target behaviors, and problem-solve as needed.
7. Repeat Steps 2–6 for each of the remaining exposure tasks the client completed.

Exposure Recording Forms are described in Table 11.1. If clients completed *in vivo* exposure but did not fill out the forms, then you will need to ask questions to try to get a sense of how the exposure went (e.g., "How intense was your distress? Did it change at all across the times that you did the task?"). In addition, barriers to completing the Exposure Recording Form should be assessed and problem-solved. Similarly, if clients did not complete any *in vivo* exposure homework, or completed less than was assigned, you should assess and problem-solve what interfered. This can typically be done with a relatively brief missing links analysis (see Chapter 14 for details on addressing homework noncompliance).

3. Orient to the Rationale for Imaginal Exposure and Processing

The rationale for imaginal exposure and processing can be a particularly challenging one to deliver. While you may be earnestly sharing important information about these core treatment procedures, clients may be anxiously counting down the minutes until imaginal exposure will begin. Therefore, you may need to work extra hard to make this final rationale compelling and engaging, which can be achieved by making this a highly interactive discussion, eliciting examples from the client, using metaphors to illustrate important concepts, and tailoring the information to apply to the client's experiences. Overall, the goal of this orienting discussion is for clients to understand (1) the role of cognitive avoidance in maintaining PTSD and (2) how imaginal exposure and processing work to reduce PTSD.

By Session 3, clients should be quite familiar with how PTSD is maintained and have some knowledge of how imaginal exposure and processing work. Given this, you may be able to elicit some or most of this information from clients by asking questions that encourage them to think critically about what they have already learned. During this discussion, it is helpful to use a metaphor to further clarify why it is important to process trauma. A vivid metaphor can capture clients' attention and hold it in a way that a description of the theory underlying imaginal exposure and processing does not. Ideally, a well-crafted metaphor will create a powerful and lasting image that clients will remember and use to help them stick with the challenging work of trauma processing. You should feel free to create your own metaphors or use one of the examples provided later in this section. The key points to cover in orienting to the rationale for imaginal exposure and processing are shown in Table 11.2.

TABLE 11.2. Key Points in Orienting to the Rationale for Imaginal Exposure and Processing

1. Cognitive avoidance (i.e., of trauma memories and thoughts) works temporarily to reduce distress but maintains PTSD in the long run by preventing new learning about the trauma.

2. Imaginal exposure and processing work to reduce PTSD by:
   a. Learning that thinking and talking about the trauma is safe
   b. Organizing the trauma memory into a coherent narrative
   c. Increasing the ability to tolerate intense emotions
   d. Reducing the intensity of distress over time (habituation)
   e. Building mastery and enhancing control
   f. Gaining a new and more helpful perspective on the trauma and its meaning

Case Example: Orienting Maria to the Rationale for Imaginal Exposure and Processing

THERAPIST: Before we do imaginal exposure, I want to make sure you're clear on why we're going to do it and how it works. Can you tell me why you think it's important to do imaginal exposure?

MARIA: Because I haven't ever really let myself think about what happened to me and it's kept me stuck as a result.

THERAPIST: That's right. Avoiding thinking about your trauma actually keeps PTSD going because it prevents you from processing what happened to you.

MARIA: It's just so hard to think about.

THERAPIST: It is hard, and it makes total sense that people try to avoid thinking about their traumatic experiences. I mean, who wants to sit around and think about really painful things if they don't have to?

MARIA: Not me.

THERAPIST: Well, that makes you completely normal! I imagine you also got that advice from people. For example, you said that your mother encouraged you not to think about your father's abuse and to just put it behind you, right?

MARIA: Yeah, she seemed to think that not thinking or talking about it would just make it go away, but that hasn't worked.

THERAPIST: That's because it doesn't work for anyone. Avoiding thinking about your trauma only works to reduce distress in the short run, but in the long run those memories are still there, and they are just as distressing when they come up. Often the harder you try not to think about your trauma, the more frequently the memories come into your mind.

MARIA: I think about the bad things that have happened to me all the time. The memories are always coming into my head—I'm not really able to avoid it. So how will imaginal exposure be different?

THERAPIST: I agree that you are not able to avoid thinking about your trauma completely, and you may even think about it repeatedly throughout your day. But what do you typically do when a trauma memory comes into your mind?

MARIA: I try to push it out of my head as soon as I can.

THERAPIST: Right. That's what most people with PTSD do. Imaginal exposure will be different because you will invite the trauma memory into your mind and you will not push it away. Instead, you will allow yourself to think about it fully and in detail.

MARIA: That will be different.

THERAPIST: Trauma memories are like scary monsters that are lurking outside your house. The monsters are knocking on your door, looking in your windows, and making loud noises at night that wake you up. They keep telling you that they need to talk to you, and they won't go away no matter how much you try to ignore them. In fact, the more you try to act like they are not there, the louder they get. Eventually, it's hard to get any moments of peace and quiet because the monsters are constantly banging on your door.

MARIA: That's what it feels like now. I can't get these thoughts about my trauma to leave me alone.

THERAPIST: Exactly, so instead of ignoring them, we need you to give them some attention. Imaginal exposure is going to be like letting the scary monsters into your house so you can listen to what they need to tell you. And rather than having them show up unexpectedly, you're going to pick a time to invite them in to have a conversation. You're also not going to do this alone. I am going to be there with you to face these monsters and hear what they have to say. And once we've heard their story, you will ask them to leave and the visit will end. They are not going to stay forever and become permanent houseguests.

MARIA: But what if they won't leave?

THERAPIST: They won't leave forever, but they will leave for a while. And once the visit is over, you and I will talk about what you think and feel about what they told you and we'll work together to make sense of their story.

MARIA: Will I have to invite them in again?

THERAPIST: Yes, you will need to keep inviting them back for more visits until they feel like you really understand their story and have compassion for what they have experienced. And the more time you spend with these monsters, the less scary they will be because you will get used to them and will learn that they are not going to harm you. These are just poor monsters with a sad story to tell who need someone to listen to them so that they will feel better.

MARIA: I guess I need to face my monsters, don't I?

THERAPIST: Yes, you do. That is how we are going to get them to stop bothering you so much. Eventually, the memories will leave you alone unless you decide to invite them in for a visit. The goal is for you to have control over the memories rather than the memories having control over you.

MARIA: That makes sense to me, but it still feels dangerous to think about what my father did to me. It's almost like I'm being traumatized all over again.

THERAPIST: That's a really common fear and is probably a major reason that you have not allowed yourself to think about your abuse in detail. Imaginal exposure will help you to learn that you can talk and think about what happened to you and it is not dangerous. There is a big difference between remembering being abused and being abused again.

MARIA: OK.

THERAPIST: So that's one reason that imaginal exposure works. Why else do you think it works to reduce PTSD?

MARIA: Well, by talking about what happened over and over again it will make it easier to talk about because you kind of get used to hearing it and it's not as scary anymore.

THERAPIST: That's right. The more you let yourself talk about what happened and think about it without avoiding, the less distressing it will be over time.

MARIA: Do you think it will get easier today?

THERAPIST: It may, but I wouldn't count on it. Often people's emotions stay quite high the first several times they do imaginal exposure. It usually takes some repetition for it to start getting less distressing.

MARIA: That sucks.

THERAPIST: I hear you, and I think there's some benefit to that, because this is going to give you the opportunity to practice tolerating really intense emotions. So if your emotions don't decrease today, then you'll find out that you can experience intense emotions and nothing terrible is going to happen. You don't have to push them away, or numb out, or hurt yourself to get the emotions to stop. Instead, you can just experience them because they are safe and they won't last forever.

MARIA: It doesn't feel that way.

THERAPIST: I know. You're worried you won't be able to tolerate the emotions, right?

MARIA: Yeah, I feel like it's going to destroy me, like I'm too weak to do this.

THERAPIST: Well, that is another reason that imaginal exposure works. It will help you to learn that you're a lot more competent than you give yourself credit for. You absolutely can do this, and you're going to feel more and more confident in your ability to do hard things the more you do imaginal exposure.

MARIA: I'm counting on that to make me feel better after I'm done.

THERAPIST: Me too, and I will be your biggest cheerleader! Now, you mentioned before that you feel like you don't know the full story of the event we're going to be focusing on. Does it feel like the memory is kind of in pieces or you're not entirely sure what order things happened in?

MARIA: Yeah, there's missing parts. Like I don't know how I got from here to there, but I did.

THERAPIST: That's very common. Imaginal exposure will also help to organize your memory so that you are clearer about what happened and have a more coherent narrative about this event. This can really help you to see things in a different way than you have before, as you might notice details you hadn't really thought about before or piece things together in a way that brings you new insights. For example, you've said that you blame yourself almost entirely for your father's abuse because you think you were a bad kid.

MARIA: Yeah, I always messed things up and then he would punish me.

THERAPIST: Well, by getting clearer about what exactly happened in a moment-to-moment kind of way, you might discover that there are other ways you could interpret the situation that aren't so self-blaming. The processing part of the session, which happens after the imaginal exposure, will help with getting those kinds of new perspectives. That's when we'll sit back together and look at the story and talk about what you think about it and what it means. We'll also evaluate whether the beliefs you have about this event fit the facts of what actually happened.

MARIA: That sounds helpful.

THERAPIST: During processing, we're also going to help you make meaning of your father's abuse in the context of your life. Imaginal exposure is like using a zoom lens to focus in on the minute details of a single event. However, processing is like using a wide-angle lens to see the broader context in which this event happened and how it has affected you in your life.

MARIA: Does that mean that we won't only talk about this one event?

THERAPIST: Right. You'll describe just that one event during imaginal exposure, but during processing we'll talk about the bigger picture of your abuse and the impact it had on you. The goal is to help you better understand the unhelpful beliefs and behaviors you developed as a result of the abuse and to replace these with new ways of thinking and behaving that will reduce misery and increase joy in your life.

MARIA: I would like that.

THERAPIST: Me too. Do you have any other questions about imaginal exposure and processing and how they work?

MARIA: What if there are parts that I don't remember? Will imaginal exposure still work?

THERAPIST: Yes, it can absolutely work. You don't have to remember every single detail—most people don't.

MARIA: Is it normal for it come back? For people to be like, "Oh wait, that's what happened!"

THERAPIST: Yes, that often happens, which makes sense. If I don't let myself think about something for a long time it's going to become less vivid and I'll forget pieces of it. And then if I let myself really, really think about it, I'll likely remember more again. So it's not unusual to remember more details, but at the same time that's not our goal. Our goal is to get the memories that you do have to be less distressing. In that process, it naturally happens that a lot of people start to remember more details than they used to, and it's also totally fine if you don't.

CASE EXAMPLE DISCUSSION

In this example, the therapist covered the key points of the rationale for imaginal exposure and processing in a conversational manner while keeping Maria engaged in the discussion. The therapist used questions to draw her into the conversation, stimulate critical thinking about the material, and elicit examples of her own experiences. In addition, a metaphor was used that appeared to add to Maria's understanding of the importance of processing her trauma. The therapist also consistently validated Maria's experiences, assuring her that her responses were normal and understandable. Maria asked several common questions during this discussion, such as how imaginal exposure differs from intrusive reexperiencing of trauma and whether she would be likely to remember more about her trauma. The therapist responded by providing her with information to address her question in a manner that conveyed that it was both reasonable to ask and not something she needed to worry about. In general, when Maria expressed concerns, the therapist maintained an unwavering stance of believing in her ability to do imaginal exposure and in the effectiveness of the treatment itself. Overall, the therapist balanced acceptance strategies, such as warmth and validation, with a consistent push for and steady march forward to the heavily change-focused strategy of imaginal exposure. As with the other rationales, you should feel free to personalize your delivery of this information to fit your own style and the client's needs, while being sure to clearly and accurately cover the key points outlined in Table 11.2. Additional examples of metaphors that can be used are provided below.

> **CLINICAL TIP**
> ### Example Metaphors for Trauma Processing
>
> 1. *Reading a scary book.* A trauma memory is like a scary book that keeps falling open to the most terrifying parts of the story. If the book is quickly closed and put away, then only the scariest moments will be remembered. If instead the book is read from start to finish, it will be possible to understand the entire story and gain a fuller perspective on what happened. If the book is read repeatedly, it will eventually stop being so scary and it will be possible to put the book away on a bookshelf and have it stay there. The book can still be taken out and read when it is useful, but it will no longer fall open unpredictably.
>
> 2. *Receiving physical therapy.* When someone has a physical injury, they often avoid doing activities that increase pain in the short term even though this makes their body less able to function in the long run. To address this, physical therapy requires people to do exercises that stretch and move the specific muscles that are most sore and tense. These exercises are often quite painful but get easier over time as the muscles get stronger and more flexible. In the long run, physical therapy will help people to have less pain and be able to function, move, and live better. (*Note:* Similar metaphors can be used for other medical treatments that increase pain in the short term, such as cleaning out an infected wound, receiving chemotherapy for cancer, or debriding a burn.)

4. Give Instructions on How to Do Imaginal Exposure

The next step is to provide instructions about how to do imaginal exposure. The goal of this discussion is to ensure that clients are clear about what they will be expected to do, as well as what you will do during imaginal exposure. Making these procedures as clear and predictable as possible in advance can help to increase clients' sense of control and reduce the likelihood that they are caught by surprise by something that happens during imaginal exposure.

Orienting to the Client's Role during Imaginal Exposure

At first blush, imaginal exposure sounds like a straightforward, albeit exceptionally challenging, thing to do: you just talk about your trauma. However, there are specific ways in which imaginal exposure is done that are intended to optimize its effectiveness and clients will need to be oriented to these procedures before they begin.

- *Tell the story in detail.* Clients are asked to tell the complete story of the traumatic event from the start to end points that were identified in the Trauma Interview in Session 1. This description should be as detailed as possible, including external details of the situation (e.g., what other people said and did; things they could see, hear, or smell), as well as internal details of their own experience (e.g., their thoughts, emotions, and physical sensations at the time of the trauma). The goal is for clients to describe out loud everything they remember about the traumatic event and to not leave anything out.

- *Eyes closed and present tense.* During imaginal exposure, clients are asked to keep their eyes closed and describe the traumatic event in the present tense. These strategies are designed to increase the vividness of the trauma memory, facilitate emotional engagement, and help clients mindfully focus on the memory.

- *Repeat the story.* Clients are expected to repeat the story multiple times in the session. This means that when they get to the end of the trauma narrative they should go back to the beginning and start over. Clients should be instructed to continue imaginal exposure for a specific amount of time (e.g., 30–45 minutes) and to complete whatever number of repetitions fit within that time period.

- *Stick to the facts.* As much as possible, imaginal exposure should be a description of the facts of the traumatic event, including what exactly happened and what clients were thinking and feeling at the time it was happening. During imaginal exposure, clients should try not to editorialize (e.g., express opinions about what happened, wonder aloud about whether their memory is accurate) or talk about things that may be related to the trauma but are not a description of the event itself (e.g., a friend's reaction to learning about the trauma several weeks later). Clients' can be assured that their thoughts and opinions about the trauma, as well as other related experiences, will be discussed during processing.

- *Avoid avoidance.* Clients should be quite familiar with the expectation that they are to minimize avoidance during exposure, but it is nonetheless useful to remind them of this before starting. Clients should be encouraged to allow themselves to fully experience the emotions that arise during imaginal exposure and to be on the lookout for and work to prevent other forms of avoidance.

Orienting to the Therapist's Role during Imaginal Exposure

It is critical to orient clients in advance to what they can expect us to say and do during imaginal exposure. Clients are used to us behaving in certain ways while delivering DBT and our behavior during imaginal exposure is radically different. During DBT, we are highly interactive, respond freely and genuinely to the client, and guide the pace and content of the session. During imaginal exposure, we are largely silent, do not respond to what clients say, and sit back and allow them to lead the way. Without prior orientation, clients are likely to interpret this shift from directive to nondirective therapy as meaning that we have been shocked into silence or are so disgusted by them that we cannot even speak. To prevent these kinds of misattributions, it is important to prepare clients for this change in our behavior while also reassuring them that we will resume being interactive and respond to the content of what they have shared during processing after the imaginal exposure is complete.

Although the degree to which we interact with and respond to clients is greatly reduced during imaginal exposure, we are also not completely silent. There are three main ways in which clients should expect us to interact during imaginal exposure:

- *Assess SUDS.* You will ask the client to provide a SUDS rating about every 5 minutes during imaginal exposure by asking a quick question, such as "What are your SUDS?" The goal is to monitor the level of distress the client is experiencing without significantly interrupting the flow of the imaginal exposure. Thus, clients should be instructed to provide the SUDS ratings quickly without spending a lot of time thinking about it and then to immediately resume their narration of the trauma.

- *Provide cheerleading.* You will also make reinforcing comments during imaginal exposure, which often includes offering encouragement and praising the client's efforts.

• *Prompt and coach.* You may also prompt clients with brief questions designed to elicit additional details in the trauma narrative or help them to continue if they have paused in their retelling. In addition, you may provide coaching when needed to reduce avoidance and help clients complete imaginal exposure as effectively as possible.

Case Example: Giving Maria Instructions

THERAPIST: Before we start, I want to make sure you're clear on what you and I are each going to be doing during the imaginal exposure. The first thing is that I want you to tell the entire story from start to finish. Based on what we discussed during the Trauma Interview, this means that you will start from the point at which you were sitting on the floor playing with your toys and end after you had been hiding in your closet for a few minutes.

MARIA: What if there are parts I don't remember?

THERAPIST: Good question. If you don't remember a part, that's totally fine. You can just skip from the last thing you remember to the next thing you remember. I don't want you to try to fill in the gaps if you don't remember what happened. So just say whatever you do remember and it's completely fine if there are holes—there usually are.

MARIA: OK.

THERAPIST: When you're telling the story I also want you to describe everything you can remember about what happened without leaving out any details. This means that you should describe anything that was going on around you that you could see, hear, or smell, as well as anything that was going on inside of you, such as your thoughts, emotions, and sensations. We want the description to be as detailed and vivid as possible, almost like a movie that we are watching in high definition.

MARIA: That sounds intense.

THERAPIST: It will be intense and allowing yourself to remember what happened in vivid detail without avoiding is what is going to make this memory less distressing in the long run.

MARIA: OK.

THERAPIST: It's also going to be important that you describe exactly what your father did to you and your mom during this event, including the details of the physical and sexual abuse. For example, you should describe where he touched you on your body and what kinds of sexual behavior he forced on you so that it is clear what happened. We're going to shine a light in all the dark corners of this memory so nothing remains hidden. That's how we're going to get this memory to stop haunting you by confronting all of it without avoiding. So if you see it in your mind, just say it out loud.

MARIA: But you're going to think I'm bad and gross when you find out what happened!

THERAPIST: That is a very common worry and I completely understand why it would be hard to talk about those kinds of details. At the same time, believing you are bad and gross, and assuming other people will think similarly about you, are PTSD-related beliefs that we need to disconfirm. I know you believe I am going to think you're gross, but the only way to find out is to tell me the story and see what reaction I actually have. My prediction is that I'm going to have even more respect for you once I learn more about what you have survived, but there's only one way to know for sure which one of us is correct.

MARIA: This is going to be hard.

THERAPIST: Yes, it will be, and I totally believe that you can do it. While you are telling the story I also want you to keep your eyes closed and describe what happened in the present tense as if it is happening now. So instead of saying, "I was sitting on the floor playing with my toys," you would say, "I am sitting on the floor playing with my toys." The reason we do it with your eyes closed and in the present tense is that we want to make the memory as vivid as we can in your mind's eye. And saying it with your eyes open or in the past tense keeps you more detached from the memory and may make it harder to be emotionally engaged. OK?

MARIA: Uhhh . . .

THERAPIST: What are you thinking?

MARIA: I'm thinking that no matter what you say it's not going to sound great!

THERAPIST: All right. I'm just going to keep pushing forward then! We're also going to have you tell the story repeatedly. That means that when you get to the end of the story you will just go right back to the beginning and do it again.

MARIA: I have to do it again?

THERAPIST: Yes, it's done in repetition.

MARIA: How many times?

THERAPIST: It's not about the number of times, it's more about doing it for a long enough period of time. We're going to aim for 30–45 minutes. We want it to be long enough that when you're done you don't come out of the experience saying, "I made it because it was only 5 minutes and I couldn't have stood another minute of that!" That's another one of those beliefs that we have to disprove, that you can't tolerate thinking about it for very long. So just keep repeating it for 30–45 minutes and we'll see how many repetitions you get through in that amount of time.

MARIA: OK.

THERAPIST: The last thing I want you to do is to stay focused on just telling the story of this one event. While you're telling the story, you are likely to have other thoughts come up, such as your beliefs about the abuse now or thoughts about other times the abuse happened. Those kinds of thoughts and insights are what we're going to talk about during processing once the imaginal exposure is done. But during the imaginal exposure, the focus is going to be on just describing the facts of what happened this particular time that your father abused you.

MARIA: What if I mess up and say something that isn't just the story of what happened?

THERAPIST: First of all, that's not messing up and it's completely normal for that to happen. For example, you might make a comment about something that came to you and then go right back to telling the story and that would be totally fine. I will also make a note of anything like that that comes up to be sure we go back and talk about it during processing. In general, I am mostly going to be taking notes and paying close attention while you tell the story, and I will not be saying very much. This means that I am suddenly not going to seem like your normal DBT therapist. Imaginal exposure is not meant to be a conversation, it is an experience you are having that I am witnessing with you. And it's important that you know in advance that my silence will have nothing to do with what you're telling me or anything about you. It's just because I don't want to distract you from the memory and the emotions it is bringing up.

MARIA: Are you going to be totally silent?

THERAPIST: No. I will ask you to give me a SUDS rating about every 5 minutes. When I do, just give me a number as quickly as you can and then get right back into telling the story. I will also give you encouragement as you are doing it, and I may ask a quick question here or there or provide some brief coaching to help you do the exposure as effectively as possible. But I won't be responding to the details of what you are sharing. I am going to wait to do that until you're done with the imaginal exposure and we move into processing. Then I will become your familiar DBT therapist again and we'll talk about your reactions and my reactions to what you shared. Do you have any questions about the actual procedures?

MARIA: No, but I wish I had more questions.

THERAPIST: All right, let's get started then. You're going to do great!

CASE EXAMPLE DISCUSSION

In this example, the therapist provided clear instructions about how Maria should do the imaginal exposure. Of note, because sexual trauma survivors often avoid describing the sexually explicit details of their trauma, the therapist preemptively coached her to include these details in the narrative. The therapist also described what she would be doing during the imaginal exposure and oriented Maria to the shift in her behavior that would occur. During these instructions, Maria asked several common questions about the procedures and expressed some concerns about what she was expected to do. In several instances, her questions stemmed from problematic beliefs that were maintaining her PTSD, such as that the therapist would think she was bad and gross once she learned about what had happened. The therapist responded by highlighting that these were PTSD-related beliefs, providing brief corrective feedback, and suggesting imaginal exposure as the solution that would help her to disconfirm these beliefs. As is typical, Maria appeared anxious and apprehensive about doing the imaginal exposure, including expressing urges to delay starting. The therapist briefly validated and addressed the concerns Maria raised, expressed faith in her ability to do the imaginal exposure, and continued to move forward confidently. In general, the therapist balanced being warm and validating with a matter-of-fact style that conveyed unwavering certainty that they were on the right path.

5. Conduct Imaginal Exposure

The primary goal of the first imaginal exposure is simply to complete it. We do not expect emotions to significantly decrease or beliefs to radically shift in this first retelling. Instead, the miraculous and celebration-worthy change is that clients are approaching and talking about their trauma rather than avoiding it. Given that this is the first time that clients have done imaginal exposure, you should offer extra encouragement and reinforcement as you guide them through it.

Complete the Exposure Recording Form

Before beginning, clients are asked to complete the "before" ratings on the Exposure Recording Form to indicate their current thoughts, emotions, and urges as they anticipate doing imaginal exposure for the first time. Common feared outcomes of the first imaginal exposure include concerns about doing the imaginal exposure incorrectly, not being able to tolerate the emotions it will elicit, losing behavioral control, and being rejected by you. Clients often begin their first imaginal exposure with high urges to engage in problem behaviors, moderate to high levels of state dissociation, and low levels of radical acceptance of the trauma. Typically, clients' ratings of overall distress (SUDS) and unjustified emotions (e.g., fear, shame, guilt, disgust) are high, whereas the justified emotions (e.g., sadness, anger) are low to moderate. After clients complete these initial ratings, you should collect and scan the form to get a sense of the client's current state, but we typically say little if anything about the ratings before moving forward to start the imaginal exposure.

> **CLINICAL TIP**
> **Recording the Imaginal Exposure**
>
> As is true for all DBT PE sessions, Session 3 should be recorded in its entirety. However, clients may wish to record the imaginal exposure separately from the rest of the session to make it easier to locate and listen to for homework. If using a digital recording device, this means that the client should stop the overall session recording and start a new recording right before imaginal exposure. This way clients will not have to search through the session recording to find the starting point of the imaginal exposure when doing their homework.

Conduct the Imaginal Exposure

During imaginal exposure, clients take a very active role as they repeatedly describe their trauma out loud. Although therapists may appear rather passive, we are also quite active during imaginal exposure, albeit in ways that are often less overt. In particular, we are engaged in three primary tasks during imaginal exposure: observing, cheerleading, and coaching.

Observing

For therapists, imaginal exposure is like a mindfulness practice that is focused on using our senses to carefully observe all aspects of clients' behavior as they recount their trauma. Similar to scientific observation, we gather information by closely observing what occurs during imaginal exposure, recording these observations using the *Therapist Imaginal Exposure Recording Form (Therapist Form 3* in Appendix B), and using this information to formulate hypotheses about what needs to change in order for PTSD to improve. This requires you to focus your attention not only on what clients are saying but also on how they are saying it. By mindfully observing both content and process, you can gain critical information about the traumatic event itself, as well as the trauma-related emotions and beliefs that are contributing to the client's ongoing suffering.

As a starting point, you need to pay close attention to the description of the traumatic event. To help clients gain a new perspective on their trauma, you need to first develop a clear and detailed understanding of exactly what happened before, during, and immediately after the traumatic event. This requires you to balance attending to the moment-to-moment details of the trauma with stepping back and considering the clarity and coherency of the trauma narrative as a whole. For example, are there certain parts of the story that are vague or confusing? Are there details that are clearly being left out? Do the details come together to form an organized and complete narrative? Is the sequence of events clear?

You should also listen to the content of the trauma narrative with the goal of identifying the problematic beliefs and emotions that may be maintaining the client's PTSD. For example, the narrative should include a description of the emotions and thoughts that clients had during the traumatic event, which are often the same as those that clients continue to experience in the present (e.g., the thought "I should have known better" occurred during the trauma and is still believed now). In other cases, there may be a discrepancy between past and current emotions and thoughts that is important to understand and process (e.g., feeling happiness or love while being sexually abused as a child and feeling shame and disgust about it now). In addition, themes related to safety, trust, power, control, self-competence, and intimacy are often evident in the trauma narrative and can provide clues about unhelpful beliefs and emotions that are keeping clients stuck.

Another key element of mindful observing is to be awake to clients' in-session emotions and behavior as they are engaged in the imaginal exposure. The most obvious way in which this is done is by asking clients to provide a SUDS rating about every 5 minutes and tracking these ratings on the *Therapist Imaginal Exposure Recording Form*. This allows you to directly monitor the intensity of clients' in-session emotions and ensures that you remain aware of clients' internal experience of distress even when it may not be readily observable. In addition, you should closely attend to clients' nonverbal behavior during imaginal exposure, such as facial expressions; gestures; posture; body movements; and voice tone, volume, and speed. These forms of nonverbal communication can also provide important information about what clients are feeling and thinking as they recount their trauma.

Within and across repetitions of the trauma narrative, you should also take note of changes in clients' emotion, behavior, and description of the trauma. These changes may be obvious (e.g., sobbing after previously being emotionally flat) or subtle (e.g., changing a word in the trauma narrative). Abrupt changes in emotional intensity are particularly important to attend to: Sudden increases often signal hot spots in the trauma memory, whereas sudden decreases may be a sign of avoidance. Similarly, changes in the trauma narrative over time, such as adding in or leaving out details, altering the words that are used, or comments indicative of a shift in perspective, can provide important information about clients' progress.

The ability to mindfully observe clients' behavior as they engage in imaginal exposure is therefore a critical skill for you to develop. Mindfully observing anything for up to 45 minutes is a challenging task, let alone mindfully observing someone who may be in intense emotional distress as they recount horrifying trauma details. Your attention is likely to wander during imaginal exposure and at times you may even intentionally distract yourself from the upsetting trauma details that clients are sharing. In addition, you may have your own emotional reactions to the traumas that clients are describing that can pull your attention away from the client and onto your own experience. The ability to attend during imaginal exposure therefore requires a corresponding ability to step back and observe the client without becoming overly reactive or overwhelmed by what they are sharing. As in mindfulness in general, this requires repeated practice of noticing when your mind has wandered, not judging yourself for becoming distracted, and gently returning your attention again and again to the task of observing the client engage in this incredibly meaningful and challenging work.

Cheerleading

Clients often approach imaginal exposure with expectations of failure. They assume they will do it incorrectly, won't be able to tolerate the distress it evokes, and will slip back into old problem behaviors. At the same time, they often hold themselves to unrealistic standards, making it nearly inevitable that they will fail in their own mind. As a result, they are quick to criticize themselves, get discouraged, and want to quit. Given this, another key task of therapists during imaginal exposure is to keep clients' morale high and inspire them to keep going. In short, we cheerlead. Most often this is done by praising clients' efforts (e.g., "You're doing great!") and providing encouragement (e.g., "You can do this!"). These brief reinforcing comments are typically timed to minimize interruption (e.g., at the end of a repetition of the narrative) or are provided in moments when clients are struggling to continue (e.g., when they have paused in the retelling). Early in treatment—and particularly the first time clients engage in imaginal exposure—frequent praise and encouragement may be needed. As clients' ability to do imaginal exposure increases, your cheerleading can gradually be reduced, and ideally, replaced by clients encouraging and reinforcing themselves.

CLINICAL TIP

Differentiating between Cheerleading and Reassuring

Many clients will seek reassurance that imaginal exposure is safe and will not result in their anticipated negative outcomes. In addition, many therapists will feel compelled to provide reassurance (whether or not clients ask for it) by, for example, telling clients how unlikely it is that their feared outcomes will occur. Although some reassurance is reasonable, particularly early in treatment, repeatedly reassuring clients is likely to interfere with progress. For example, if a client believes they are likely to have a heart attack if they think and talk about their trauma, early in treatment you may provide them with corrective information about the actual physiological consequences of experiencing intense emotion—however, this type of reassurance needs to stop as treatment progresses. Repeated reassurance is likely to interfere with exposure because it prevents clients from fully exposing themselves to the feared stimulus, including being uncertain about whether the things they are afraid of will happen.

How can you cheerlead clients without reassuring them? It is important to understand the difference between cheerleading, which involves encouraging clients to engage in exposure and praising them for doing it, and reassuring clients that their feared outcomes will not occur. Whereas reassurance functions to lessen or remove clients' doubts or fears, cheerleading is focused on inspiring clients to do imaginal exposure even though they are afraid and doubtful. Although cheerleading can at times include some reassurance, this is typically limited to reassuring clients that they are capable of doing imaginal exposure as opposed to reassuring them about the likely outcomes of the exposure.

Avoid Reassuring	*Instead Cheerlead*
"Nothing bad is going to happen."	"You can cope with whatever happens."
"Don't worry, it's very unlikely [your feared outcome] will occur."	"It may or may not occur, and I think it's worth doing the exposure to find out."
"There's no need to be afraid."	"It's OK to be afraid."
"You are not in danger."	"I have faith that you will get through this."

Coaching

The final task therapists engage in during imaginal exposure is to provide coaching to shape and refine clients' behavior. As with any new behavior, clients need coaching to improve their skillfulness during imaginal exposure. In Session 3, it is typical for the trauma narrative to be lacking in detail and for clients to be engaging in a variety of avoidance behaviors as they describe what happened. In addition, clients may struggle at first to achieve effective levels of emotional engagement during imaginal exposure. Ultimately, the goal is for clients to describe their trauma in full detail, experience the emotions this elicits, and refrain from behaviors that function to prevent, escape, or minimize distress. However, given that this is the first time clients are doing imaginal exposure, you should primarily focus on reinforcing their efforts and encouraging them to continue, and not on trying to change the way in which they are doing imaginal exposure.

The main exception is that you may remind clients of the procedures if needed (e.g., to keep their eyes closed, use the present tense, and repeat the story once they have reached the end). In addition, if the initial trauma narrative is exceptionally brief or vague (e.g., "I went in the room and bad things happened"), you may ask clients to add at least some description of the traumatic event itself. Beyond this, you generally do not request changes during this first imaginal exposure and instead are thrilled at whatever clients are able to do. As treatment progresses, there will be plenty of time to provide coaching and corrective feedback—this is described in more detail in Chapter 12.

CLINICAL TIP
Taking Care of Yourself

While providing trauma-focused treatment can be very meaningful and rewarding, it can also be emotionally taxing. Therapists are expected to be open to hearing painful trauma details, and to appear calm and unflappable as clients describe their experiences of violence, abuse, and mistreatment. This can be challenging for any therapist and is likely to be particularly difficult if you are newer to this work or have a personal trauma history. You may feel overwhelmed, angry, and drained; become preoccupied with thoughts about clients and their traumas outside of work; and notice changes in your own beliefs about safety, trust, intimacy, and control. Below are some tips for coping with these reactions if they occur:

1. *Maintain self-awareness.* Recognize and monitor your own signs of stress. Don't ignore signs of increasing burnout, emotional distress, or avoidance.

2. *Remind yourself of what you tell your clients.* Trauma memories are not dangerous, and exposure works for therapists too. If you stick with it, it will get easier.

3. *Prioritize self-care.* Take mindful breaks during your workday. Find soothing, relaxing, and pleasurable activities to engage in outside of work. Reduce your vulnerability to stress by exercising, eating healthily, and getting enough sleep.

4. *Schedule wisely.* Be strategic about when you schedule DBT PE sessions. Consider scheduling breaks after these sessions, limiting the number of sessions you have in a day, or avoiding back-to-back DBT PE sessions.

5. *Accept your reactions.* Validate and normalize your emotional reactions. Don't judge your reactions for being too intense or not intense enough. Accept your reactions and be compassionate toward yourself.

6. *Get support.* Don't try to manage your reactions on your own. Get support from your consultation team during and between team meetings. Consider seeking your own personal therapy if needed.

7. *Use your skills.* Practice skills during imaginal exposure to help yourself stay focused on the client without becoming overwhelmed. Try paced breathing, sip a cold drink, encourage yourself, or use any other skill that helps you to stay present.

8. *Observe your limits.* Figure out your personal limits, such as the number of DBT PE clients you can treat at one time and the types of trauma that you will treat. Also, remember that doing trauma-focused treatment is not for everyone.

Complete the Exposure Recording Form (Peak and After Ratings)

As soon as the imaginal exposure is complete, clients are reinforced for doing the imaginal exposure and then asked to fill out the peak and after ratings on the Exposure Recording Form. Given that this is the first imaginal exposure, typically there is little evidence of change from pre- to post-exposure. Often probability and cost estimates remain inflated, urges to engage in problem behaviors are still present, emotions (particularly the unjustified ones) continue to be intense, and radical acceptance of the trauma is low. These ratings will be used to inform targeting during processing.

Case Example: Maria's First Imaginal Exposure

Maria's Exposure Recording Form is shown in Figure 11.1. Before starting imaginal exposure, her feared outcomes were that she would be unable to do the imaginal exposure (100% probability/100% cost), she would hate herself (100% probability/100% cost), and her therapist would think she was bad and gross (85% probability/100% cost). Before she started the imaginal exposure, she was having moderate urges to kill herself (2/5) and self-harm (3/5), and high urges to quit therapy (4/5). She rated her SUDS, fear, guilt, shame, and disgust as 100, whereas the justified emotions of sadness and anger, as well as radical acceptance, were low (0–20). Her therapist scanned these ratings but did not comment on them prior to starting the imaginal exposure.

Maria began the imaginal exposure quite tentatively, speaking softly and slowly with frequent pauses. She initially lapsed into the past tense when describing what happened and her therapist gently reminded her a few times to use the present tense. The first repetition of the narrative took about 8 minutes and Maria reported her SUDS were 100 the entire time. In total she completed four repetitions over 40 minutes and her SUDS decreased to an 85 by the end. Throughout the imaginal exposure she was visibly quite distressed, including crying at times, covering her face with her hands, and curling up in a ball in her chair. Her therapist offered frequent encouragement both during and at the end of each repetition, including telling Maria that she was doing a great job and to keep going. Although it was clear that Maria was avoiding at times (e.g., leaving out details in the trauma narrative), her therapist did not coach her to make any changes and instead focused on reinforcing her efforts.

Maria's description of the abusive episode included a lot of external details, such as the layout of the living room, the show that was playing on the TV, and the color of her father's shirt. As is typical in the early sessions, her description of the actual abuse itself was quite vague. She described some details of the physical violence that occurred, such as her father punching her mother in the stomach and slapping Maria in the face, as well as what her father had said to her, such as calling her a "bad child" and telling her she "deserved to be punished." After making her mother leave to go buy him more beer, Maria said that her father had taken her pants off to spank her. Although it was clear that he had also sexually abused her while he was spanking her, she did not specifically describe what he had done and instead said general things, such as "he touched me down there." The narrative included some description of Maria's behavior, including that she was crying and begging him to stop, but included few details about her internal experience except that she had been afraid and in physical pain. There were also several points when Maria said that she could not remember exactly what happened, but she kept going and focused on describing what she could remember.

Name: _Maria_   Date: _2/13_

Time started: _3:10_   Time stopped: _3:45_

Situation practiced: _Dad abused me and mom after I spilled his beer_

Exposure type (circle one): (Imaginal) / In vivo   Location (circle one): (In session) / Homework

Probability and Cost Estimates

What is the worst that could happen in this situation? (Be as specific as possible.)	How likely is it that this will happen? (0–100)		How bad would it be if this happened? (0–100)		Did this happen?
	Before	After	Before	After	Y or N
1. It will be too hard and I won't be able to do it	100	90	100	100	N
2. I will hate myself	100	100	100	100	Y
3. You will think I'm bad and gross	85	70	100	100	?

SUDS, Urges, and Dissociation

	SUDS (0–100)	Urge to kill myself (0–5)	Urge to self-harm (0–5)	Urge to quit therapy (0–5)	Urge to use substances (0–5)	Dissociation (0–100)
Before	100	2	3	4	0	20
Peak	100	3	5	5	0	50
After	85	2	4	3	0	30

Specific Emotions and Radical Acceptance

	Fear (0–100)	Guilt (0–100)	Shame (0–100)	Disgust (0–100)	Anger (0–100)	Sadness (0–100)	Joy (0–100)	Radical acceptance (0–100)
Before	100	100	100	100	0	20	0	20
After	60	100	100	100	5	30	10	30

What Did You Learn during This Exposure Task? _I was able to do it!_

FIGURE 11.1. Exposure Recording Form for Maria.

At the end of the imaginal exposure, her therapist immediately congratulated Maria on finishing, saying, "You did it! That was incredibly hard and I'm so proud of you!" She then handed Maria the Exposure Recording Form to complete the peak and after ratings (see Figure 11.1). Maria reported minimal changes in SUDS or the probability and cost estimates of her feared outcomes. Her urges to kill herself, self-harm, and quit therapy, as well as her state dissociation, had each increased during imaginal exposure before decreasing to lower levels at the end. Although her fear decreased from 100 to 60, the other unjustified emotions all remained at 100 at the end of imaginal exposure. She reported small increases in sadness, anger, and radical acceptance, as well as some joy for having succeeded at completing the imaginal exposure. Maria's therapist briefly scanned these ratings and then moved directly into processing.

CASE EXAMPLE DISCUSSION

Maria's experience was quite typical for the first session of imaginal exposure. Emotional distress remained high throughout the imaginal exposure, there were no notable shifts in her predictions about the likely outcomes of imaginal exposure, and urges to engage in problem behaviors were moderate to high. This lack of change is common in the first session: Corrective learning is typically gradual and requires multiple repetitions of imaginal exposure and processing. In addition, although Maria did a fantastic job of sticking with the imaginal exposure for the allotted time and allowing herself to experience intense emotions, there were clearly areas that could be targeted for improvement. For example, as is typical for the first imaginal exposure, Maria's trauma narrative included more external than internal details and was generally lacking in specificity, particularly in the most difficult moments. In addition, there were clear signs of avoidance at times, such as frequently pausing, speaking quietly, and covering her face with her hands.

As is expected for the first session of imaginal exposure, her therapist did not coach her to make any changes beyond reminding her to use the present tense. Instead, the therapist focused on cheerleading, reinforcing Maria's efforts, and paying close attention to both the content and process of the imaginal exposure while taking notes on the *Therapist Imaginal Exposure Recording Form*. These observations help to inform the coaching that will be provided in subsequent sessions as the therapist works to help Maria complete the imaginal exposure more and more effectively. In addition, the therapist gained critical information about the details of the abuse itself that provided her with additional insight into the potential beliefs and emotions fueling Maria's PTSD. For example, upon hearing that her father had called her a "bad child" and told her she deserved to be punished, the therapist began to more clearly understand how Maria came to view herself and her abuse in this way. In addition, the therapist listened to the trauma narrative for evidence that might help to disconfirm Maria's beliefs. For example, because she knew that Maria believed she was a bad child, the therapist took careful notes about how Maria had behaved effectively after she accidentally spilled her father's drink, such as by apologizing and helping to clean up the mess. These types of observations can often be used during processing to help clients reevaluate and challenge their beliefs to better fit the facts of what occurred. Overall, Maria's first imaginal exposure was a success as she achieved the goal of getting through the story, which is considered a triumph in the first session.

6. Conduct Processing of the Imaginal Exposure

Once imaginal exposure is complete, the next task of the session is to conduct processing. As with imaginal exposure, the overall goal of processing is to promote change in the problematic emotions and beliefs that are maintaining PTSD. However, these two procedures follow different pathways to achieve this goal. Imaginal exposure typically puts clients in emotion mind by eliciting intense emotions related to the trauma. In emotion mind, problematic trauma-related beliefs that are congruent with the current emotional state are present and it is difficult to think logically about the facts of the trauma. In contrast, processing involves activating reasonable mind by helping clients approach the trauma intellectually, analyze what happened, and reflect on what it means about themselves, others, and the world. Together the two procedures are used to help clients find their wise mind by integrating emotion and reason to find a balanced perspective on their trauma that reduces suffering.

In effect, processing can be thought of as DBT that is targeting trauma-related emotions and beliefs that are increasing misery and maintaining PTSD. Like DBT, processing is conducted in a principle-driven manner: There is considerable flexibility in terms of what is discussed and in what order, and therapists select strategies from DBT based on the theories underlying the treatment and the in-the-moment responses of the client. In the remainder of this chapter, I discuss the goals, common targets, general structure, and most common DBT therapist strategies that are used during processing.

The Function of Processing

Overall, the task of processing in DBT PE is conceptualized as emotion regulation—that is, the goal is to change the intensity of trauma-related emotions to levels that are justified and effective by helping clients to develop a more accurate and balanced perspective about the meaning of their trauma. At times, emotions change as a direct result of imaginal exposure without the need for targeting via processing. For example, imaginal exposure often provides information to directly disconfirm fear-related beliefs, such as that talking about trauma is dangerous and intense emotions will result in loss of behavioral control. For these types of beliefs, repeated imaginal exposure to the trauma memory may be all that is needed for the beliefs to change and fear to eventually dissipate.

Imaginal exposure alone is not always sufficient to change emotions, however, particularly those that are being driven by erroneous interpretations about the trauma, such as guilt, shame, and self-directed disgust. For these types of emotions, imaginal exposure is likely to activate the emotion and associated beliefs but may not provide information that directly disconfirms it. For example, simply describing a trauma out loud rarely leads clients to suddenly recognize that the trauma was not their fault or to stop viewing themselves as bad and disgusting people. Instead, these types of beliefs and the emotions they cause must be actively targeted during processing. Most often this is done by helping clients challenge their erroneous interpretations and acquire more accurate perspectives about their own and others' behavior during and after the trauma. Once new, more adaptive beliefs are present—even if only tenuously—therapists move to strengthen this new learning. This can be done by highlighting and reinforcing adaptive beliefs that clients generate, asking clients to elaborate on new insights, and giving feedback to shape and expand on new beliefs. Finally, it is not assumed that new learning will necessarily generalize to other traumas clients have experienced or to their life outside of therapy. Therefore, therapists also work to help clients actively apply new learning to make sense of other traumas and their life narrative more broadly, as well as to rehearse new learning outside of therapy.

In sum, processing functions to move clients along a path from initial *acquisition* of new learning (which may or may not develop as a direct result of imaginal exposure), to *strengthening* of this new learning so that it becomes more likely to be activated than previously held PTSD-related beliefs, and ultimately to *generalization* of new learning to all relevant contexts in the client's life. As an example, a client I treated who had been traumatically invalidated by her church community began DBT PE with the belief "I am bad because I questioned their values and was not faithful enough," which caused her to feel intense guilt and shame. Over the course of treatment, this belief initially shifted to "It's OK that my values were different than their values," before strengthening to "I didn't do anything wrong and I'm glad I stood up for what I believe in," and then generalizing to the more global belief "I'm proud of my values." These cognitive shifts each led to reductions in guilt and shame until eventually this memory no longer activated those emotions at all.

The Targets of Processing

The specific trauma-related emotions and beliefs that are targeted during processing are individually determined based on the content of the trauma narrative, ratings on the Exposure Recording Form, the client's in-session behavior, and the case formulation. Although the specific beliefs that clients hold vary, there are often more commonalities than differences in the ways that people with PTSD have interpreted their traumas. Table 11.3 includes common themes, specific beliefs, and associated emotions that are often targeted during processing.

The Structure of Processing

While there is considerable flexibility in processing, there is a general order in which things tend to occur during this portion of the session (see Table 11.4). Processing typically begins by reinforcing clients for completing the imaginal exposure and giving them positive feedback about their performance. The exact way in which this is done varies depending on what clients find to be reinforcing and may range from a brief "Nice work!" to more effusive praise, cheering, and high-fiving. If clients are experiencing extreme emotions that are likely to interfere with their ability to participate effectively in the more cognitive tasks of processing, you may also coach clients to use DBT skills to reduce arousal (e.g., TIP, self-soothe). If skills coaching is needed, it should be brief (e.g., a minute or two of paced breathing) with the goal of beginning processing as soon as possible. In most cases, skills coaching is not needed and clients are able to transition directly from imaginal exposure into processing. Before beginning the processing discussion, you should also review the client's ratings on the Exposure Recording Form and you may briefly comment on ratings that stand out in one way or another. A more in-depth discussion of the ratings is typically reserved until later in the processing discussion.

Processing typically begins by providing clients with an opportunity to share their reactions to the imaginal exposure and working to elicit the client's thoughts and emotions about the trauma. This is typically done by asking open-ended questions, such as "What did you notice during the imaginal exposure?"; "How do you feel about this event now?"; and "What stands out to you after telling that story today?" Clients' responses to these initial open-ended questions typically provide useful information about the trauma-related beliefs and emotions that are causing distress. For example, clients may say, "I just keep thinking that it was my fault," "I feel really ashamed," or "I'm so mad at myself for freezing." You can then use a wide range of DBT strategies to target the factors that are believed to be maintaining PTSD. As in DBT, there is no "right" way to respond and you will often have to use multiple strategies before finding one that is effective in helping clients begin to shift their perspective.

Once clients have had an opportunity to share their reactions, therapists typically become more directive in guiding the content of the processing discussion. This usually involves sharing your own observations and asking focused questions to test hypotheses about the mechanisms underlying the client's PTSD. For example, you may ask about moments in the trauma narrative when the client appeared particularly distressed (e.g., "You began to cry when you were describing what your mother said to you. What is it about that moment that is particularly upsetting?"), highlight problematic beliefs that were present in the client's description (e.g., "At

TABLE 11.3. Common Targets during Processing

Themes	Example beliefs	Common emotions
	Beliefs about others and the world	
Danger	• "The world is dangerous." • "I am likely to be attacked or assaulted." • "I have to be on guard all the time."	Fear, anger
Trust	• "People can't be trusted." • "If I trust someone, they will take advantage of me." • "You can never tell who will harm you."	Fear, anger
Intimacy	• "If I get close to someone, they will leave." • "People only want me for sex." • "I'm better off alone."	Fear, anger, sadness
Power	• "People always try to control me." • "I can't stop bad things from happening to me." • "There is no point in trying to stand up for myself."	Fear, anger, sadness
Judgment	• "People are bad and evil." • "Certain types of people (e.g., men, police) are bad and evil." • "People are selfish and only look out for themselves."	Anger, disgust
	Beliefs about the self	
Blame	• "I am responsible for causing the trauma." • "I blame myself for something I did during the trauma." • "I should have known better."	Guilt, anger
Loathing	• "I hate the kind of person I am." • "There is something innately wrong with me." • "I deserve to suffer."	Shame, anger
Disgust	• "I am dirty and gross." • "My body is repulsive." • "I am physically contaminated because of what happened."	Disgust, shame
Esteem	• "I am stupid, incompetent, and weak." • "I am worthless and don't deserve to be treated well." • "If I am not perfect all the time, I am a failure."	Shame, disgust
	Beliefs about emotions	
Control	• "I have to keep my emotions under control all the time." • "If I get upset, I will lose control over my behavior." • "I can't control my emotions."	Fear, shame
Tolerance	• "Feeling emotions is unbearable." • "I can't handle feeling distressed or upset." • "If I let myself have emotions, I won't be able to function."	Fear, shame
Duration	• "If I get upset, I will feel that way for a very long time." • "If I let myself feel something, it will never stop." • "If I think about my trauma, it will mess up my entire week."	Fear

TABLE 11.4. The Structure of Processing

1. Reinforce the client for completing imaginal exposure.
2. Coach the client to use DBT skills to reduce arousal (if needed).
3. Review the Exposure Recording Form and briefly comment on the ratings.
4. Ask open-ended questions to elicit the client's reactions to the imaginal exposure and target any problematic emotions and beliefs evident in their responses.
5. Ask focused questions to identify and target other problematic emotions and beliefs that are hypothesized to be maintaining PTSD based on ratings on the Exposure Recording Form and/or your own observations.
6. Consolidate new learning.

one point you said that you should have known better than to trust them. What did you mean by that?"), or comment on specific emotion ratings from the Exposure Recording Form (e.g., "Your shame is at 95. What are you feeling ashamed about?"). Once problematic trauma-related beliefs and emotions are identified, you will target them using a variety of DBT strategies to promote change (see below).

At some point during processing, therapists also discuss the ratings on the Exposure Recording Form in more detail, including explicitly commenting on the changes (or lack thereof) that occurred from pre- to post-exposure on key ratings with the goal of consolidating learning. For example, if SUDS remained high throughout the imaginal exposure, you may highlight this and reinforce learning about clients' ability to tolerate intense distress. Alternatively, if certain emotions reduced in intensity during imaginal exposure, you may point out these changes and emphasize that emotions will eventually decrease when not avoided. If feared outcomes did not occur, you may call attention to the discrepancy between the predicted and actual outcomes of exposure. On the other hand, if feared outcomes did occur, you may highlight that they were not as catastrophic as expected and clients were able to cope effectively with them. Essentially, no matter what occurs during imaginal exposure, it provides an opportunity for new learning that you can then reinforce and consolidate during processing.

The Strategies of Processing

Processing is typically the component of DBT PE that therapists feel least confident in delivering. This is due in large part to the fact that there are many DBT strategies that could be used, none of which are required and many of which may be reasonable depending on the context of the processing discussion. Whereas the rest of DBT PE is like a recipe that clearly specifies the ingredients and provides step-by-step instructions on how to mix them together, processing is like a choose-your-own adventure story with an infinite number of paths that could be followed and no way to know in advance which ones will lead to dead ends versus positive outcomes. Therefore, you have to choose strategies that you think will be most likely to help the client reach their desired destination, and when a dead end is reached, alter your course and try a different path forward.

Importantly, therapists do not select strategies at random or throw out comments arbitrarily. Although many strategies may be tried, processing is a targeted intervention during which you maintain a laser focus on identifying and addressing the problematic beliefs and emotions that are hypothesized to be maintaining the client's PTSD. Strategies are selected that are expected to produce change in these targets and many combinations of DBT strategies can be effective in producing the desired outcome. Therefore, it is less important which exact strategy is used in any given moment and more important that it is selected strategically to target the specific factors that are believed to be fueling the client's PTSD.

For some therapists, this description of the strategies of processing may be quite satisfying and provide you with a sufficiently clear idea of what to do and how to proceed. For others who (like me) prefer things to be more concrete, this description may feel overly vague and ambiguous. When I was first learning to conduct processing, its nebulousness felt overwhelming. I generally understood that the goal was to process the client's thoughts and emotions about their trauma, but what exactly did this mean? And what exactly was I supposed to do? In an effort to make processing more concrete, early in the development of DBT PE I completed DBT adherence coding on the processing portions of the DBT PE sessions that my team members and I were conducting. My goal was to identify the specific DBT strategies that we used most often and that seemed most effective in promoting change. After many hours spent watching and coding sessions, I discovered not only that processing in DBT PE *is* DBT (i.e., we were adherent to DBT while conducting processing) but that we were using and balancing many strategies from all three of DBT's paradigms: change, acceptance, and dialectics.

Next, I describe the DBT strategies that tend to be used most often during processing and then provide an example of how to apply strategies from each paradigm to a specific scenario.

Acceptance Strategies

Acceptance strategies form the foundation of processing and permeate all aspects of our interventions. If clients do not feel accepted and understood, particularly when they are being asked to discuss the most painful moments of their lives with us, processing is likely to grind to a halt. Thus, acceptance strategies are used early and often throughout processing to keep clients engaged in this challenging discussion and willing to work toward change.

Validation

All six levels of validation are regularly used to convey acceptance of the client and communicate that their reactions make sense. Therapists pay close attention to both the content and process of what clients are saying and doing (validation level 1) and use accurate reflection to communicate understanding of the client's experiences (validation level 2). Mind reading (validation level 3) may be used to bring unstated (and perhaps avoided) thoughts, emotions, and urges into the open so they can be discussed. For example, if you suspect clients are leaving out relevant details from the narrative, you can use mind reading to assess this (e.g., "Listening to you today made me wonder if you might have wanted your mom to suffer so that she would know what it was like to feel the way you were feeling"). When accurate, mind reading can be a profound experience for the client of feeling understood.

The higher levels of validation are often used to actively counteract clients' tendency to invalidate themselves and their experiences. For example, clients almost always judge the ways in which they responded at the time of their trauma. Validation level 4 can be used to highlight how these responses were understandable given their prior learning history (e.g., having been raised to believe that children should obey adults would predispose a child to comply with an adult abuser's demands) and biology (e.g., sexual arousal is a normal biological response to genital stimulation). Validation level 5 can be used to communicate that clients' responses are normal and make sense given the situation they were in at the time of the trauma (e.g., most people do not leave abusive relationships right away), as well as currently (e.g., many people find it embarrassing to talk about sex). Finally, you should strive to behave in a radically genuine manner by sharing your authentic reactions, treating clients as equals, and not adopting an overly professional or detached stance (validation level 6). For example, you might respond to a client's description of being ignored when they disclosed their sexual abuse to their mother by saying, "I can't begin to tell you how much I hate that you got that response! I really wish she had paid attention and given you the help you needed."

Reciprocal Communication

In terms of style, our default approach is to be warm, nurturing, and nonjudgmental. This includes being awake to clients' reactions, taking their perspectives seriously, and working collaboratively to decide how to move forward. In addition, we often use self-disclosure to strategically share our reactions with clients and model adaptive ways of thinking. For example, you may counteract clients' self-blame by sharing your own perspective on why the trauma was not the client's fault. In addition, therapists often disclose their thoughts and feelings when clients ask about them, and doing so would facilitate change. For example, if a client asks, "Do you feel disgusted by me?" you may disclose your feelings to disconfirm this expectation (e.g., "No, I respect you even more now that I know what you have been through"). As these examples illustrate, reciprocal communication strategies, although based in acceptance, can also lead to change by providing clients with a corrective learning experience. In particular, responding to clients with warmth, caring, and acceptance, especially after they have shared the details of their traumas, can help to actively correct some of the harm of prior negative disclosure experiences and invalidating environments more broadly.

Change Strategies

Although therapists often lead with acceptance, ultimately the goal is to help clients change the trauma-related emotions and beliefs that are keeping them stuck. To that end, therapists also utilize a variety of DBT change strategies during processing.

Problem Assessment

Before a problem can be changed, it must first be carefully assessed to ensure that it is accurately understood and specifically defined. In processing, this means that therapists often ask relevant questions to identify and clarify the specific emotions and problematic beliefs that clients have about their trauma. For example, if a client says something that seems indicative of a problematic belief (e.g., "I encouraged the abuse"), your first response is often to ask assessment questions, such as "How do you think you encouraged it?" These types of questions typically continue until you clearly understand and can describe the client's problematic belief and the reasons why they view it as accurate. For example, if the client above responds to the first question with "Because I consented," then you might ask another question, such as "What exactly did you consent to?" and so on until the client's way of thinking is clearly understood. In addition, therapists may generate and test hypotheses about the specific beliefs that are maintaining

PTSD. For example, you might respond to the above statement with a hypothesis, such as "By any chance did your abuser tell you that you encouraged him to do what he did to you?" Another commonly used assessment strategy is to highlight patterns of recurring thoughts and responses that are contributing to PTSD. For example, you might say, "Have you noticed how often you find ways to hold yourself and not your abuser responsible for your abuse?"

Problem Solving

Once a target has been assessed and is clearly defined, therapists then move to try to change it using standard DBT problem-solving strategies. This often includes providing clients with didactic information about topics relevant to the problem to increase knowledge and insight about their own experiences. You might impart knowledge via discussion and/or by providing clients with articles or books to read, podcasts to listen to, or videos to watch on topics such as sibling incest, sexual functioning in sexual trauma survivors, and common abusive tactics used by intimate partners. When a problem is identified (e.g., intense shame), you can help the client to generate and evaluate potential solutions (e.g., the skill of opposite action) and drag out new behavior (e.g., ask clients to practice this skill in session). Knowledge and solutions discussed in session are then actively generalized to relevant contexts in the client's life, such as by asking the client to implement the solution in multiple settings. Homework assignments, including *in vivo* exposure tasks and listening to the imaginal exposure, also function to help generalize new learning to the client's life more broadly.

Cognitive Modification

Of the core problem-solving strategies in DBT, cognitive modification tends to be used most often during processing given the focus on changing maladaptive trauma-related beliefs. A necessary first step is to help the client become aware of their own cognitions and styles of thinking. You can do this by asking clients to observe and describe their thoughts and beliefs and highlighting maladaptive beliefs when they arise. When a problematic belief is identified, you can actively help the client to reevaluate their thinking and challenge their belief. This may be done in any number of ways, such as by calling the client's attention to disconfirming information (e.g., facts in the trauma narrative that don't match the client's interpretations), using the Socratic method (e.g., asking questions to help clients evaluate the accuracy of their thoughts), providing corrective information (e.g., via psychoeducation), and selling more adaptive thinking styles (e.g., highlighting the pros and cons of changing their way of thinking).

The final step is to help clients generate new, more adaptive beliefs to replace the old problematic ones. Whenever possible, it is preferable for clients to generate new beliefs themselves as these are likely to be more believable and personally meaningful. However, when clients are unable to identify more adaptive ways of thinking, therapists may eventually directly suggest more functional beliefs. This more directive approach to cognitive modification is often needed when clients lack any prior experience or model that would enable them to conceive of a different perspective. For example, many clients do not have any experiences to draw upon that would help them to view themselves as competent, lovable, and worthwhile people. In such cases, we may initially need to directly suggest more validating ways of thinking about themselves. However, this should be titrated as treatment progresses and clients should be increasingly expected to self-generate new ways of thinking.

Irreverent Communication

Although our default style during processing is reciprocal warmth and responsiveness, irreverent communication strategies are also used and serve an important function. Therapists use a very matter-of-fact manner to discuss all aspects of clients' trauma, including the details of the event itself, the client's responses during the event, and their present-day reactions to what occurred. For example, you will need to "plunge in where angels fear to tread" with straightforward questions and responses to discuss potentially sensitive topics, such as the sexually explicit details of a rape and the ways in which clients may have increased their risk of experiencing trauma. The function of being matter-of-fact when talking about sensitive topics is to convey that there is nothing too difficult to talk about: We are not shocked by clients' experiences and clients are not too fragile to talk about them.

In addition, therapists sometimes directly confront dysfunctional thoughts, behaviors, and emotional responses. This direct confrontation functions to get the client's attention, highlight the seriousness of the problem, and communicate a sense of urgency to change it. For example, you might say, "Constantly saying you are stupid is completely unhelpful and makes you miserable—you have got to stop talking about yourself that way!" Unorthodox irreverence is also used at times to address particularly entrenched beliefs and associated emotions (e.g., intense self-loathing and shame) by saying something unexpected, extreme, or humorous in response. For example, if a client who was forced to perform oral sex on her brother says, "I'm disgusting because I made my brother orgasm," an irreverent response could be "Thank God you were able to make him orgasm! Think how much longer it would have lasted if he hadn't!" Such irreverent responses function to help the client see a completely different point of view and get unstuck from styles of thinking that are particularly resistant to change. It is important to remember that irreverence is typically balanced with validation, requires a strong therapeutic relationship, and is often reserved for problems that are particularly intractable.

Dialectical Strategies

During processing, therapists maintain an overall balanced and dialectical approach while also using specific dialectical strategies to create movement when the client is stuck, transform rigid and extreme positions into more flexible and balanced ones, and highlight and synthesize opposites when they arise.

Dialectical Approach

As in DBT, therapists remain balanced between change and acceptance during processing, including balancing acceptance of clients' problematic beliefs and emotions as they are with efforts to change them. This means that within each topic area, and across the session as a whole, both acceptance- and change-oriented strategies are used. For example, when a problematic belief is identified, you may initially respond with validation before moving to try to change it. In addition, therapists maintain a balanced style that involves using both reciprocal and irreverent communication strategies. Overall, therapists move with speed and flow during processing, utilizing a variety of strategies and styles, alternating quickly between them as needed, and keeping the client slightly off balance to promote change.

Specific Dialectical Strategies

Given the chronic and overlearned nature of most of our clients' trauma-related beliefs, it is to be expected that impasses will be reached when attempting to change them. For example, clients may hold rigidly to beliefs that are clearly dysfunctional and you and your clients may become polarized over whose view of reality is more accurate. When such impasses occur, dialectical strategies that magnify the tension between opposites can help to get unstuck and create movement toward a less extreme position. For example, you might use devil's advocate (i.e., arguing in favor of a maladaptive belief in an extreme way that pulls for the client to argue against it), extending (i.e., taking the client's statement literally and more seriously than they do), activating wise mind (e.g., asking the client what they know to be true in their own wise mind), and making lemonade out of lemons (e.g., turning something that seems problematic into a strength). You can also use metaphors, analogies, and stories to reframe a problem and open up new possibilities for change. When polarities arise, you should model dialectical thinking by acknowledging the validity in both sides of the issue, searching for what is left out, and working to find a synthesis.

Table 11.5 provides an example of how multiple DBT strategies could be used during processing to target a particular problematic belief.

Case Example: Maria's First Processing

Below is an excerpt from the processing discussion between Maria and her therapist that occurred after she completed her first imaginal exposure. The DBT strategies that are used are specified in parentheses.

THERAPIST: I'm so impressed with you for sticking with the exposure and really allowing yourself to experience some very intense emotions! What was that experience like for you? (*reinforcement, asks relevant question*)

MARIA: It was really hard, and I really wanted to stop, especially the first time I told the story. I'm surprised I was able to keep going and do it.

THERAPIST: That's actually one of the things you were afraid of—that it would be too hard and you wouldn't be able to do it. What do you think now? (*assesses cognitions*)

MARIA: I guess I'm stronger than I thought I was. There were some moments when I really thought I couldn't take it anymore, but then I just kept going. By the third and fourth time it started to get a little bit easier.

THERAPIST: It sounds like you learned two really important things already. One is that you were more able to tolerate thinking and talking about your abuse than you thought you would be. And the other is that by sticking with it rather than avoiding, it got a little bit easier by the end. (*consolidates learning*)

MARIA: Yes, I guess that's true.

THERAPIST: It looks like what really changed was your fear, which dropped from 100 to 60. What made your fear come down? (*emotion focus, asks relevant question*)

MARIA: I was really afraid of doing it since I hadn't ever done it before. I thought I was going to go crazy or something. But after I told it a few times and nothing terrible happened, then it wasn't as scary.

TABLE 11.5. Applying DBT Strategies during Processing

The scenario

The client is an adult woman who was sexually abused by her stepfather from the ages of 6 to 12. For most of the time she was being abused, the client did not view the abuse as a problem because it was done in a nonviolent and seemingly caring way. She first began to realize the abuse was a problem when she was 12 and was exposed to information about sex in school and from peers. She then began to protest against her stepfather's advances, which led him to stop abusing her. During processing, the client expresses the following belief: "I should have realized sooner that what we were doing was wrong."

Potential DBT strategies

Below are examples of strategies that could be used to respond to the client in this scenario. Keep in mind that there is no right answer: Any of these strategies (as well as many others), applied alone or in combination, could be a reasonable way to target this problematic belief.

Acceptance strategies

"You think you should have been aware at a younger age that what your stepfather was doing to you was not OK." (*Validation Level 2*)

"It must be really painful to think that if you had realized sooner that the abuse was wrong that you might have been able to stop it earlier." (*Validation Level 3*)

"It is understandable that you didn't know it was wrong given your history of being told by your stepfather that it was normal and not a problem." (*Validation Level 4*)

"It is really common for children who are being sexually abused to not realize the abuse is a problem until they are older." (*Validation Level 5*)

"I didn't learn about sex until I took a sex education class in school in sixth grade. I wouldn't have known it was wrong before then either." (*self-disclosure*)

Change strategies

"Why do you think you should have known it was wrong?" (*assesses cognitions*)

"How is it understandable that you didn't realize it was a problem until you were 12?" (*generates new cognitions*)

"You were a child who had been taught to believe it was OK by an adult you trusted. How in the world could you have known it was wrong?" (*challenges cognitions*)

"In the United States, the legal age that people can consent to sex varies from 16 to 18 across states. These laws exist because younger children are not mature enough to know whether sex is right or wrong." (*provides didactic information*)

"Your elementary school must have had very advanced sex education!" (*irreverence*)

Dialectical strategies

"You think that as a child you should have known it was wrong and at the same time you don't seem to think that your stepfather who was an adult should have known it was wrong. How does that make sense?" (*magnifies tension*)

"Thinking you should have known the abuse was wrong when your stepfather told you it was OK is like thinking that children should not believe in Santa Claus when their parents tell them he exists." (*metaphor/analogy*)

THERAPIST: Well, that's another great thing to have learned! Feeling intense emotions can be really hard, but it's not dangerous. So, what are you thinking about this event now as you look back on what happened? (*reinforcement, assesses cognitions*)

MARIA: I just feel like it was my fault. If I had been more careful, none of this would have happened.

THERAPIST: So, you're blaming yourself for what happened. Is that why your guilt is so high—a 100? (*observes and describes cognition, emotion focus*)

MARIA: Yes.

THERAPIST: What do you mean when you say you should have been more careful? (*assesses cognitions*)

MARIA: I should have been more careful not to bump into the table. If I hadn't spilled his drink, he wouldn't have hit my mom or abused me.

THERAPIST: OK, so the reason you think this was your fault is because you accidentally spilled his drink, which led him to get angry and violent. (*validation level 2*)

MARIA: Yes.

THERAPIST: Did the spill cause a lot of damage? (*asks relevant question*)

MARIA: No. It spilled on the floor, but I cleaned it up and it didn't leave any stains or anything.

THERAPIST: So, it was an accident, it didn't cause any serious damage, and you immediately repaired the mistake by cleaning it up. (*validation level 2*)

MARIA: Yes, but I still think I deserved to be punished for making a mess.

THERAPIST: Do you think beating and sexually abusing a child is a reasonable punishment for accidentally spilling a drink? (*challenges cognitions*)

MARIA: No, I guess not when you say it like that.

THERAPIST: What do you think would have been a reasonable punishment for spilling a drink? (*generates new cognitions*)

MARIA: Maybe making me go to my room or giving me extra chores.

THERAPIST: That sounds more reasonable to me. Although personally, I'm not convinced that any punishment was needed. If one of my kids spilled a drink on accident, I would be satisfied if they did exactly what you did: apologize and clean it up. (*reinforcement, self-disclosure, challenges cognitions*)

MARIA: Really?

THERAPIST: Yes. It is normal for kids to make messes. And when it is minor and an accident, I don't think it necessarily has to be punished. (*validation level 5, challenges cognitions*)

MARIA: Well, I still feel like if I hadn't made the mess, then none of this would have happened.

THERAPIST: I can see why you would think that. It does seem like spilling your dad's drink is what prompted him to get angry in that moment. (*validation level 5*)

MARIA: So how is it not my fault then?

THERAPIST: Did you intend to cause him to hurt you and your mom? (*asks relevant question*)

MARIA: No, of course not!

THERAPIST: Do you think your dad intended to hurt you? (*asks relevant question*)

MARIA: Yes, he said we deserved to be punished.

THERAPIST: So, if he hurt you on purpose and you didn't intend for him to do that, it doesn't seem reasonable to blame yourself for his behavior. (*direct confrontation*)

MARIA: Maybe not, but I just wish I hadn't provoked him.

THERAPIST: That makes sense to me too. I bet you tried really hard not to upset him. (*validation levels 5 and 3*)

MARIA: I always tried to be good, but I always ended up doing something wrong and then he would get mad at me.

THERAPIST: He sounds kind of like a jack-in-the-box. At some point you knew he was going to jump out and scare you, but you never knew exactly when it was going to happen. Was it hard to predict when your dad would get angry or abusive? (*metaphor, asks relevant question*)

MARIA: Sometimes it happened out of the blue, especially when he was drinking. But other times it would happen because my mom or I did something to upset him.

THERAPIST: No wonder you felt like you had to be perfect all the time! Even a small mistake like spilling a drink could trigger him to extreme violence. Do you think it's possible he would have gotten violent that day even if you hadn't spilled his drink? (*validation level 5, challenges cognition*)

MARIA: I guess it's possible. The more he drank, the more likely he was to get violent. And he had already been drinking for awhile when this happened.

THERAPIST: It sounds like there really wasn't any foolproof way to prevent him from abusing you and your mom on this day or in general. (*challenges cognition*)

MARIA: I just hate thinking that though.

THERAPIST: Why do you hate thinking that? (*assesses cognitions*)

MARIA: Because I'd rather believe that I could have done something to prevent it than think that it was unavoidable.

THERAPIST: I get that. In some ways it feels better to think you had some control over your dad's behavior, even when it makes you feel guilty and terrible about yourself, than it does to accept that you couldn't stop him from abusing you and your mom. (*validation level 5, clarifies contingencies*)

MARIA: Yeah, I don't like thinking that I was powerless to protect myself.

THERAPIST: Well, that's the other extreme, right? Either you always should have been able to prevent your dad from hurting you or you were completely powerless and unable to protect yourself. What would be a more balanced perspective? (*highlighting polarities, working for a synthesis*)

MARIA: Sometimes I was able to stop my dad from getting angry and violent and sometimes I was not.

THERAPIST: That sounds more accurate. And why do you think you couldn't prevent him from getting angry and violent in this event? (*reinforcement, generates new cognitions*)

MARIA: Because what I did was an accident, I didn't mean to do it. And he was drunk, which made it more likely that he would escalate.

THERAPIST: I agree. You did not intend to upset him and it sounds like even small things could make him angry and violent, particularly when he was drunk. Also, as you said earlier, physical and sexual abuse is not an appropriate punishment for spilling a drink. In my opinion, abusing children is never appropriate under any circumstance. (*reinforcement, strengthens cognition*)

MARIA: I hear what you're saying, and I can see why it might not be my fault, but it still feels like it's my fault.

THERAPIST: That's understandable. You've been blaming yourself for this for years and I don't expect that to change in one session. I'm just glad that you're starting to see that there may be other ways to view this situation, even if you're not yet sure you believe them. (*validation level 5, shaping*)

CASE EXAMPLE DISCUSSION

This excerpt provides an example of the general structure, goals, targets, and strategies of processing. The therapist began with reinforcing Maria for completing the imaginal exposure and then asking an open-ended question about her experience. As is common in Session 3, Maria responded by talking about how difficult it had been to do imaginal exposure for the first time. The therapist validated the difficulty of the task and then highlighted and strengthened the new learning that had occurred. In particular, she called attention to the discrepancy between Maria's prediction that she wouldn't be able to tolerate doing imaginal exposure and what had actually occurred. In addition, she highlighted how approaching rather than avoiding the trauma memory had resulted in some habituation of fear and that nothing bad or dangerous had happened.

After debriefing the experience of doing imaginal exposure, the therapist asked a second, more targeted question to elicit Maria's thoughts about the trauma itself. This resulted in Maria expressing a problematic belief—namely, that it had been her fault that her father had abused her and her mother, and she should have been able to prevent it. The therapist initially responded by labeling the belief as self-blaming and linking it to Maria's high rating of guilt on the Exposure Recording Form. She then assessed the belief in more detail, asking a relevant question to identify exactly why Maria thought it was her fault. Once the problematic belief was clearly defined, the therapist began to work to help Maria reevaluate her thinking. Rather than directly confronting the belief or suggesting alternatives, the therapist started by asking a series of Socratic questions (e.g., "Do you think beating and sexually abusing a child is a reasonable punishment for accidentally spilling a drink?") to stimulate Maria to think more critically about what had actually happened. As Maria began to generate more adaptive beliefs (e.g., identifying less severe forms of punishment that may have been appropriate), the therapist strengthened these beliefs by sharing her own perspective (e.g., "That sounds more reasonable to me"). The therapist also used self-disclosure to further stimulate Maria's thinking by sharing what they would have done with their own kids. After building the case against Maria's belief, the therapist then directly confronted and challenged the belief by saying, "So, if he hurt you on purpose, and you didn't intend for him to do that, it doesn't seem reasonable to blame yourself for his behavior."

When presented with this alternative perspective, Maria expressed reluctance to let go of her self-blaming belief because she thought she had provoked her father's violence. When this impasse was reached, the therapist shifted from her heavily change-oriented approach to acceptance by validating how Maria's efforts to not provoke her father made sense. She then began using dialectical strategies to try to get her unstuck, including using a metaphor of a jack-in-the-box to illustrate the unpredictability of her father's behavior, as well as highlighting and synthesizing the extremes of always being able to prevent him from hurting her versus being completely powerless to protect herself. By the end of this discussion, Maria was beginning to see that there might be another way to view this situation, even though she still felt as if it was her fault. The therapist normalized this difficulty changing a long-held belief and reinforced Maria's willingness to consider other potential perspectives.

Overall, this example illustrates how processing is a targeted intervention that aims to identify and change problematic trauma-related beliefs and emotions that are contributing to maintaining PTSD. In this process, therapists use a variety of change, acceptance, and dialectical strategies from DBT in a balanced and principle-driven manner to promote change.

7. Assign Homework

After processing is complete, the final task of the session is to assign homework. In Session 3, it is typical for the *in vivo* exposure tasks that were assigned in Session 2 to still be eliciting moderate to high levels of distress. As a result, clients are often assigned the same tasks to continue working on as homework, but you and the client may select one or more new tasks if desired (to increase variability and/or if habituation has occurred). In addition, clients are asked to listen to the imaginal exposure recording daily and to the entire session recording once, and to use skills from their Post-Exposure Skills Plan as needed. You can review the client's plan for what they are going to do after this first imaginal exposure session and potentially schedule a phone check-in for later in the day. It may also be helpful to plan to check in via phone at other times before the next session to discuss and reinforce progress with homework.

SESSION 3 HOMEWORK ASSIGNMENTS

1. Listen to the recording of the imaginal exposure (ideally daily).*

2. Continue *in vivo* exposure (at least two tasks, ideally doing one per day).

3. Use the Post-Exposure Skills Plan as needed.

4. Listen to the entire session recording one time.

*Note. It may also be useful for the client to listen to the processing discussion.

CHAPTER 12

Intermediate Sessions (Sessions 4+)

SESSIONS 4+ COMPONENTS AND TIME ESTIMATES

	60-minute session	90-minute session
Review the DBT diary card and set the session agenda	3 min.	3–5 min.
Review homework	5–10 min.	10–15 min.
Orient to the imaginal exposure planned for the session	3 min.	3–5 min.
Conduct imaginal exposure	20–30 min.	30–45 min.
Conduct processing of the imaginal exposure	20–30 min.	30–45 min
Assign homework	3–5 min.	5–10 min.

From Session 4 until the final session of DBT PE, each session includes the same components and most of the time is spent conducting repeated imaginal exposure and processing. Although these intermediate sessions are identical in structure, the topics that are addressed vary based on the exposure tasks that are being completed and the trauma-related emotions and beliefs that are being processed. Nonetheless, these sessions can feel repetitive and clients' morale is likely to wax and wane, often increasing as the beneficial effects of treatment become apparent and decreasing in moments when change is slow or certain emotions and insights are particularly painful. Thus, you need to be prepared to boost your clients' morale when it flags and keep them motivated to continue until they achieve their goals. Across these sessions, you also need to closely monitor your client's progress and make data-driven adjustments to tailor your interventions to most effectively target the factors that are maintaining their PTSD. In this chapter, I discuss the progression of imaginal exposure and processing across the intermediate sessions, highlight key clinical decisions that must be made, and describe the typical course of change. A session checklist is provided in Appendix C.

1. Review the DBT Diary Card and Set the Session Agenda

Each session begins with a brief review of the DBT diary card that is primarily focused on ensuring that no higher-priority behaviors have occurred that would warrant pausing the treatment (see Chapter 14 for details). During the first several weeks of imaginal exposure, it is not unusual for clients to report increases in various urges, emotions, and PTSD symptoms that may be tracked on the diary card. If these kinds of initial exacerbations occur, clients can be reassured that this is not unusual and usually lasts no more than a few weeks until the treatment begins to work. As DBT PE progresses, it is typical to see urges and problem behaviors decline to levels that are lower than they were before DBT PE. After reviewing the diary card, an agenda is quickly set that specifies the planned components of the session.

> **CLINICAL TIP**
> ### Outcome Monitoring
>
> You should continue to monitor outcomes throughout the intermediate sessions. At a minimum, this includes having clients complete a PTSD measure (e.g., the PTSD Checklist) every other week (e.g., Sessions 5, 7, 9). In addition, you may ask clients to complete a measure of another relevant outcome (e.g., posttraumatic cognitions, trauma-related shame) on alternate weeks (e.g., Sessions 4, 6, 8). These outcome measures are typically given to clients prior to the session and then briefly reviewed along with the DBT diary card. A list of potential measures can be found in Appendix D.

2. Review Homework

Starting in Session 4 and continuing throughout the intermediate sessions, homework review involves discussing *in vivo* and imaginal exposure tasks that were completed since the last session. Assuming at least moderate levels of homework completion, you need to review multiple homework assignments and completed Exposure Recording Forms in the 5–15 minutes allotted for this in each session. In the prior chapter, I reviewed strategies for how to review homework efficiently and effectively and I now focus on the functions of homework review in the intermediate sessions.

Contingency Management

It is important to emphasize that a large majority of the exposure tasks that clients complete during DBT PE are done as homework outside of session. Thus, for clients to get a sufficient dose of exposure for PTSD to improve, they must complete homework consistently. Allotting time at the beginning of each session to review homework functions both to hold clients accountable for homework assignments and to provide an opportunity to reinforce homework completion. If clients are completing little homework and their overall progress in treatment is minimal or slow, then increasing the level of homework completion is likely to be an important intervention to improve outcomes (see Chapter 14).

> ### CLINICAL TIP
> #### How Much Exposure Homework Is Enough?
>
> The standard homework assignments in PE involve asking clients to complete daily *in vivo* and imaginal exposure. This means that perfect adherence to homework would require clients to complete at least two exposure tasks per day, which would likely involve spending an hour or more doing exposure. I'm sure it will not come as a surprise to learn that few clients complete this much exposure homework. The good news is that perfect homework adherence is not necessary for the treatment to work. For example, a study of standard PE found that clients who were at least moderately adherent to imaginal exposure homework assignments (two to five times per week) reported more improvement than those who completed fewer assignments (zero to one time per week), but did not differ from those with higher adherence (six to seven times per week) (Cooper et al., 2017). This suggests that you should continue to ask for and reinforce high levels of homework completion *and* be satisfied as long as clients are moderately adherent to homework and showing steady improvement in PTSD.

Progress Monitoring

As the intermediate sessions progress, you should review homework with an eye toward determining the degree to which the mechanisms that are hypothesized to be maintaining the client's PTSD are changing. Is overall distress (SUDS) getting lower across repeated trials of the same task? Are unjustified emotions (e.g., fear, guilt, shame) decreasing in intensity over time? Are probability and cost estimates of feared outcomes being corrected? This information is obtained during homework review and plays a key role in monitoring progress and determining when changes to the interventions may be needed.

Coaching

Therapists also provide coaching during homework review to help clients improve the skillfulness with which they are completing their between-session exposure tasks, particularly if progress is slow. To do this, you need to ask clients to specifically describe what they are doing as they complete homework tasks. This may include asking clients to describe the task itself (e.g., What exactly is the cue they are approaching? Where are they doing the task? How long are they doing it for?), their own behaviors (e.g., Are their eyes open or closed? Are they engaging in any safety behaviors?), and their internal experience (e.g., What are they thinking about while they do the task? What emotions or physical sensations are they aware of?). Armed with these behavioral assessment data, you can then provide specific coaching to help clients improve the effectiveness of their between-session exposure.

3. Orient to the Imaginal Exposure Planned for the Session

In each session, you will briefly orient the client to the imaginal exposure that is planned for that session. This typically includes specifying the memory or hot spot you would like the client to focus on and, when needed, reminding how imaginal exposure is done (e.g., eyes closed, present tense). Prior to starting imaginal exposure, therapists also typically give coaching feedback to help clients improve the effectiveness of this core treatment procedure. (Information about how to provide coaching is included in the next section.) Overall, the goal is for clients to be clear about what they are being asked to do prior to starting imaginal exposure.

4. Conduct Imaginal Exposure

In the intermediate sessions, clients continue to complete imaginal exposure while you provide coaching and reinforcement to help them do so with increasing skillfulness. As clients progress through these sessions, several key clinical decisions need to be made, including when to (1) transition from the full trauma narrative to hot spots, (2) switch from one trauma memory to another, and (3) move to the final session of DBT PE.

Improving the Effectiveness of Imaginal Exposure

In contrast to Session 3 in which therapists largely refrain from providing coaching, in the intermediate sessions you will provide clients with feedback to shape and improve the skillfulness with which they complete imaginal exposure. The ultimate goal is for clients to describe their trauma in full detail while allowing themselves to experience the emotions this elicits without avoiding. In the early sessions, most clients struggle to do imaginal exposure in an optimal way, and it is through direct and behaviorally specific coaching paired with reinforcement that clients improve their skillfulness over time. It is also important to note that many clients require minimal coaching to do imaginal exposure effectively and you should generally adopt a "less is more" approach, allowing the client to direct the focus and pace of the imaginal exposure as much as possible, while providing corrective feedback when needed to address issues likely to significantly impede progress.

What to Target for Coaching

There are two main areas in which therapists provide coaching to improve the effectiveness of imaginal exposure: (1) increasing the amount of detail in the trauma narrative and (2) reducing avoidance. In some cases, additional coaching may also be needed to address specific problems that may arise during imaginal exposure (e.g., difficulties with emotional engagement)—this is discussed in detail in Chapter 14.

1. Filling in the Details

It is the norm rather than the exception for the trauma narrative to initially be lacking in detail, to have obvious gaps, and/or to be hard to follow in some sections. This may be due to a variety of factors, such as the client's uncertainty about how to do imaginal exposure, avoidance of details that are particularly distressing, and fragmented trauma memories. As treatment progresses, the goal is for clients to fully describe everything they can remember about the traumatic event in a moment-to-moment fashion without leaving anything out. By recounting the trauma in detail, clients learn that they can tolerate thinking about all aspects of their experience and they are likely to develop new insights about what happened to them. The progression from a vague and disjointed to a detailed and coherent trauma narrative is often achieved by providing coaching.

In the early sessions of imaginal exposure, it is often obvious that pieces are being left out of the trauma narrative and these omissions typically occur in the most difficult moments of the event. For example, a client who was raped may describe in detail the events leading up to and following the rape—however, the rape itself may only be briefly described (e.g., "He started having sex with me. This went on for a while until he stopped"). In addition, clients often leave out details of their internal experience (emotions, thoughts, physical sensations) and instead focus primarily on describing the external situation. When the trauma narrative is less detailed than desired, this is usually resolved by providing specific instructions to add the missing details, as well as by asking brief questions during the imaginal exposure to elicit these details when needed (e.g., "What emotion are you having in that moment?" or "Where did he touch you?").

CLINICAL TIP
What If the Trauma Narrative Is Too Long?

There is no way to know in advance how long it will take clients to describe the full trauma narrative and you may discover that the narrative is longer than would be ideal (e.g., it takes 30 minutes to get through one iteration). This is particularly likely to occur for clients who experienced a trauma that lasted multiple hours. If it is necessary to shorten the trauma narrative, it is typically preferable to choose a later start point and/or an earlier end point rather than asking clients to be less detailed. Once you have heard the full story, it may be clearer how the narrative could be trimmed without removing any central elements. For example, if a client went to a bar with friends and left several hours later with a man who took her to his apartment and raped her, it may be reasonable to shorten the narrative to leave out a description of what occurred in the bar and instead start when she entered his apartment. Alternatively, if the narrative includes a description of events that happened after the acute trauma was over (e.g., after raping her the perpetrator drove the client back to the bar to rejoin her friends), then the end point could be moved closer to when the acute trauma ended. In some cases, the event may include two or more separate events that are connected and both traumatic, but that occurred hours apart (e.g., a rape followed by being forced to make a report to the police later that night). In these cases, you may need to divide the narrative into two events and target them separately (or address one via imaginal exposure and the other during processing). If the narrative is shortened, the portion that is retained should include the most distressing moments, as well as the most significant meaning elements (i.e., the details most associated with the client's primary problematic beliefs and emotions about the event).

At times, it can be hard to determine whether clients are leaving out details. For example, the client may be vividly describing the trauma and there may not be any clear gaps or missing pieces. However, you may have a gut feeling that something is being left out or the pieces don't seem to quite add up. In addition, if the client is not improving as much as desired, this can be a sign that an important detail is being omitted. When you suspect something is being left out, it can be challenging to address due to fear of invalidating clients' efforts or appearing to doubt the accuracy of what they are sharing. However, it is a disservice to clients to allow this type of avoidance to go on without intervention as it is likely to limit the effectiveness of treatment. Thus, you need to directly ask clients whether they are leaving something out in a nonjudgmental way, while also offering validation as to why they may be motivated to do so.

CLINICAL TIP

What If My Client Can't Remember Some Details of What Happened?

The amount of detail that clients remember about their traumas varies widely with some clients having a nearly photographic memory of the entire event from start to finish, whereas others may remember only a few bits and pieces of what occurred. Most clients fall somewhere in the middle: They can clearly recall many details of the event and there are some pieces they do not remember clearly or at all. Difficulty recalling aspects of a traumatic event can be caused by things such as the amount of time that has passed since the trauma occurred, where they focused their attention during the trauma, the presence of factors likely to disrupt memory encoding (e.g., dissociation, intoxication, head injury), and chronic efforts to avoid thinking about the trauma.

Given that a common avoidance strategy during imaginal exposure is to omit details that are particularly upsetting, it is important that you first assess whether missing pieces in the trauma narrative are due to avoidance versus forgetting. If the issue is that clients do not remember certain details, do not attempt to get them to fill in these gaps in the trauma narrative—instead, encourage them to describe only what they can recall. It may also be helpful to normalize the inability to remember some details as a common PTSD symptom, and to remind clients that the goal is to help them be able to live with the details they do remember. At times, clients will attempt to fill in holes in the trauma narrative by describing things they do not remember, such as their assumptions about what happened or details that other people told them about later. If you discover that clients have included elements in the trauma narrative that they do not actually remember, then you should instruct them to take out these elements and describe only what they directly recall.

It is also important to note that over the course of imaginal exposure most clients do remember more details about what happened. Although imaginal exposure is not intended to help clients remember forgotten details of their trauma, additional details often naturally emerge as clients allow themselves to fully think about the trauma memory. Sometimes these newly remembered details are peripheral to the event (e.g., the color of the carpet) and sometimes they are central to understanding what occurred (e.g., realizing that the perpetrator made them promise not to tell anyone what had happened). When new details are remembered, clients should be instructed to add them to the trauma narrative to make the story as complete as possible.

Case Example

As described in Chapter 11, when Maria first completed imaginal exposure the trauma narrative clearly lacked details, particularly about the sexual abuse, as well as her internal experience throughout the event. In Session 4, her therapist decided to focus first on increasing her description of the details of her internal experience, and to wait until subsequent sessions to target increasing her use of behaviorally specific language when describing the sexual abuse. Below is a brief excerpt in which the therapist provided coaching to Maria prior to starting imaginal exposure in Session 4.

THERAPIST: You truly did an amazing job last week with the imaginal exposure! I was so impressed at how much you shared about what happened, as well as the fact that you stuck with it for 40 minutes even though it was incredibly distressing.

MARIA: Thank you, it was really, really hard.

THERAPIST: Yes it was and you did great! Today I want you to keep doing what you did last time, including describing the event in as much detail as possible while allowing yourself to experience the emotions that this will bring up. I also want you to try to include even more details about your internal experience during this event, such as the emotions you were having, the thoughts that went through your mind, and any physical sensations you remember experiencing.

MARIA: Did I not do that last time?

THERAPIST: You did describe some internal details, like you talked about feeling afraid when your father first got angry and feeling pain when he hit you. So, you definitely had some details in there. What I'm asking is for you to try to include even more of those kinds of details in your description, as this often really helps to make the event more vivid and to understand better what your experience was at the time.

MARIA: What if I can't remember what I was feeling? I think I was numb for a lot of it.

THERAPIST: That's completely fine. I just want you to describe whatever you can remember. If what you remember is feeling numb, then just describe that. And if there are parts of the event where you don't have any idea what you were thinking or feeling, then you don't have to try to put in those details. What I'm hoping is that you can describe more about the emotions, thoughts, and physical sensations that you do remember having, whatever those were. Is that clear?

MARIA: Yes. I can't say I'm excited to do that, but I'll do my best.

With this additional coaching, Maria readily included more description of her internal experience in the trauma narrative. To illustrate these differences, below is an excerpt from the beginning of the trauma narrative in Session 3 versus Session 4.

SESSION 3

"I am playing with my toys on the floor near where he is sitting and watching TV. I bump into the table and his beer spills onto the floor. I'm afraid he's going to get mad, so I apologize but it doesn't matter. He gets mad anyway and yells at me for being such a bad kid. Then he slaps me in the face, which hurts a lot, and tells me to clean up the mess I made. I run to get paper towels and start to clean it up."

SESSION 4

"I am playing with my toys on the floor near where he is sitting. I'm trying to be quiet because he's watching TV and I know he doesn't like it if I make noise. But I'm not careful enough and I bump into the table and his beer spills onto the floor. I immediately feel afraid and my heart starts pounding because I know he is going to get mad at me. I tell him, 'I'm sorry, I didn't mean to. I'll clean it up.' But it's too late, he's already angry. He yells at me and calls me a bad kid. I think he's right because I always mess things up and now I've done it again. It makes me hate myself. Then he slaps me hard on my face and the sound is really loud. My cheek hurts and my eyes start watering, but I try not to cry because I know he doesn't like it when I cry. I don't move because I'm scared, and I don't know what he's going to do next. But then he yells at me for just standing there and tells me to clean up the mess I made. I run to the kitchen to get some paper towels. I think that if I do a really good job cleaning it up that maybe he will calm back down and nothing else will happen."

CASE EXAMPLE DISCUSSION

As this example illustrates, the inclusion of internal details in the trauma narrative really brings Maria's story to life in a much more vivid way by, for example, describing her emotions (e.g., fear) and physical sensations (e.g., racing heart, watering eyes). In addition, including her thoughts in the narrative provided useful insights that helped her to make sense of her experience. For example, Maria had always blamed herself for provoking her father to violence. By adding in her thoughts at the time it became clear that she had been trying very hard to do the opposite. From the beginning of this event, she had been acutely aware of the potential for upsetting her father and had done several things that were intended to placate him. This helped her to recognize that she could not control his anger and violence even when she tried hard to do so. With this more detailed description, it also became clear that Maria's belief that she was bad and always messed things up preexisted this event and was reinforced by it. This allowed for continued processing of this self-critical belief, including how it had developed due to her father's invalidation and may have affected her responses at the time of this particular event.

2. Reducing Avoidance

I do not think it is an exaggeration to say that all clients will engage in avoidance at some point during imaginal exposure. Clients avoid in a multitude of ways that are sometimes overt and easy to recognize (e.g., leaving exposure sessions early) and other times are covert and harder to detect (e.g., thinking about suicide while describing their trauma). Avoidance may also include things clients are doing (e.g., wearing sunglasses) and not doing (e.g., not crying when feeling intense sadness), which requires you to pay attention to both the presence and absence of behaviors during imaginal exposure. Avoidance behaviors are also likely to vary considerably across clients, making it important to understand each client's typical ways of avoiding. Moreover, the same behavior (e.g., pausing while recounting one's trauma) may function as avoidance for some clients (e.g., by helping them to distract from the trauma memory), whereas it may help to counteract avoidance for others (e.g., by helping them to better focus on the emotions that have been elicited by exposure). The only certainty is that avoidance will occur at some point for each client, and if it is pervasive or persistent, will reduce the effectiveness of imaginal exposure. When avoidance is significantly interfering with progress, you will therefore need to provide coaching to help clients notice and change behaviors that are functioning to artificially reduce distress. (See Table 12.1 for examples of common avoidance behaviors.)

When addressing avoidance, it is important not to assume that clients are aware they are avoiding. While there are certainly times that clients engage in avoidance intentionally, at other times clients may not realize that something they are doing is functioning as avoidance. At times, you may also not be aware that clients are avoiding, or you may suspect avoidance is occurring but not know exactly what clients are doing to avoid. Thus, the first step in addressing avoidance is to identify and specifically define the avoidance behavior. When avoidance is occurring in obvious ways, this may involve simply highlighting the behavior and labeling it as avoidance. When it is unclear if or how clients are avoiding, you will need to carefully assess potential emotional, cognitive, and behavioral strategies that clients may be using to reduce

TABLE 12.1. Examples of Avoidance Behaviors during Imaginal Exposure

- Avoiding certain words or leaving out important details in the trauma narrative
- Distracting oneself by thinking about other things (e.g., target behaviors, positive events)
- Focusing on certain emotions (e.g., anger) and blocking others (e.g., fear, sadness)
- Doing another activity at the same time (e.g., playing with a fidget toy)
- Taking antianxiety medications or using alcohol or drugs prior to session
- Attempting to hide (e.g., covering one's face, turning away, curling into a ball)
- Refusing to do exposure or stopping prematurely
- Editorializing (e.g., talking about one's thoughts about the trauma rather than describing the trauma itself)
- Dissociating
- Shutting off emotions or intentionally inducing emotional numbness
- Speaking quietly or with long pauses
- Bringing comforting or soothing items to session (e.g., pets, blankets, scented lotion)
- Seeking reassurance from the therapist
- Carrying something that increases one's sense of safety (e.g., weapons, medication)
- Inconsistent attendance (e.g., frequently canceling or no-showing exposure sessions)

distress during exposure. This typically involves asking direct questions (e.g., "What are you thinking about while you are telling the story?") and testing hypotheses (e.g., "When you wear a lot of makeup, does that make it feel easier to do the imaginal exposure?").

Once an avoidance behavior is identified, you should provide coaching about what to do that would be more effective. This typically includes asking the client to stop the avoidance behavior and dragging out new behavior to replace it. For example, clients may be asked to stop speaking quietly and instead to talk at their normal volume, or to stop fidgeting and instead to hold their hands still in their lap. Ideally, clients will be active collaborators in identifying and eliminating avoidance behaviors and will agree to make changes that are requested even when they would prefer not to. At times, however, clients may express unwillingness to stop the avoidance behavior or may engage in the new behavior only temporarily before resuming the avoidance. If this occurs, it can be helpful to validate clients' urges to avoid and briefly remind them of the rationale for exposure. If an avoidance behavior persists over multiple sessions despite repeated coaching and feedback, this will likely need to be targeted using DBT's standard protocol for addressing therapy-interfering behavior.

CLINICAL TIP

Is Using DBT Skills during Exposure Avoidance?

Often therapists (and clients) will ask whether using DBT skills during exposure is considered avoidance and should be discouraged. As with many things in DBT PE, the answer is "it depends." Largely this determination depends on the function of the skill. Is it working to escape the avoided cue and reduce distress? Or is it helping to approach the avoided cue and fully experience emotion? For example, DBT crisis survival skills function to distract from stressors and soothe during times of high emotion and are therefore usually discouraged during exposure. In contrast, DBT mindfulness and reality acceptance skills function to promote approach and acceptance of painful emotions and may help to make exposure more effective. Therefore, you should work with your client to determine which DBT skills may be detrimental versus beneficial in helping them to experience the emotions elicited by exposure without avoiding. Of note, there may also be times when clients are coached to use DBT skills to change (rather than accept) their emotions during imaginal exposure (e.g., to address overengagement)—this is discussed in detail in Chapter 14.

Case Example

Over the course of the first several imaginal exposure sessions, Maria's therapist coached her to continue adding details to the trauma narrative, including explicit details of the sexual abuse itself, and to reduce avoidance behaviors that were clearly occurring, such as dissociating, pausing frequently, speaking quietly, and covering her face with her hands. By the end of Session 5, Maria was describing the trauma in vivid detail, including both internal and external details of the event, and there was no longer any overt avoidance occurring during imaginal exposure. As a result, she was beginning to show some evidence of between-session habituation (e.g., her fear had decreased to 40 and guilt to 65). However, her SUDS were still quite high (75+), which led her therapist to begin to wonder whether some type of avoidance was still present that was interfering with achieving greater reductions in distress.

At the beginning of Session 6, her therapist raised this possibility to Maria and asked for her help in thinking through whether there might be anything she was doing during the imaginal exposure, intentionally or unintentionally, that could be functioning to reduce distress. Maria said that while she was listening to her imaginal exposure recording over the past week, she had realized that she was not saying it was her father who had done this to her and instead was just saying "he" or "him." She said that she hadn't been doing this on purpose but wondered if maybe this was avoidance. Her therapist thanked her for suggesting this and asked her what she had called her father at the age the trauma occurred. Maria said she used to call him "daddy," so her therapist asked her to refer to him using that name when she recounted the trauma. Maria agreed to do this and, when she first said "daddy" during imaginal exposure, she began to sob. After multiple repetitions of the imaginal exposure with his name included, Maria's SUDS eventually decreased to a 60 for the first time. At the same time, her anger increased to a 60 and her guilt decreased to a 45.

CASE EXAMPLE DISCUSSION

As this example illustrates, it is often challenging to identify avoidance, particularly when it involves the absence of a behavior. This highlights the importance of enlisting clients to be active collaborators in ferreting out avoidance. In this case, Maria's recent awareness that she was not explicitly saying it was her father who had done this to her provided a clear path forward for intervention and coaching her to stop this avoidance had a quick and noticeable effect in facilitating further decreases in overall distress and guilt. During processing, Maria talked about how saying "daddy" made him feel more like a real person. This also led to a discussion about her feelings of intense betrayal that her father, who was supposed to love and protect her, had instead actively harmed her. As a result, Maria began to experience significant anger toward her father for the first time and to blame him more for the abuse than she blamed herself, both clear signs of progress that were facilitated by eliminating this avoidance behavior.

How to Provide Coaching

When there are multiple behaviors that need to change to maximize the effectiveness of imaginal exposure, you need to make decisions about which behaviors to target and in what order, as well as when to provide this coaching. On the one hand, it is important to not be excessively demanding by expecting clients to eliminate all avoidance immediately. On the other hand, it is important not to ignore behaviors that are likely to interfere with imaginal exposure or to treat clients as if they are fragile and unable to make needed changes. The synthesis typically involves applying the principles of shaping—that is, breaking the desired behavior into small steps that are within the client's current capability and reinforcing each gradual approximation toward the goal of describing the trauma in full detail without avoidance. Coaching must also be balanced with reinforcement of clients' effective behaviors to keep them motivated to continue and reduce the likelihood that they will feel as if they are "failing" at imaginal exposure. In addition, it is important to be nonjudgmental when providing coaching and validate the understandable reasons why clients may have difficulty doing imaginal exposure in optimal ways.

When corrective feedback is given, it should be behaviorally specific so that clients are clear about exactly what needs to be changed to improve skillfulness. General instructions, such as "Please be more detailed when you describe what happened," should be avoided and instead behaviorally specific instructions should be given, such as "When you get to the part where you thought he was going to kill you, slow down and describe exactly what you were thinking and feeling." Similarly, if coaching is provided to reduce avoidance, you should specifically describe what behaviors to stop and what to do instead. For example, if a client who is experiencing intense shame is avoiding by covering their face and sitting curled up in a ball during imaginal exposure, it would likely not be sufficient to tell the client to "do opposite action." Instead, behaviorally specific instructions should be given, such as "I'd like you to stop covering your face and sitting curled up in a ball. Instead, I want you to practice opposite action to shame by keeping your hands down, sitting up straight, and putting your feet on the floor."

When coaching feedback is given, it should be timed to be as nonintrusive as possible. Feedback is typically given before imaginal exposure begins rather than interrupting clients during imaginal exposure. If clients do not incorporate the requested changes, you may briefly provide coaching again at the end of a repetition of the trauma narrative (e.g., "You're doing great. Next time remember to describe the physical sensations you were feeling as this was happening"). If these between-repetition prompts still do not elicit the requested change, then coaching may be provided in the middle of imaginal exposure, such as by asking brief questions to elicit additional details (e.g., "What are you feeling in your body?"). In general, however, you should refrain from providing lengthy instructions or teaching a new skill in the middle of imaginal exposure. If longer or more detailed corrective feedback is needed, this is typically done during processing after imaginal exposure is complete and/or prior to starting imaginal exposure in the subsequent session.

The Progression of Imaginal Exposure

Over the course of the intermediate sessions, imaginal exposure progresses in a structured way that begins with the client recounting the full story of a trauma, then shifts to describing the most distressing moments of that trauma ("hot spots"), and eventually returns to telling the full story to determine whether a trauma has been sufficiently treated. Once one trauma memory has been fully resolved, then other trauma memories may be targeted if needed using this same sequence of steps until no trauma memories remain that continue to cause significant distress and PTSD. The exact timing of these shifts within and across trauma memories, as well as the number of trauma memories that are targeted, varies across clients. Decisions about when and how to move forward are made collaboratively with clients based on their progress and treatment goals. The typical progression of imaginal exposure over the course of the intermediate sessions is shown in Figure 12.1 and described in detail below.

1. Telling the Full Story

Imaginal exposure begins in Session 3 with clients telling the full story of a traumatic event from a specified start point (typically right before anything upsetting started to happen) until an end point (usually after the client was out of immediate danger). In the initial intermediate

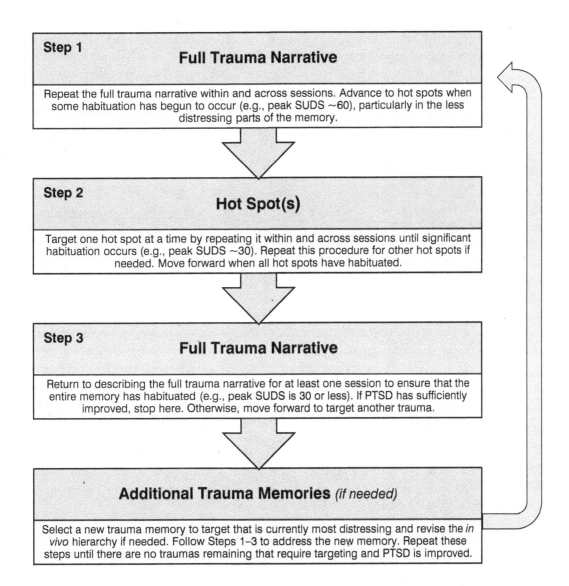

FIGURE 12.1. The progression of imaginal exposure in the intermediate sessions.

sessions, clients continue to describe this traumatic event in its entirety while working to fill in the details and reduce avoidance behaviors. Once the trauma narrative is more fully elaborated (e.g., it now includes all of the key details about the trauma) and habituation has begun to occur, particularly for the less distressing parts of the memory (e.g., peak SUDS are about 60), then the imaginal exposure shifts to focus on hot spots. The exact timing of this progression varies across clients, but typically occurs after about three to four sessions of imaginal exposure and processing (i.e., by Session 6 or 7).

2. Hot Spots Procedure

The first step in implementing the hot spots procedure is to orient clients to the rationale for narrowing the focus of the imaginal exposure to just the most painful moment(s) of the trauma. I like to use a metaphor of this being similar to receiving a full body massage. Although the massage therapist addresses each part of your body, they spend the most time massaging the muscles that are particularly sore and tense to help you achieve maximum relief. Similarly, the primary reason for focusing on hot spots is to give extra attention to the parts of the memory that are causing the most distress, thereby ensuring that those particularly painful moments are directly and thoroughly treated. This is likely to result in faster habituation of the most distressing moments than if they were embedded in a longer narrative, and will therefore provide the client with the most rapid relief. It may also be useful to highlight that starting with the full trauma narrative before shifting to hot spots facilitates a gradual approach to imaginal exposure while ensuring that both you and the client are aware of the full context of a traumatic event before narrowing in to focus only on one part of it.

After orienting to this rationale, you and your client will collaboratively identify hot spots. Often you will have a reasonably clear idea of what the hot spots are based on observing the client's behavior during imaginal exposure and seeing the points in the trauma narrative at which they appear to reliably experience higher distress. Clients' SUDS ratings during imaginal exposure may also provide useful information about which moments in the trauma narrative are most distressing. Most of the time, however, hot spots can be quickly identified simply by asking the client a straightforward question, such as "What moment or moments in this trauma currently bother you the most?" Clients are typically well aware of the moments they find most painful, which are often those that they view as the strongest proof that they are bad, disgusting, unlovable, and/or to blame for what occurred.

Some clients may identify more than one hot spot—however, only one hot spot is targeted at a time. Similar to the process of selecting the first target trauma during the Trauma Interview in Session 1, clients are encouraged to begin by focusing on the hot spot that is currently causing the most distress. Once the first hot spot is selected, imaginal exposure resumes with the client describing just that one hot spot over and over. Given that hot spots are briefer than the full trauma narrative, they are often repeated many more times within a session. It is also typical for distress to be higher during the first hot spot session than in the prior session in which the full trauma narrative was recounted, and the client's distress typically resumes a downward trajectory in subsequent sessions.

The client continues to describe the same hot spot for as many sessions as it takes for sufficient habituation to occur, usually until peak SUDS are about 30. At that point, a second hot spot can be targeted if needed, and so on. Typically, only one or two hot spots need to be targeted and this takes about three or four sessions (i.e., until Session 9 or 10) to complete. When there are no more hot spots that require targeting, the client then returns to recounting the entire trauma narrative from start to finish for at least one more session. This enables the client to put all the pieces back together, consider the hot spot(s) in the context of the larger trauma, and ensure that there are no parts of the memory that continue to elicit significant distress. Typically, clients discover that the entire trauma memory is now habituated (e.g., peak SUDS is 30 or less) and they no longer find it very difficult to talk about that traumatic event in detail.

3. Switching to a New Trauma Memory

Given that clients in DBT PE typically have complex trauma histories, their PTSD is rarely sufficiently treated by targeting only one trauma memory. On average, two to three trauma memories are targeted before clients remit from PTSD. Thus, after one trauma memory has been sufficiently treated, it is important to assess whether other traumas continue to cause high distress. In addition, if PTSD symptoms have decreased but remain elevated, this likely signals a need to target other traumas. If more treatment is needed, you and the client must decide which trauma memory to target next. In cases where the first trauma memory was part of a chronic trauma type (e.g., repeated sexual abuse by the same perpetrator), then it should first be determined whether there are other memories from this same trauma type that continue to cause significant distress. Often a chronic trauma can be addressed by targeting one event, but this is not always sufficient. If other events from within the same chronic trauma type continue to be highly distressing, it is recommended that you pick the event that is now most distressing from that chronic trauma type to target next. If there are no longer any events from that chronic trauma type that are distressing and/or if the first trauma was a one-time event, then the client should pick the memory that is currently most distressing from a new trauma type.

As a reminder, during the Trauma Interview in Session 1 the top three most distressing trauma memories at that time were identified and ordered for targeting. You should review this original treatment plan with the client to determine whether it still makes sense to follow, but you do not need to hold rigidly to it if things have shifted. For example, some memories that were originally identified may no longer be as distressing due to generalization or clients may now be willing to target traumas that they initially refused to put on the list. Once a second trauma memory has been selected, it may also be useful to redo the portions of the Trauma Interview that focus on gathering information about a specific target trauma (i.e., Sections 3 and 4) before beginning with a new memory. In addition, you should review the *in vivo* exposure hierarchy that was created in Session 2 and consider whether new items need to be added to more directly target avoided situations related to the next trauma memory. In some cases, an entirely new *in vivo* exposure hierarchy may be needed if the next trauma that will be targeted is a totally different type than the first (e.g., the first memory was child sexual abuse and the second is a mugging).

Typically, the first memory that is targeted in treatment takes the longest to improve and often requires seven or more sessions of imaginal exposure and processing before it is sufficiently treated. However, subsequent memories typically progress more quickly, often taking only three to five sessions to resolve. This is because much of the corrective learning that occurred when targeting earlier traumas (e.g., that emotions can be tolerated, that the client is not to blame for others' behavior) will generalize to other traumas in a way that makes them less difficult to talk and think about from the start. Often what has to be resolved with other traumas are beliefs that are specific to those events (e.g., ways in which the client thinks the trauma proves that they are inherently bad). When a second trauma memory is complete, then you and the client should again evaluate whether there are any additional traumas that continue to cause significant distress and PTSD symptoms. If so, another memory can be targeted, and if not, the client can progress to the final session of DBT PE. (The decision about when to end DBT PE is discussed in greater detail later in this chapter.)

5. Conduct Processing of the Imaginal Exposure

In each intermediate session, processing is conducted after imaginal exposure is complete. In Chapter 11, I describe the general structure, common targets, and typical DBT strategies used during processing. I focus now on how processing progresses over the course of the intermediate sessions using an emotion regulation framework in which emotions are used to identify targets, monitor progress, and select interventions likely to promote change. Strategies for targeting specific trauma-related emotions during processing are discussed in detail in Chapter 15.

An Emotion Regulation Approach to Processing

Although processing aims to change problematic trauma-related beliefs, this is done in the service of regulating emotions: belief change is not the end goal. Therefore, in DBT PE, processing is done through an emotion-focused lens in which specific emotions that are unjustified or ineffective are targeted for change using a variety of DBT strategies. This emotion-focused approach is consistent with DBT, which formulates clients' problems in terms of emotions (not cognitions) and views helping clients learn to regulate their emotions as a central component of treatment. The steps involved in regulating emotions in DBT are explained in detail in other sources (e.g., Dunkley, 2020; Linehan, 2015), and are briefly reviewed here as they are applied during processing.

Step 1. Identify and Label Emotions

Before an emotion can be changed, it first must be accurately identified. In DBT PE, this is done by asking clients to identify and rate the intensity of seven specific emotions—fear, sadness, anger, guilt, shame, disgust, and joy—immediately before and after every exposure task they complete. Of note, research suggests that simply labeling emotions can help to downregulate them (e.g., Fitzpatrick, Ip, Krantz, Zeifman, & Kuo, 2019) and when this is done in the context of exposure therapy, it may enhance outcomes (e.g., Kircanski, Lieberman, & Craske, 2012). Thus, the first thing clients are asked to do after imaginal exposure is to complete the *Exposure Recording Form* (*DBT PE Handout 8/8A* in Appendix A), which includes labeling and rating the intensity of the specific emotions that have been activated by the exposure.

Step 2. Select an Emotion to Regulate

With the completed Exposure Recording Form in hand, therapists then begin the processing discussion by asking clients open-ended questions about their experience (e.g., "What stands out for you today after telling that story?"). Clients' responses to these initial questions often include expressions of problematic trauma-related emotions and beliefs. When this occurs, you will typically follow the client's lead and address whatever is most salient to them in that moment. After the client has had an opportunity to discuss their reactions, therapists shift to asking more targeted questions to identify specific emotions to regulate based on the ratings on the Exposure

Recording Form and/or their observations during imaginal exposure. For example, you might say, "You sounded angry while you were telling the story today and you rated your anger at a 90. What are you feeling angry about?" Of note, multiple emotions may be targeted during a single processing conversation, but only one emotion can be regulated at a time.

When selecting an emotion to regulate, you must first determine whether the emotion is justified or unjustified. In DBT, emotions are considered unjustified if they do not fit the facts of the situation (e.g., fear that occurs in the absence of an actual threat), whereas emotions that are consistent with the reality of the situation are justified (e.g., anger toward the person who perpetrated one's abuse). It is important not to confuse the determination of whether an emotion is justified with whether it is understandable: Unjustified emotions can always be understood and validated even if they are unhelpful or do not fit the facts of the situation. Table 12.2 describes the situations in which the emotions tracked on the Exposure Recording Form are considered justified.

Overall, the goal is to help clients reduce the intensity of unjustified emotions to a level that fits the facts of the current situation while also ensuring that justified emotions are at a level that is effective (neither insufficiently nor excessively intense). For most clients, the trauma-related emotions of fear, guilt, shame, and self-directed disgust are unjustified and need to be decreased. For example, clients often feel afraid when not in danger, guilty about things they did during the trauma that do not violate their values, ashamed about characteristics that are unlikely to cause rejection, and disgust at themselves when they are not physically contaminated. In contrast, sadness (e.g., about the losses caused by past trauma), as well as anger and other-directed disgust (e.g., toward perpetrators), are justified and may need to be increased or decreased to a level that is effective. This is consistent with research on DBT PE that has found that fear, guilt, shame, and disgust (i.e., the typical unjustified emotions) significantly decrease from the first to the last imaginal exposure session, whereas the justified emotions of sadness and anger do not significantly change (Harned et al., 2015).

TABLE 12.2. Determining When Emotions Are Justified

Emotion	When the emotion fits the facts
Fear	• You or someone you care about are in danger. • Your well-being or that of someone you care about is being threatened.
Guilt	• Your behavior violates group norms that are important to you. • You have done something that violates your own values.
Shame	• You have done something that will cause people you care about to reject you if it is revealed.
Disgust	• You or something you are in contact with is physically dirty or contaminated. • You are near people who you strongly dislike because of their harmful or offensive behavior.
Anger	• You or someone you care about are harmed, threatened, or insulted. • An important goal is blocked or threatened.
Sadness	• You have lost someone or something important to you. • Your life is not the way you would like it to be.
Joy	• An activity is pleasurable. • A person or activity improves your well-being or quality of life.

Step 3. Select and Implement Tailored Interventions

Once an emotion has been selected to regulate, the next step is to implement tailored interventions that will increase or decrease its intensity to a level that is effective and appropriate to the situation. Importantly, regulating an emotion is not the same as applying general strategies to reduce arousal (e.g., TIP skills)—different emotions require different regulation strategies. In DBT, emotions are conceptualized as being activated by a prompting event and the person's interpretations about the event, which lead to a full system response that includes biological changes, physical sensations, action urges, facial expressions, body language, words, and actions. The strategies that are likely to be most effective for regulating an emotion depend on the event and interpretations that are prompting it, as well as how it is experienced and expressed by the client. Thus, targeting typically begins by assessing the various components of the client's emotion to determine what may be causing and maintaining it. This may include questions such as:

- Are there certain beliefs you have about the trauma that make you feel [emotion]?
- Is there something specific that happened during or after the trauma that causes you to feel [emotion]?
- Where do you feel [emotion] in your body?
- What urges do you have when you are feeling [emotion]?

Once the factors contributing to the client's emotion are understood, the therapist shifts to identifying tailored interventions that are likely to change the intensity of the emotion in the desired direction. Often emotions are changed by helping clients correct erroneous interpretations and beliefs about the trauma (i.e., the prompting event). However, DBT includes multiple strategies that can be used to change emotions that extend beyond cognitive interventions and involve changing other aspects of the emotional response (e.g., physiology, body language, actions). This full-system approach to changing emotions is often necessary when the beliefs that drive the emotion are particularly entrenched and difficult to change. Chapter 15 provides detailed information about how to apply DBT strategies to the task of regulating trauma-related fear, guilt, anger, shame, disgust, and sadness.

Case Example: Targeting Maria's Disgust

Maria reported high disgust toward herself from the start of DBT PE, and her therapist began to actively target this emotion during processing in Session 7. To start, her therapist highlighted that Maria had rated disgust at a 90 and asked her what it was about the memory that made her feel disgust. Maria said that thinking about her father touching her sexually made her feel like she was disgusting and dirty. Her therapist validated Maria's reaction and said it was understandable given that sexual contact with family members is viewed as disgusting by most people. However, since Maria's disgust at herself was not justified, her therapist suggested they work on reducing it, and Maria agreed. She then began working to help Maria shift from feeling unjustified disgust at herself to feeling justified disgust at her father and his abusive behavior. To that end, she used cognitive modification strategies to help Maria recognize that she had not willingly participated in the sexual behavior that disgusted her and it was forced on her by her father. Given the progress Maria had already made in reducing self-blame for her abuse, she was able to acknowledge in wise mind that it was her father who had engaged in inappropriate and disgusting behavior, not her. Nonetheless, she said that she continued to feel as if she was disgusting even though she recognized it did not fit the facts.

At that point, her therapist began to assess for other factors that were contributing to Maria's disgust beyond her negative interpretations of herself. She asked Maria what she had urges to do when she felt self-disgust. Maria said that she typically had urges to avoid looking at her body or being seen by others, and that she often wanted to wash herself. Her therapist asked if she ever acted on these urges. Maria said that after she listened to her imaginal exposure recording, she usually took a shower and then stayed in her room for the rest of the night to avoid having to be near her mother. Her therapist then hypothesized that these behaviors may be contributing to Maria's ongoing high levels of disgust and suggested that she use opposite action instead to engage in behaviors that are inconsistent with disgust-related urges. After agreeing to give this a try, Maria and her therapist made a plan that after listening to her imaginal exposure recording she would not shower and would instead interact with her mother, ideally while being physically close to her (e.g., sitting next to her).

Additionally, her therapist suggested this would be a good time to have her start working on *in vivo* exposure practices that would target her disgust about her body. After reviewing her hierarchy, Maria decided she would work on looking at herself in a full-length mirror while clothed. Her therapist instructed her to use opposite action while doing this *in vivo* exposure practice. Specifically, she coached her to look at herself without acting disgusted, which might include things like turning away, curling up her lips, scrunching her nose, or shuddering. Instead, she encouraged Maria to look directly at her body without avoiding any parts of it, describe what she saw without judgment, and keep her face and posture relaxed as she did this. Maria agreed she would do this four times for 20 minutes each in the coming week. With these interventions, Maria's disgust at herself decreased to 30 in the next session and she was instead feeling appropriate disgust toward her father (post = 70).

CASE EXAMPLE DISCUSSION

As this example illustrates, regulating emotions requires careful assessment and an individualized approach to tailor interventions to the specific emotion and the factors that are maintaining it. In Maria's case, her disgust was being fueled by negative interpretations about herself related to her father's sexual abuse (e.g., that she was dirty), as well as behaviors she was engaging in that were consistent with disgust (e.g., showering, isolating herself from others). During processing, her therapist assessed these maintaining factors, generated solutions, and implemented several interventions designed to reduce her self-directed disgust. These included cognitive strategies (e.g., evaluating whether disgust fit the facts of her behavior vs. her father's behavior), opposite action to disgust (e.g., not showering after exposure), and *in vivo* exposure (to looking at herself in the mirror). As was the case with Maria, it is often necessary to target both the cognitions and behaviors that are maintaining an emotion to get an unjustified emotion to change, and this typically requires multiple strategies that are implemented both in and out of session.

The Typical Progression of Processing

Processing is a flexible and principle-driven intervention that uses DBT strategies to target the problematic emotions and beliefs that are maintaining clients' PTSD. As such, the targets that are addressed during processing are not predetermined and there is no way to know in advance exactly what will be addressed in any given session. Adding to this complexity is the fact that multiple emotions and associated beliefs are typically targeted within the same session, pursuing one for a period of time, ideally until it begins to shift in some way, and then moving forward with speed and flow to target another. However, targeting during processing is not entirely unpredictable: Most clients follow a similar overall trajectory of change in emotions across these intermediate sessions. Therefore, being familiar with this typical pattern can help you to know what to expect in terms of the order in which emotions and their associated beliefs are likely to change.

As shown in Figure 12.2, clients typically begin treatment with high levels of the unjustified emotions of fear, guilt, shame, and self-directed disgust, and low to moderate levels of the justified emotions of anger and sadness. In the early sessions, fear typically decreases via repeated imaginal exposure, whereas guilt is often reduced due to direct targeting of self-blaming beliefs during processing. In the middle portion of treatment, anger toward perpetrators and others involved in the trauma often increases as a result of reducing guilt and self-blame. Processing typically shifts to focus on shame and self-directed disgust—the two unjustified emotions that are often still high at this point in treatment. This typically includes focusing on clients' negative beliefs about themselves (e.g., as bad, worthless, and repulsive) and working to increase self-compassion and positive esteem. For clients with intense and problematic anger, targeting may also include working to decrease anger during processing by reducing judgments and increasing acceptance of people who were involved in the trauma.

In the later treatment sessions, anger typically subsides and is replaced by justified disgust toward others, whereas the self-directed emotions of shame and disgust both decrease to low levels. Sadness is often particularly intense during the later portion of treatment as clients reach a place of radical acceptance of their past traumas and shift to grieving the losses and suffering caused by these extremely painful experiences. At the end of treatment, fear, guilt, shame, self-directed disgust, and anger are typically low, whereas justified sadness and other-directed disgust may be moderate to high. Overall, this typical pattern of change in emotions

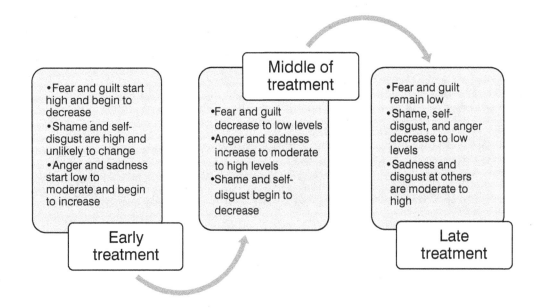

FIGURE 12.2. The typical course of change in emotions in the intermediate sessions.

Why Is So Much Focus Placed on Processing in DBT PE?

Processing in DBT PE differs substantially from how it is typically conducted in standard PE. In standard PE, imaginal exposure is viewed as the primary agent of change and processing is a less targeted and often briefer intervention, with the amount of time spent engaged in processing often decreasing across the intermediate sessions (Foa et al., 2019). In contrast, in DBT PE imaginal exposure and processing are viewed as equally important in achieving change, and comparable amounts of time are devoted to each. In addition, rather than being an informal discussion, processing is a formal and targeted intervention that is primarily used to address nonfear emotions that are not sufficiently changed by imaginal exposure alone. The greater emphasis on processing in DBT PE reflects the client population with whom the treatment is used. For these complex clients, fear is typically the least problematic and easiest to change trauma-related emotion. Instead, guilt, shame, and self-disgust are often at the core of their suffering and quite difficult to change. Although imaginal exposure can help to reduce these negative self-directed emotions, it is often not sufficient to fully modify the long-standing and entrenched self-critical thinking styles that fuel them. Thus, processing was modified in DBT PE to enable more formal and direct targeting of the full range of clients' trauma-related emotions by "doing DBT." Specifically, processing in DBT PE *is* DBT that is used to target specific trauma-related emotions for up- or down-regulation as needed (see Chapter 15).

across the course of DBT PE reflects important progress in modifying trauma-related beliefs to more accurately fit the facts of past traumas and their impact. The *Therapist Imaginal Exposure Progress Monitoring Form* (*Therapist Form 4* in Appendix B) can be used to track progress in changing these emotions over the course of treatment.

Case Example: Maria's Course of Treatment

To provide an illustration of how the intermediate sessions progress, the *Imaginal Exposure Progress Monitoring Form* for Maria is shown in Figure 12.3. As described earlier in this chapter, Maria's Sessions 3–5 focused on describing the full story of the episode of her father's abuse with increasing detail and less avoidance. After including her name for her father ("daddy") in the trauma narrative in Session 6, Maria began to experience greater habituation. At the beginning of Session 7, review of her imaginal exposure homework indicated that her SUDS had peaked at 60 in her last two homework practices. Given this progress, her therapist decided to advance to hot spots in Session 7. After orienting her to the rationale for hot spots, Maria identified one hot spot in the memory: when her father told her she was bad and deserved to be punished while he was spanking her and penetrating her vagina with his fingers. As Maria had successfully eliminated avoidance at this point, only two sessions were needed before this hot spot habituated to a peak SUDS of 50 in Session 8 and 30 in the homework she completed before Session 9. Thus, in Session 9, they returned to describing the full memory of the abusive episode to ensure that there was nothing about it that continued to cause high distress, and when there was not, they agreed that no further imaginal exposure was needed on this first trauma memory.

Across the seven sessions in which her father's abuse was addressed, the emotions targeted for regulation during processing were consistent with the typical pattern of change, with the early sessions focused on guilt and self-blame before targeting switched to focus on shame,

Client: *Maria*

Session #	Memory #	Description of the Imaginal Exposure	Primary Targets in Processing	Peak SUDS	Post Fear	Post Guilt	Post Shame	Post Disgust	Post Anger	Post Sad	Post RA	PTSD Score
3	1	Full narrative	Fear, guilt	100	60	100	100	100	5	30	30	68
4	1	Full narrative	Guilt	90	50	90	100	100	10	50	45	–
5	1	Full narrative	Guilt, shame	80	40	65	90	90	15	60	50	62
6	1	Full narrative	Shame, anger	70	20	45	80	75	60	60	65	–
7	1	Hot spot 1	Disgust, shame	85	20	25	85	90	100	70	75	57
8	1	Hot spot 1	Anger	50	0	5	40	70	90	80	100	–
9	1	Full narrative	Sadness	30	0	0	15	50	30	100	100	47
10	2	Hot spot 1	Guilt	70	20	70	100	80	70	60	70	–
11	2	Full narrative	Shame	50	0	20	80	75	65	70	85	38
12	2	Hot spot 1	Disgust, shame	40	0	0	50	75	50	80	100	–
13	2	Full narrative	Sadness, anger	25	0	0	10	60	50	75	100	31
14	3	Full narrative	Guilt, shame	80	0	60	80	50	60	50	90	–
15	3	Hot spot 1	Anger	45	0	10	25	20	70	50	100	11
16	3	Full narrative	Sadness	20	0	5	5	50	10	60	100	–

Note. RA = radical acceptance. PTSD score = PTSD Checklist for DSM-5 (PCL-5) score.

FIGURE 12.3. Imaginal Exposure Progress Monitoring Form for Maria.

self-directed disgust, and eventually anger and sadness. Although Maria's PTSD significantly decreased across these sessions (her score on the PTSD Checklist for DSM-5 [PCL-5; Weathers et al., 2013] changed from 68 to 47), she continued to have significant PTSD symptoms, and therefore she and her therapist decided to target a second trauma memory. Since Maria reported that there were no other memories of her father's abuse that continued to cause her intense distress, she decided to focus on a different trauma type for the second memory: the rape by her ex-boyfriend.

In Session 10, Maria completed her first imaginal exposure to this second trauma memory. Her SUDS were high (peak = 70), but not as high as they had been with the first memory because a lot of the earlier learning readily generalized to this second trauma. For example, Maria already believed that she could do imaginal exposure and tolerate her emotions, and she was more able to identify ways in which the rape was not her fault based on the new perspectives she had developed when processing her father's abuse. Overall, it was much faster to target this second memory and only four sessions were needed, including two hot spot sessions. In addition, processing focused primarily on continued targeting of shame and disgust, particularly related to her beliefs about being worthless and dirty. During the sessions in which this second memory was targeted, her PTSD decreased even further (PCL-5 = 31) but continued to cause her some distress. Thus, Maria and her therapist decided to target a third memory with the goal of achieving full remission of her PTSD.

In Session 14, they began targeting a third trauma involving bullying by peers in high school. This event was quick to process, requiring only three sessions before habituation fully occurred and Maria no longer met criteria for PTSD (PCL-5 = 11). At this point, she and her therapist decided that no further exposure sessions were needed, and they agreed to advance to the final session of DBT PE. In sum, the DBT PE portion of Maria's treatment took 17 sessions (including 14 exposure sessions) during which three distinct trauma memories were targeted before she achieved remission from PTSD.

CLINICAL TIP
How Many Intermediate Sessions Are Needed?

In DBT PE, the number of intermediate sessions is flexible and individually determined based on regular monitoring of the client's progress. The key indicators of progress that are typically considered when making this decision include:

1. *PTSD symptoms.* The goal is for clients to achieve a clinically significant improvement in PTSD symptoms, ideally to the level of diagnostic remission.
2. *Peak SUDS.* The goal is for clients to experience no more than mild distress during imaginal and *in vivo* exposure.
3. *Specific emotions.* The goal is for unjustified emotions to have decreased to a level that fits the facts, and for justified emotions to be at a level that is effective.
4. *Problematic beliefs.* The goal is for problematic trauma-related beliefs about the self, others, and emotions to have been replaced by more adaptive beliefs.

As with most clinical decisions in DBT PE, the decision about whether more intermediate sessions are needed is made collaboratively with the client. In addition to the indicators listed above, it is critical that clients feel a sense of "doneness"—that is, that they have learned what they needed to learn and now feel as if they can live with the trauma memories and the emotions they cause. Often this decision is relatively easy to make because the improvements clients have experienced are so dramatic that it is quite clear that more sessions are not needed. However, not all clients will achieve an optimal level of improvement during DBT PE and the decision to stop the intermediate sessions may be due to other factors, such as lack of progress or having reached the end of the treatment contract. Whatever the reason, once it has been decided that no more intermediate sessions will be delivered, you will advance to the final session of DBT PE (see Chapter 13).

6. Assign Homework

The final task of every intermediate session is to assign homework, which always includes repeated listening to the most recent recording of the in-session imaginal exposure, completing multiple *in vivo* exposure practices, and listening to the entire session recording one time. At times, you may also ask clients to repeatedly listen to the processing discussion to further consolidate important new learning that occurred in that portion of the session. As discussed at the beginning of this chapter, clients are typically asked to complete both imaginal and *in vivo* exposure daily, although completing them less often (e.g., three to four times per week) may be sufficient for progress to occur. The frequency with which clients are asked to complete both types of exposure should be based on careful monitoring of their progress; clients who are making slower progress may be asked to increase the frequency of exposure homework to achieve more rapid gains.

When assigning homework, you and the client need to decide when they are ready to move to new *in vivo* exposure tasks, and if so, which task(s) should be assigned next. Traditionally, *in vivo* exposure has been conducted using a gradual and linear approach in which clients begin with tasks that elicit a moderate degree of distress, complete each task repeatedly until habituation occurs, and then progress up the hierarchy to the next most distressing item. More recently, research has suggested that conducting variable exposure may improve retention and retrieval of learned information (Craske et al., 2014). Variable exposure typically begins with a less distressing task to increase treatment compliance, but then involves selecting items from the hierarchy in random order rather than using a linear approach. This means that once clients have made sufficient progress with one *in vivo* task, they can choose a task that they wish to work on next regardless of its position on the hierarchy. Thus, as treatment progresses, clients are likely to be simultaneously working on *in vivo* exposure tasks that elicit varying degrees of distress.

SESSIONS 4+ HOMEWORK ASSIGNMENTS

1. Listen to the recording of the imaginal exposure (ideally daily).*
2. Continue *in vivo* exposure (at least two tasks, ideally doing one per day).
3. Use the Post-Exposure Skills Plan as needed.
4. Listen to the entire session recording one time.

*Note. It may also be useful for the client to listen to the processing discussion.

CHAPTER 13

The Final Session

FINAL SESSION COMPONENTS AND TIME ESTIMATES

	60-minute session	90-minute session
1. Review the DBT diary card and set the session agenda.	3 min.	3–5 min.
2. Conduct brief imaginal exposure and review progress.	10–15 min.	15–20 min.
3. Rerate the *in vivo* exposure hierarchy and review progress.	5–10 min.	10–15 min.
4. Teach relapse prevention and management skills.	30–45 min.	45–60 min.
5. Assign homework.	2 min.	2–5 min.

The final session of DBT PE provides clients and therapists with an opportunity to both consolidate and celebrate the often tremendous changes that have occurred over the course of treatment. Whereas clients typically begin DBT PE with serious doubts about their ability to do the treatment, by the final session they have accumulated undeniable evidence that they are competent and strong people who can succeed at doing very difficult things. As a result of their hard work, most clients will have achieved significant improvements in their PTSD, as well as a wide variety of other problems that were being exacerbated by unresolved trauma. Clients are often no longer haunted by intrusive trauma memories, are regularly engaging in activities they find meaningful, have an increased sense of connection to the people in their lives, and are generally feeling more at ease in the world. The negative beliefs clients held about themselves, and the shame and self-hatred they caused, have usually subsided and a more positive self-construct has begun to take root. Perhaps most notably, clients who were previously chronically suicidal typically no longer wish to be dead, and instead believe, often for the first time, that it is possible to have a life that feels worth living.

Although the degree and type of change that clients experience by the final session varies, there is always something to be celebrated, and for many clients, these changes have been truly transformative. The final session provides an opportunity to reflect upon the changes that have occurred by reviewing clients' progress and discussing how they can maintain and even increase these gains in the future by teaching them relapse prevention and management skills. In addition, this session often provides information that can be useful in helping clients begin to identify goals they wish to pursue in Stage 3 after DBT PE is complete. All client handouts for the session are in Appendix A and a session checklist is provided in Appendix C.

1. Review the DBT Diary Card and Set the Session Agenda

Unlike prior sessions, the primary function of reviewing the diary card in the final session is to highlight and reinforce progress that has occurred over the course of DBT PE that is now evident in their daily lives. In particular, you should explicitly comment on how the ratings on the diary card have changed during DBT PE. Typically, prior target behaviors, as well as urges to engage in them, are greatly reduced if not completely absent. If positive or desired behaviors are being tracked on the diary card, these are likely to have increased. Whereas clients often begin DBT PE with high daily ratings of emotional misery and specific painful emotions, such as shame, by the final session ratings of negative emotions are often quite low and may even have been surpassed by positive emotions, such as joy. Overall, the review of the diary card in the final session provides a valuable opportunity to discuss and celebrate how the work that clients have done in DBT PE has contributed to positive and often far-reaching changes in the urges, emotions, and behaviors they now experience in their day-to-day life. Once this review of the diary card is complete, you can briefly set the session agenda to orient clients to the remaining components of the final session (see above).

2. Conduct Brief Imaginal Exposure and Review Progress

After discussing the changes clients have experienced in their lives more broadly, the next task is to review their progress with imaginal exposure and processing specifically. To facilitate this discussion, the client is asked to complete imaginal exposure one final time by recounting the full narrative of the last trauma memory that was targeted. Rather than repeating the narrative multiple times, however, the client is only asked to tell the story one time from start to finish, which will ideally be relatively brief (10 minutes or less). As in the earlier exposure sessions, clients should be asked to complete the Exposure Recording Form immediately before and after this single repetition of the trauma narrative. While the client is completing the imaginal exposure, you should pay close attention to their verbal description of the trauma, nonverbal behavior, and general affect with an eye toward identifying specific changes that have occurred compared to earlier in treatment.

Once the imaginal exposure is complete, therapists typically start the consolidation discussion by asking an open-ended question to elicit the client's perspective on what has changed, such as "What is it like now when you tell that story compared to the first time you told it?" Clients often respond with statements about how it has gotten easier, that it no longer really bothers them to think about their trauma, and that they now view what happened in a very different light. You can also share your own observations of changes in the client's verbal and nonverbal behavior during imaginal exposure. For example, the trauma narrative in the final session often includes adaptive beliefs that have formed over the course of treatment (e.g., "I did the best I could to fight him off, but he was a lot stronger than me"), which can be compared to earlier versions of the narrative that included unhelpful ways of thinking about what had happened (e.g., "I should have been able to stop him").

In addition, the ratings on the Exposure Recording Form often provide a useful framework to discuss progress in changing the specific trauma-related beliefs and emotions that were maintaining the client's PTSD. Important changes in clients' beliefs are often reflected in the probability and cost estimates associated with doing imaginal exposure. For example, many clients begin treatment predicting that they will be unable to tolerate thinking and talking about their trauma, and doing so will put them in danger. By the final session, clients generally believe that nothing bad will happen if they allow themselves to think about their trauma and they can cope effectively with whatever it brings up. Similarly, the type and intensity of emotions that clients currently experience during imaginal exposure can be contrasted with their emotions earlier in treatment, which can be reviewed using the *Imaginal Exposure Progress Monitoring Form (Therapist Handout 4)*. Changes in emotions can be linked to shifts in the way clients now think about themselves and the traumas they have experienced. Finally, it may also be useful to comment on changes that are evident in urges to engage in problem behaviors and state dissociation during imaginal exposure, as well as their radical acceptance of the trauma.

In addition to identifying and reinforcing the specific improvements that have occurred related to imaginal exposure and processing, it is also important to clarify what worked to achieve these gains. Clients can be asked to share their own perspective on what worked in general (e.g., "Why do you think imaginal exposure and processing helped?"), as well as what worked to achieve specific changes (e.g., "Why do you think your guilt is now zero when it used to be 100?"). Often clients' explanations for their progress reflect the primary mechanisms of change in the treatment, including extinction/habituation (e.g., "It got less scary the more I talked about it") and belief change (e.g., "I don't feel guilty because I no longer think it was my fault"). You can reinforce and expand on the explanations that clients provide to further consolidate their learning about what works to reduce PTSD-related suffering.

Case Example

In the final session, Maria completed one repetition of imaginal exposure to the last memory she had been addressing in treatment: the episode of bullying in high school. It took Maria about 7 minutes to tell the full story of this event, after which she and her therapist reviewed her progress.

THERAPIST: Congratulations on completing your last imaginal exposure!

MARIA: Thank you!

THERAPIST: What is it like to do that now compared to the first time you did imaginal exposure?

MARIA: It's so different! The first time I did it I really thought I wasn't going to survive. And now it hardly bothers me at all.

THERAPIST: Isn't it amazing? You have worked so hard to get to this place where it now feels totally manageable to think and talk about the traumas you have experienced.

MARIA: I'm not afraid of these memories anymore. They're things that happened to me in the past and they were terrible, but they don't have to interfere with my life anymore.

THERAPIST: That makes me so happy to hear!

MARIA: (*smiling*) I know you said this would happen, but I have to admit that I had doubts about whether you were right.

THERAPIST: I'm so glad you trusted me enough to do this even though you had doubts. And I'm very glad that I turned out to be right!

MARIA: (*laughs*) Me too!

THERAPIST: Besides being easier to think and talk about, what has changed for you about how you think about the traumas you have experienced?

MARIA: I think one of the biggest things that has changed across all the traumas is that I no longer view them as my fault. With my father, I now see how abusive he was to both me and my mother. He used violence to control us and we were terrified of him all the time. But it wasn't my fault or my mother's fault that he was abusive, even though he tried to blame us for his behavior. He is responsible for his own actions.

THERAPIST: I completely agree.

MARIA: And the kids that bullied me in high school are the ones who have something to feel guilty about, not me. I may have had sex with more people than the average high school kid, but that was because I was messed up by what my father had done to me. It didn't make it OK for people to spread rumors about me or call me names or constantly make offensive comments to me.

THERAPIST: Again, I couldn't agree more.

MARIA: With the rape, I really thought that it was my fault because I had talked to that guy at the party even though I knew it would make my boyfriend jealous. But now I realize that does not make rape OK, and he was wrong to be so controlling of me.

THERAPIST: This is like music to my ears! Do you remember your guilt was at 100 for each of these traumas when we started? And now it's gone.

MARIA: I know! I don't feel guilty anymore. It's pretty wonderful!

THERAPIST: Yes, it is. So how do you feel about yourself now that you've gotten such a different perspective on these traumas?

MARIA: I think that's what has changed the most. Since I was a little kid, I have always viewed myself as bad and thought I deserved to be treated poorly. Through this treatment I realized how those beliefs got started because of the way my father treated me. He taught me to believe that I was worthless and that nothing I did was ever good enough. He made me think that I deserved to be abused by him because I was always doing things wrong. It was like he brainwashed me into viewing the world his way so that he was always right and I was always wrong.

THERAPIST: He really did have a profound impact on the way you viewed yourself.

MARIA: Yes, and because he made me think I was such a bad person, that affected the way I thought about the things that happened to me later with the bullying and the rape. I just filed those into the same category and assumed they were further proof that I was bad and deserved to be mistreated. But now I see things so differently, it's like the brainwashing has been undone. I can honestly say I feel good about who I am as a person, and I never would have said that before.

THERAPIST: I think that is the change I am most excited about for you. Believing that you are fundamentally a good and valid person who deserves to be treated well is going to change the way you lead your life in so many positive ways.

MARIA: I agree!

THERAPIST: So, you have clearly experienced some big improvements as a result of this treatment. How do you think imaginal exposure and processing worked to help you achieve these changes?

MARIA: I had never really let myself think about the traumas I had experienced because they made me feel so guilty and ashamed. Having to think and talk about them in detail was really hard, but it helped me to more clearly understand what happened and reconsider some of the ways I had always thought about these events. It also really helped to hear your perspective on what I had been through. I remember I was so shocked the first time you said to me that I didn't deserve my father's abuse, because I had always been told the opposite was true.

THERAPIST: Right, so rather than avoiding your trauma memories and keeping them hidden, by thinking and talking about them you were able to develop a different and much more validating perspective on what happened to you.

MARIA: And the more I did it, it got a lot easier to think about all these events, so I no longer feel like I have to avoid them. I mean, they are still not fun to think about, but they don't make me feel totally overwhelmed anymore.

THERAPIST: Well, that's a perfect summary of how imaginal exposure and processing works! And it has certainly worked for you.

CASE EXAMPLE DISCUSSION

As this excerpt shows, this discussion focused on consolidating the learning that occurred as a result of imaginal exposure and processing, and often invokes a sense of amazement and pride in both the client and therapist. Very often the changes that have occurred are quite profound, spanning not only changes in clients' beliefs about specific traumatic events but also the way clients view themselves and the world more globally. In Maria's case, the most significant changes were related to her self-blaming beliefs about the traumas she had experienced, as well as her negative beliefs about herself as a person. In this excerpt, the therapist worked to elicit and strengthen the most significant new beliefs that Maria had developed during treatment. Throughout this discussion, both the therapist and Maria joined in acknowledging and celebrating the important changes that had occurred, while also using this as an opportunity to highlight exactly how and why imaginal exposure and processing had worked to achieve these changes.

3. Rerate the *In Vivo* Exposure Hierarchy and Review Progress

After discussing the progress related to imaginal exposure, the session then moves on to review the client's progress with *in vivo* exposure. To facilitate this discussion, you will ask the client to provide a current SUDS estimate for each of the tasks on the original In Vivo *Exposure Hierarchy* (DBT PE Handout 7), which you can then write down in the "Final Session" column. After all the *in vivo* exposure tasks have been rerated, you and the client can review and discuss the differences between the SUDS ratings from the beginning of treatment (in the "Session 2" column) and their current ratings. Typically, this comparison indicates that many previously avoided situations and activities are now much less distressing than they used to be, which is yet another cause for pride and celebration. Often clients are shocked to see how high their original SUDS ratings were, as many of the activities on the hierarchy have become routine parts of their lives that no longer elicit much if any distress. At the same time, this review of the hierarchy often reveals some *in vivo* exposure tasks that may require additional practice as SUDS ratings remain moderate to high. When this occurs, clients can be reassured that this is normal, as there is often not enough time to repeatedly practice every item on the hierarchy during the time it takes to complete DBT PE, and that part of the discussion of relapse prevention later in the session will include identifying specific *in vivo* exposure tasks that they want to continue practicing.

Similar to the discussion of progress in imaginal exposure, you should then consolidate clients' learning about what worked to achieve reductions in distress associated with the situations included on the hierarchy. Often these explanations can be elicited from clients and then reinforced and strengthened by you. Again, the overall goal is for clients to clearly recognize that repeatedly approaching rather than avoiding safe but distressing situations made it possible to achieve long-term reductions in distress by facilitating corrective learning. In this discussion, you should highlight key areas of new learning that occurred as a result of *in vivo* exposure that will enable them to have fuller and more meaningful lives.

Case Example

Maria's final session ratings of the items on her *in vivo* exposure hierarchy are shown below. Each situation on the hierarchy had gotten considerably less distressing, and most were now rated as 20 or less. Maria was particularly surprised to remember that she had originally rated taking a shower with the lights on as 99, as she no longer experienced this as distressing at all (SUDS = 0). She had even started taking baths to relax, something she now did regularly and enjoyed. In the consolidation discussion, Maria and her therapist talked about how *in vivo* exposure had contributed to significant changes in Maria's beliefs, particularly about the likelihood that men would harm her and that she needed to be perfect all the time. Although Maria's shame about her body had decreased significantly (e.g., she now felt comfortable wearing shorts and going to the gym), she still found it moderately difficult to look at herself naked in the mirror (SUDS = 50). She had also recently joined a women's sexual trauma support group and was still feeling somewhat uncomfortable in the group (SUDS = 40). Her therapist normalized these remaining areas of difficulty and said they would talk more about these later in the session to decide whether Maria would like to continue working on them.

Maria's *In Vivo* Exposure Hierarchy		
Exposure task	SUDS (Session 2)	SUDS (Final session)
1. Looking at body naked in a full-length mirror	100	50
2. Taking a shower with the lights on	99	0
3. Leaving chores undone that affect mom (e.g., dirty dishes in sink, not sweeping kitchen floor)	90	20

Exposure task	SUDS (Session 2)	SUDS (Final session)
4. Being late	90	5
5. Going to a women's sexual trauma support group	85	40
6. Wearing shorts in public	80	10
7. Going to the gym	80	5
8. Taking a break before chores are done	75	0
9. Getting a pedicure or manicure	75	10
10. Looking at body while clothed in full-length mirror	70	20
11. Sitting next to a man on a bus	70	15
12. Talking to a male employee in a store	65	10
13. Looking at face in mirror	55	5
14. Leaving chores undone that don't affect mom (e.g., not making bed, leaving dirty clothes on bedroom floor)	45	0
15. Making eye contact with men in public	40	0

CLINICAL TIP

What If My Client Has Not Significantly Improved?

In some cases, clients will finish DBT PE without having experienced notable improvements. This may occur if a problem arose that significantly interfered with treatment or made it necessary to stop DBT PE prematurely. In such cases, there may be little progress to review in the final session. However, there are typically at least some achievements that can be highlighted and reinforced, such as that the client was willing to initiate such a challenging treatment, succeeded in completing at least some amount of exposure, and may have learned something beneficial in the process. You can also use this review as an opportunity to generate hope for the future, including emphasizing that the problems the client continues to struggle with are treatable and that it is possible for them to achieve more significant gains in the future when they are in a better place to continue with DBT PE or another evidence-based PTSD treatment.

4. Teach Relapse Prevention and Management Skills

The majority of the final session is spent teaching clients a set of skills intended to prevent PTSD from increasing in the future and to effectively manage an increase in PTSD if it does occur. These relapse prevention and management skills are not part of standard PE and were added to DBT PE due to concerns that relapses of PTSD may be more common among individuals with borderline personality disorder (BPD; e.g., Zanarini et al., 2011). Therefore, clients are taught a set of skills that will help them maintain the gains they have worked so hard to achieve during DBT PE. These relapse prevention and management skills are described in a series of handouts (see Appendix A) that are reviewed with clients in the final session and are described in detail below.

Goals of Relapse Prevention

The overall goal of relapse prevention is a dialectical one: to reduce the likelihood of a future relapse of PTSD while at the same time being prepared to respond effectively if a relapse does occur. You can start by providing a brief overview of this set of skills by reviewing *DBT PE Handout 11* (*Goals of Relapse Prevention*). The first three goals focus on how to prevent relapses by continuing to practice formal exposure tasks, adopting an exposure lifestyle that involves regularly engaging in informal exposure, and identifying and reducing factors that are likely to contribute to a relapse. The fourth goal addresses how to manage potential increases in PTSD by applying the skills and knowledge they have learned in treatment to the task of reducing PTSD again if needed. Overall, the aim is to empower clients to know what they can do to help prevent a recurrence of PTSD, normalize increases in PTSD that may occur despite these efforts, and recognize that they have the skills and knowledge needed to minimize the duration and impact of a relapse if it does occur.

Continue Doing Exposure: Become Your Own Exposure Therapist

The first relapse prevention strategy is to continue to periodically do formal *in vivo* and imaginal exposure. Formal exposure refers to doing exposure in a planned, structured, repeated, and prolonged manner—just as it was done during DBT PE. Clients should be encouraged to continue doing formal exposure after DBT PE for two reasons. First, formal exposure can be used to achieve even greater reductions in PTSD and associated distress by targeting trauma cues that were not fully resolved during DBT PE. Second, formal exposure can be used to ensure that the gains achieved in DBT PE are maintained after treatment is complete and to detect potential increases in distress before PTSD has a chance to return.

Clients are asked to complete *DBT PE Handout 12* (*Become Your Own Exposure Therapist*) in session by identifying specific *in vivo* and imaginal exposure tasks they will continue to practice on their own. For *in vivo* exposure, the SUDS ratings that were obtained earlier in the session for the items on the hierarchy can be reviewed to identify tasks that continue to elicit moderate or high distress that could benefit from additional practice. There may also be some situations that clients no longer find very distressing but that they are unlikely to regularly encounter in their lives (e.g., being in crowded places) that they may want to intentionally expose themselves to periodically to ensure that their gains are maintained.

For imaginal exposure, the focus is typically on maintaining gains by periodically completing imaginal exposure to the traumas that were addressed during DBT PE to ensure that distress does not increase. In some cases, there may be trauma memories that were not fully resolved in treatment that may benefit from continued exposure to achieve additional gains. When doing imaginal exposure on their own, clients can listen to recordings made during treatment, create new recordings, or describe the trauma out loud without recording it. You should also encourage clients to set specific goals for how often they will do these formal imaginal exposure tasks and help them to troubleshoot potential barriers. Clients can also engage in processing on their own, such as by journaling or making art about their thoughts and feelings about the trauma and/or by talking to a trusted support person.

By the end of DBT PE, clients have completed so much formal exposure that they are typically fully capable of designing and completing self-directed exposure tasks without the help of a therapist. *DBT PE Handout 13* (*Guidelines for Doing Exposure Effectively*) consolidates the knowledge they have gained about how to do exposure and can either be briefly reviewed with clients in session or given to them to review on their own. Overall, the goal is to equip clients to become their own exposure therapists, rather than relying on you to continue to assign, provide instructions, and monitor their completion of formal exposure. For this reason, we typically do not assign ongoing *in vivo* and imaginal exposure as homework and instead ask clients to take responsibility for deciding how to do formal exposure moving forward and to ask for coaching if they run into problems.

Adopt an Exposure Lifestyle

The second relapse prevention skill focuses on adopting an exposure lifestyle by regularly engaging in informal exposure. In contrast to formal exposure, informal exposure is often unplanned, relatively brief, and may not be repeated. Essentially, an exposure lifestyle involves constantly being on the lookout for urges to avoid and choosing to approach instead. Given that PTSD is fundamentally a disorder of avoidance in which people routinely and reflexively choose to avoid cues that elicit emotional distress, if clients instead adopt the habit of approaching things that elicit uncomfortable emotions, then PTSD will be unlikely to return. Adopting an exposure lifestyle is also intended to increase joy and meaning in clients' lives. By choosing to engage in activities and situations that are outside their comfort zone, clients are also likely to meet people and have experiences that they would otherwise not have had an opportunity to enjoy. *Adopt an Exposure Lifestyle (DBT PE Handout 14)* describes the FREE skill for living an exposure lifestyle.

1. *Fight fear.* The goal is to not let fear limit your freedom. When unjustified fear makes you want to avoid doing things that are important to you, use opposite action to fight fear by choosing to approach instead. Do things that make you afraid all the way without avoiding and repeat them over and over until fear decreases.

2. *(do) Random acts of exposure.* This involves looking for opportunities to practice exposure and seizing the moment when it arises. When you notice things in your day-to-day life that you want to avoid, spontaneously choose to confront them instead. This may include people, situations, activities, physical sensations, and thoughts that elicit a wide range of emotions, such as shame, disgust, guilt, fear, and sadness. Be sure to do exposure only to things that wise mind says are effective to approach.

3. *Expand your world.* It is important to be willing to do things that are not part of your usual routine and may make you feel uncomfortable. This can include trying activities you have not done before, exploring unfamiliar places, and looking for ways to meet new people. Adopt a "just say yes" approach to living that opens up your world to new possibilities and increases joy and meaning in your life. When trying something new, let go of self-consciousness and participate fully in the activity.

4. *Embrace emotions.* A critical part of adopting an exposure lifestyle is to embrace your emotions. Rather than trying to block or get rid of painful emotions, allow yourself to experience them fully. When doing exposure or trying something new, allow emotions to naturally come and go like a wave without pushing them away or holding on to them. Use mindfulness of current emotion to observe where you feel your emotions in your body. Remind yourself that emotional pain is an unavoidable part of life and that trying to avoid emotions prolongs suffering. Instead, radically accept your emotions to achieve freedom from suffering in the long run.

After you have taught clients the FREE skill, ask them to begin practicing the skill and to complete *DBT PE Handout 15 (Practicing the FREE Skill)* as homework. This handout includes space for clients to identify two situations that they wanted to avoid, describe what they did to use the FREE skill to approach instead, and identify the outcome of using the skill in terms of what they learned from the experience. The goal of assigning the FREE skill as homework is to have clients immediately begin to transition from DBT PE's formal and structured approach to exposure to a more informal approach to incorporating exposure into their everyday lives.

Identifying and Reducing Risk Factors for a Relapse of PTSD

The third relapse prevention skill is derived from Marlatt and Gordon's (1985) cognitive-behavioral relapse prevention model for substance use disorders. This model emphasizes the need to help clients identify factors that are likely to contribute to or precipitate relapses, including both general antecedents (e.g., lifestyle factors, ineffective coping strategies) and immediate prompting events (e.g., high-risk situations). The goal is for clients to prevent, reduce, and/or respond effectively to these contributing factors to decrease the risk of a relapse. When applying this relapse prevention model to PTSD, there are three important types of risk factors to consider that are described on *DBT PE Handout 16* (*Risk Factors for a Relapse of PTSD*) and reviewed with clients in the session. *DBT PE Handout 17* (*Reducing the Risk of a Relapse of PTSD*) is intended to be a self-monitoring tool that can be given to clients to track their use of skills that address these risk factors.

Factors That Increase Emotional Vulnerability

One way to lower the risk that PTSD will increase again in the future is to decrease factors that make people vulnerable to negative emotions, such as poor sleep, unhealthy eating, substance use, and lifestyle imbalances (e.g., many external demands and few pleasurable activities). When people are emotionally vulnerable, they are likely to be much more sensitive to events that prompt negative emotions so that things that would typically be unpleasant but manageable (e.g., a trauma reminder) become high-risk situations that prompt intense and long-lasting emotional reactions. In addition, being in a state of high emotional vulnerability often decreases our motivation to use effective strategies to cope with negative emotions and stressful events when they occur.

Consistent with the DBT approach to emotion regulation, effective relapse prevention for PTSD includes both monitoring and intervening when needed to reduce emotional vulnerability and increase resilience to stress. This is done by using the ABC PLEASE skills from DBT, including (1) Accumulating positive emotions by engaging in pleasant events and activities that are consistent with one's personal values, (2) Building mastery by doing things that make you feel competent and confident, (3) Coping ahead for stressful situations, and (4) taking care of your body by treating PhysicaL illnesses, balancing Eating, avoiding mood-Altering substances, balancing Sleep, and getting Exercise. Ideally, clients will adopt the ABC PLEASE skills as a general approach to living that will reduce their baseline level of emotional vulnerability, as well as use these skills in a targeted manner when they notice warning signs that their vulnerability is increasing.

> ✓ After discussing the need to decrease emotional vulnerability, ask clients to check off the factors on DBT PE Handout 16 that they think are most likely to increase their vulnerability to a recurrence of PTSD. Are there certain vulnerability factors that have been present at times when PTSD has increased in the past that might serve as warning signs in the future?

Avoidant Coping Strategies

A second way to reduce the risk that PTSD will increase is to minimize the use of avoidance to cope with painful emotions, thoughts, and situations. Over the course of DBT PE, clients' long-standing patterns of avoidance have typically changed to a more approach-oriented coping style and the goal is to ensure that these changes are maintained after treatment so that PTSD will be less likely to return. Given that PTSD is fueled by avoidance, overuse of avoidant coping strategies—such as suppressing emotions and thoughts, avoiding situations that cause distress, and engaging in behaviors that function to escape from emotion—may in and of themselves lead to increases in PTSD. In addition, use of avoidant coping strategies may increase the likelihood of being exposed to a high-risk situation that then prompts an increase in PTSD. For example, letting problems build up without actively solving them may lead to crises that could have been averted. Avoidant coping is also likely to interfere with both anticipating and preparing for future high-risk situations and thus make people more vulnerable to these situations when they occur. Finally, people who are in the habit of relying on avoidance to cope are likely to respond to high-risk situations (e.g., new traumas) with avoidance rather than utilizing more effective coping strategies that may help to mitigate the risk that exposure to these situations will prompt a return of PTSD.

To reduce the risk of an increase in PTSD, clients are encouraged to minimize their use of avoidant coping strategies. I often tell clients that if they do not avoid, then it will be impossible for PTSD to return. Indeed, the goal of the first two relapse prevention skills—continuing to practice formal exposure and adopting an exposure lifestyle—is to decrease the likelihood that avoidance will take over again as a way of coping. In addition, if clients notice an increase in specific avoidant coping strategies, they should intervene by using formal exposure, as well as the FREE skill to instead approach the things they are avoiding.

> ✓ On DBT PE Handout 16, ask clients to check off the avoidant coping strategies they are most likely to engage in that may increase their risk of a relapse of PTSD. Which types of avoidance contributed to their PTSD in the past that can be monitored and minimized to reduce the likelihood that PTSD will return?

High-Risk Situations

Relapses are often immediately preceded by exposure to a high-risk situation, which can be anything that causes significant stress. High-risk situations for a relapse of PTSD are often trauma related, such as anniversary dates of past traumas, contact with perpetrators or others involved in one's trauma, and encountering powerful trauma reminders. In addition, high-risk situations may include general life stressors that are unrelated to past trauma, including both negative events (e.g., a relationship breakup) and positive events (e.g., starting college). Finally, a particularly potent high-risk situation for relapse is experiencing a new traumatic event, such as a sexual or physical assault.

The goal is for clients to anticipate and prepare in advance for high-risk situations whenever possible. For example, if a client is planning a trip home to visit family and may see their previously abusive brother while there, then they would ideally plan in advance for how they will cope effectively with this high-risk situation. This may include strategies to avoid the situation entirely (e.g., asking their parents not to invite their brother to the house), as well as strategies to minimize the impact of the situation if avoidance is not possible or preferred (e.g., preparing a DEAR MAN to ask their brother to leave them alone if needed). The DBT skill of cope ahead is ideally suited to this type of advanced preparation and involves identifying specific skills and strategies that will be implemented in an upcoming difficult situation and imaginally rehearsing these skills prior to entering the situation.

> ✓ Ask clients to check off the high-risk situations on DBT PE Handout 16 that are most likely to cause increases in PTSD. Are there certain situations, stressors, or times of year that have reliably prompted increases in PTSD in the past?

Guidelines for Managing Increases in PTSD

Although the hope is that the first three sets of skills will work to prevent a return of PTSD, clients must also be prepared for the possibility that PTSD may increase again in the future, particularly in times of high stress. Clients should be encouraged to view increases in PTSD that may occur as both normal and reversible: They have already succeeded in decreasing their PTSD during treatment and they can do it again in the future if needed. The *Guidelines for Managing Increases in PTSD (DBT PE Handout 18)* are intended to function as an emergency preparedness kit that may never be needed but will provide clients with clear written instructions about what to do if they experience an increase in PTSD in the future. These strategies for managing a relapse are informed by three key principles derived from Marlatt and Gordon's (1985) model of relapse prevention.

1. *Increases in PTSD symptoms are gradual and early detection is the goal.* A relapse of PTSD is typically not a sudden or immediate event, but rather PTSD symptoms slowly increase over weeks or months before culminating in a full-blown relapse. Rather than viewing PTSD as a black-and-white state, a dialectical view is encouraged that recognizes that PTSD symptoms fall on a continuum from total absence of any symptom to severe, life-impairing PTSD. Often increases in PTSD start with only a few symptoms: The person may begin to have difficulty sleeping, notice more frequent thoughts about their trauma, or be aware that they are feeling more on guard. For many clients, the initial increase in trauma-related distress may not involve traditional symptoms of PTSD and may instead include things such as a resurgence of old ways of thinking (e.g., about themselves as bad and incompetent), falling back into trauma-related relationship patterns (e.g., requesting excessive reassurance to quell fears of abandonment), or increased feelings of numbness. Whatever the warning signs are, the goal is for clients to notice these signs early before they become more severe.

2. *Increases in PTSD symptoms do not inevitably lead to a full-blown relapse of PTSD.* When clients notice that PTSD symptoms or trauma-related distress are increasing, the goal is to respond quickly and effectively to prevent them from getting worse. Rather than ignoring or minimizing these initial increases or feeling powerless to do anything about it, clients are encouraged to move swiftly to identify and address the factors that may have contributed to the increase. If this is done, clients are likely to be able to limit the duration and impact of the initial lapse and prevent it from turning into a full-blown relapse. Overall, the goal is to empower clients to know that they can have some control over PTSD if it does begin to increase again in the future, rather than PTSD having control over them.

3. *Relapses are not personal failures and should be viewed with compassion.* PTSD symptoms wax and wane over time for most people and sometimes the stressors in one's life are more powerful than one's capacity to cope. For many people, experiencing a prolonged period of high stress or an acute stressor, such as a new traumatic event, will precipitate an increase or relapse of PTSD despite one's efforts to prevent it. In addition, relapses often occur in the context of other vulnerability factors, such as poor sleep, negative emotional states, and a low sense of competence that may reduce resilience and decrease motivation to use difficult skills like formal and informal exposure to fight the return of symptoms. Therefore, if PTSD does partially or fully return, it is important to adopt a nonjudgmental stance toward oneself and the relapse, validate the understandable reasons it has occurred, and use self-encouragement to stay motivated to manage it effectively. This compassionate approach is likely to be much more effective than judging or criticizing one's perceived failures, which will only make it harder to mount the energy and resources needed to successfully reduce PTSD again.

These three core principles of effective relapse management form the basis of the guidelines for managing an increase in PTSD described in DBT PE Handout 18 that include step-by-step instructions for what to do when an increase in PTSD has been detected.

- *Step 1.* Identify the factors that may have contributed to the increase. For example, have they been more emotionally vulnerable, relying primarily on avoidance to cope with stress, and/ or recently exposed to a high-risk situation? Whatever the likely culprits are, it is important to validate rather than judge these factors by focusing on the understandable reasons they have occurred.

- *Step 2.* Brainstorm potential solutions that could eliminate or reduce the impact of the factors that have contributed to the increase in PTSD. Use the DBT problem-solving skill to brainstorm multiple potential solutions without censoring. These could include specific skills from DBT, formal and informal exposure procedures from DBT PE, or more general solutions that may be helpful.

- *Step 3.* Select one or more solutions to work on now that are well matched to the problem, feasible to implement, and likely to be effective. When needed, solutions can be broken into small steps. Often it takes considerable time and effort to find and implement solutions that work to reduce PTSD. Therefore, if one solution doesn't work, then others should be tried until PTSD decreases again.

- *Step 4.* Identify strategies to stay motivated to keep working hard until effective solutions are found, such as self-encouragement and reinforcement of small steps toward goals. If clients are unable to find solutions that work or are otherwise having difficulty managing an increase in PTSD on their own, they may consider seeking more treatment in the future and/or return for a few booster sessions with you if possible.

DBT PE Handout 19 (Managing an Increase in PTSD) is for clients to complete in the future if they experience an increase in PTSD. The handout provides clear written instructions that walk clients through the four steps of effective relapse management. In the final session of DBT PE, you can review this with clients and help them think about where they will store this handout so that they will be able to access it in the future if needed.

Case Example

Maria and her therapist reviewed each of the relapse prevention handouts in the final session. For the first skill, Maria agreed to continue doing formal *in vivo* exposure to the two tasks from her hierarchy that still elicited moderate distress (looking at herself naked in the mirror and attending her support group), as well as to periodically listen to the imaginal exposure recordings she had created during DBT PE to ensure that the distress caused by thinking about these traumas remained low. She wrote these *in vivo* and imaginal exposure tasks, as well her current SUDS, for each of them on DBT PE Handout 12. Her therapist expressed faith that Maria now had the skills and knowledge to do formal exposure in a self-directed way and suggested that she refer to DBT PE Handout 13 for guidance if needed. Her therapist also said that she would be happy for Maria to report on her progress on these formal exposure tasks during their sessions and offered to provide consultation if she ran into any difficulties.

Maria really liked the idea of adopting an exposure lifestyle by using the FREE skill (DBT PE Handout 14) and thought this would be particularly helpful as she continued to work on building a life worth living now that she no longer had PTSD. Maria said that she could imagine using the FREE skill to address her ongoing urges to avoid interacting with men by choosing to approach or start conversations with men she happened to encounter in her day-to-day life. She was also looking for ways to meet new people, so the idea of expanding her world by using a "just say yes" approach to life also appealed to her. To help her get started with these types of informal exposure tasks, Maria's therapist assigned her homework to use the FREE skill two times and complete DBT PE Handout 15 before their next session.

They then moved on to discuss factors that often contribute to increases in PTSD. On DBT PE Handout 16, Maria checked off boxes in each section that she believed would increase the risk of PTSD returning and thus could serve as warning signs for her to monitor moving forward. In terms of emotional vulnerability, she identified not getting enough sleep, overeating, and not engaging in pleasurable activities as factors that generally made her more vulnerable to stress. Maria also thought it would be particularly important to pay attention to her use of avoidant coping strategies, as she identified with all the examples on the handout and could now readily see how these had contributed to her PTSD in the past. Finally, Maria and her therapist agreed that therapy ending in 3 months would be a significant high-risk situation that they would use cope ahead to prepare for when the time got closer. In the meantime, they agreed to be on the lookout for other high-risk situations that may arise. Maria's therapist oriented her to DBT PE Handout 17 and suggested it as a useful way for Maria to track her efforts to use skills that would reduce the risk of a relapse.

Finally, Maria's therapist reviewed DBT PE Handout 18 with her and framed it as an emergency preparedness kit for her to have available in case she ever experienced an increase in PTSD in the future. Her therapist normalized the possibility that such an increase could occur and encouraged Maria not to consider this to be a failure or catastrophe but rather a problem to be solved. She then walked her through the four steps of effective relapse management and encouraged her to keep DBT PE Handouts 18 and 19 in a place that she could easily find them in the future. Her therapist also emphasized that Maria clearly had the ability to successfully decrease her PTSD, and that she would be able to do so again in the future if needed. At the end of this discussion Maria said, "I really hope my PTSD doesn't come back, but I feel like I know what to do to decrease the chance that it will. I also feel capable of managing it effectively if it does. This really helps me feel more in control of my future."

5. Assign Homework

As described above, clients are assigned homework to use the FREE skill to begin making the shift from the formal exposure of DBT PE to an informal exposure lifestyle. Clients may also decide to continue practicing certain *in vivo* or imaginal exposure tasks on their own or they may opt to take a break from formal exposure. Clients should also be encouraged to do something to celebrate their completion of DBT PE, including the often life-changing improvements they have experienced. However, the journey does not end here. There is still work to be done to ensure that their gains are maintained and to build on these gains by setting new goals that are achievable now that the specter of PTSD is out of the way. The journey will continue in the third stage of treatment (see Chapter 18), which begins after the final session of DBT PE is complete and focuses on helping clients reach their remaining life-worth-living goals.

FINAL SESSION HOMEWORK ASSIGNMENT

Practice the FREE skill and complete DBT PE Handout 15.

PART IV

TROUBLESHOOTING AND TAILORING TREATMENT

CHAPTER 14

Troubleshooting Problems

Therapists are likely to encounter a wide variety of problems when delivering DBT PE that range from routine avoidance to extreme behavioral dysregulation. Although the list of potential problems that could arise is endless, the list of reasons why a behavior may constitute a problem is relatively short. Simply put, a behavior is a problem if it is likely to make DBT PE not work. Therefore, if clients are not sufficiently improving during DBT PE, you need to determine which conditions necessary for PTSD to decrease are missing or insufficient and identify solutions to address these specific problems. In this chapter, I present a principle-driven and step-by-step approach to troubleshooting problems that may interfere with making progress during DBT PE, as well as provide guidelines for deciding when to pause (and ideally resume) DBT PE if problems become significantly interfering.

How DBT PE Works

To successfully assess and solve problems that arise during DBT PE, you must have a clear understanding of how DBT PE works. As shown in Figure 14.1, effective treatment of PTSD requires repeated contact with internal and external trauma cues to activate the emotions and beliefs that are maintaining PTSD. For new learning to occur, information that disconfirms the client's inaccurate beliefs must be presented. Over time, repeated exposure to trauma cues in the presence of disconfirming information results in changes in problematic trauma-related beliefs and emotions that, in turn, lead to improvements in PTSD. This process is referred to as corrective learning. If problems occur that interfere with any of these key elements of the treatment, then progress in reducing PTSD will be limited. For example, behaviors that function to reduce contact with trauma cues, disrupt emotional activation, or interfere with processing disconfirming information are likely to decrease the effectiveness of DBT PE. The gray ovals in Figure 14.1 highlight general strategies that can be applied to address problems at each point in the corrective learning process—these are described in detail later in this chapter.

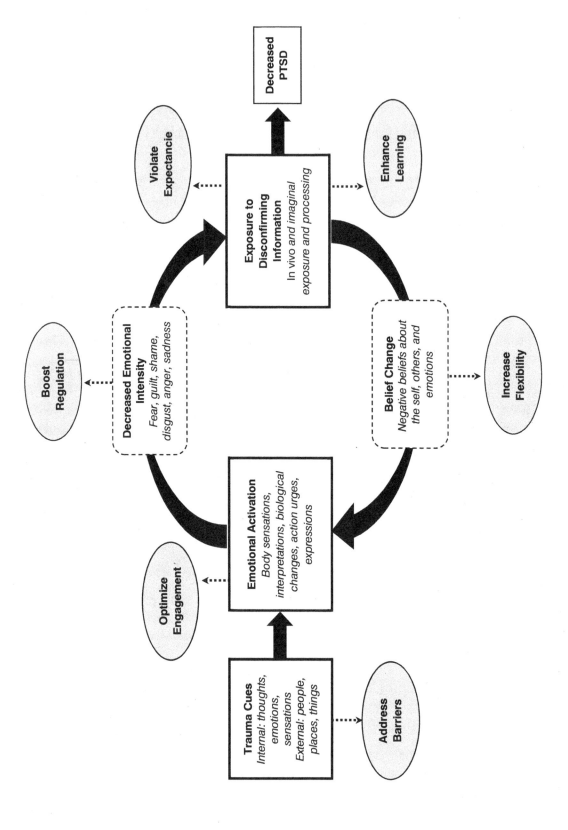

FIGURE 14.1. Addressing problems during the corrective learning process.

Using DBT's Approach to Problem Solving

When a problem occurs that is interfering with making progress, the overall approach is to use DBT problem-solving strategies to address it. There are four steps in this process, including assessing the problem, generating solutions, obtaining a commitment to implement the solution(s), and troubleshooting what might get in the way (see Table 14.1). When working to identify the problem, it is important that you consider both your own and the client's behavior as potential contributors to the lack of improvement. Therapy-interfering behaviors on the part of the therapist may include things such as providing excessive reassurance to clients during exposure, encouraging clients to engage in safety behaviors or use DBT skills that reduce the intensity of arousal when this is not needed, conducting imaginal exposure for an insufficient amount of time, frequently interrupting imaginal exposure, reinforcing rather than disconfirming clients' problematic beliefs, and not assigning enough homework. When you think that you may be contributing to the client's lack of progress, you should seek consultation from your team about how to address this.

Most often, however, problem-solving efforts are focused on helping clients change behaviors that are interfering with achieving maximal gains during DBT PE. How quickly you move to addressing problematic client behaviors will likely depend on their severity. If the behavior is clearly interfering with treatment, such as when clients come to sessions intoxicated or completely refuse to do exposure tasks, you should move rapidly to solve it. If the behavior is milder or less obviously interfering, such as low levels of dissociation during exposure or completing homework three times per week rather than daily, you may opt to take a wait-and-see approach before deciding whether it is interfering enough to limit progress and require targeting. At times, problems may be covert and difficult to detect, such that the only way to know they exist is because the client is not improving. For example, cognitive avoidance strategies, such as repeatedly counting to 10 or thinking about engaging in target behaviors, are not observable and you may not realize they are occurring until you begin to assess for interfering factors when the client is not improving. In general, my recommendation is to begin problem solving if clients do not experience at least some reduction in the intensity of their peak distress (SUDS) after about three sessions of imaginal exposure to the same memory or 3 weeks of repeatedly practicing the same *in vivo* exposure task. If we are not starting to move the needle on decreasing emotional distress after that much repetition, there is likely a problem that needs to be solved.

TABLE 14.1. What to Do When There Is a Problem

Steps in DBT problem solving	Questions to ask
1. Assess the problem	• What behaviors are interfering with corrective learning and limiting progress? • What is causing the problem and why is it not resolving?
2. Generate solutions	• What solutions might work to address the factors that are causing and maintaining the problem? • What behaviors could the client do instead that would be more effective?
3. Obtain commitment	• Is the client willing to implement the identified solutions? If not, what will help to increase motivation?
4. Troubleshoot	• What might get in the way of implementing the solutions? • How can those potential barriers be addressed?

Addressing Common Problems

When progress is slow or limited, you and the client need to collaboratively determine what is interfering with treatment and generate solutions. This can be done using *DBT PE Handout 20 (Troubleshooting Problems during DBT PE)*, which illustrates a step-by-step method for identifying where in the corrective learning process problems are occurring and what types of solutions may be helpful. Consistent with a behavioral approach to treatment, emphasis is placed on the function of potential problems (i.e., how they interfere with the corrective learning process) rather than on the specific type of problem that may occur. This is because many different behaviors can function to cause the same problem (e.g., forgetting and avoidance can each contribute to not doing enough exposure) and the same behavior (e.g., dissociation) can function to cause multiple problems (e.g., interfering with emotional activation and information processing). Given this, potential problems are organized in terms of how they interfere with the core ingredients of the treatment.

Problems with Approaching Trauma Cues

Defining the Problem

For DBT PE (or any treatment) to work, clients must receive a sufficient dose of the active ingredients of the intervention. When clients are not completing enough exposure for DBT PE to be effective, it is like taking only half the dose of a prescribed antibiotic for an infection and expecting the medication to still work. In DBT PE, dose can be defined in terms of the number of sessions received, the number of exposure tasks completed in and outside of sessions, the amount of time spent engaged in exposure, and/or the degree to which exposure tasks are completed as intended. In studies of DBT PE and PE, completing treatment is typically defined as receiving at least eight sessions, including at least six sessions of imaginal exposure—clients who meet this definition of completing treatment are more likely to experience a reliable improvement in PTSD than those who do not. However, research on PE has found that relatively few patients (28%) reach excellent response (at least a 70% reduction in PTSD severity) after eight sessions and most patients (72%) need additional sessions to achieve maximal gains (Zang, Su, McLean, & Foa, 2019). This is consistent with research indicating that the average length of DBT PE is 13 sessions when a "treat-to-remission" approach is used (Harned et al., 2012, 2014). In addition, studies have found that inconsistent attendance during trauma-focused treatment predicts less improvement in PTSD (Mills et al., 2016; Tarrier et al., 2000). Thus, it is critical that clients attend sessions regularly and complete treatment to increase the likelihood that they will achieve meaningful change in PTSD.

It is possible, however, for clients to attend sessions and still not receive a sufficient dose of the active treatment ingredients. This can occur if clients engage in behaviors during sessions that limit the time available for imaginal exposure and processing (e.g., repeatedly debating the merits of exposure, talking about other topics) or refuse to complete imaginal exposure altogether. Clients may also receive an insufficient dose of exposure due to problems with homework compliance. For example, research on PE suggests that clients who complete imaginal exposure homework less than twice per week are at particularly high risk of poor outcome (Cooper et al., 2017). Finally, not doing exposure tasks as assigned, and instead doing tasks in ways that dilute their potency, will also lead to dose problems. For example, a client may be assigned an *in vivo* exposure task to go to an unfamiliar grocery store during daytime hours, stay in the store for at least 20 minutes, and talk to the cashier while paying. If the client instead goes to the grocery store at 3:00 A.M. after researching the layout of the store online, stays in the store for less than 10 minutes, and uses the self-service line to pay, then they have essentially turned an active treatment ingredient into a placebo.

Potential Solutions

Dose problems typically involve the absence of effective behavior, such as not attending sessions, completing exposure homework, or doing exposure tasks as assigned. In DBT, if the absence of a behavior is the problem, then a missing links analysis is typically used to assess and problem-solve the factors that are getting in the way of the desired behavior occurring. Missing links analysis involves asking a series of four questions designed to determine whether the failure to engage in effective behavior is being caused by (1) not knowing what was expected, (2) not being willing to do the effective behavior, (3) not remembering to do what was expected, or (4) some other problem that got in the way of doing what was needed when the thought entered their mind.

Problems caused by not knowing what is expected are often readily solved by providing clearer instructions, having clients pay close attention when instructions are given, and encouraging clients to ask questions when they are unclear what they are supposed to do. Similarly, problems related to forgetting to do exposure are often straightforward to address by using memory aids, such as writing homework assignments on their diary card, putting alerts in their phone, or placing blank Exposure Recording Forms in a location where they will regularly see them. Finally, when clients are willing to do exposure and remember they are supposed to, the problems that interfere are often solved by helping them overcome logistical barriers (e.g., scheduling time for exposure, locating necessary supplies in advance) and use skills to avoid procrastination (e.g., self-encouragement, opposite action).

Most often, however, dose problems are caused by clients being unwilling to do exposure tasks due to PTSD-related avoidance, which can be a more challenging problem to solve. Given that avoidance is a core symptom and maintaining factor for PTSD, it should be expected that clients will at times avoid doing exposure. When this occurs, it is important to adopt a nonjudgmental stance, ideally even viewing this as an opportunity to learn more about the client's problematic beliefs and avoidance behaviors, and work with the client to collaboratively generate solutions. Depending on the specific reasons they are not completing exposure tasks as assigned, different DBT skills may be helpful, such as opposite action, radical acceptance, pros/cons, wise mind, effectiveness, and so on. General strategies to build motivation to complete exposure may also be helpful, such as linking exposure to achieving goals that are important to the client, using contingency management strategies to identify reinforcers for completing exposure, and obtaining and strengthening commitments to do exposure tasks as assigned. In some cases, solutions may involve changing exposure tasks to make them more doable, such as by shortening their duration or reducing the intensity of the stimulus. If these types of modifications are made, it is also important to set the expectation that these will be temporary changes and clients will eventually need to do the exposure task as originally designed for it to be maximally effective. If unwillingness to do exposure becomes a significant barrier and/or clients express high urges to quit DBT PE entirely, the strategies described in Chapter 5 can be used to strengthen their overall commitment to DBT PE.

Potential Solutions for Dose Problems

- Ensure that clients understand what is expected.
- Use memory aids to decrease forgetting.
- Address logistical barriers (e.g., lack of privacy, missing supplies, competing demands).
- Reiterate the rationale for why avoidance will prolong PTSD.
- Set rewards to reinforce exposure completion.
- Link completing exposure to achieving important client goals.
- Evaluate the pros and cons of doing versus not doing exposure.
- Use DBT skills that encourage approaching rather than avoiding exposure (e.g., opposite action, willingness, radical acceptance, wise mind, self-encouragement).
- Temporarily modify the exposure task to make it more doable.
- Obtain, strengthen, and troubleshoot commitments to do exposure.

Problems with Emotional Activation

Once clients are doing exposure, the next problem that can occur is that the emotions elicited by exposure cues are either insufficiently or excessively intense. On the continuum from emotional numbness to emotional flooding, there are many levels of emotional activation that are likely to be effective in facilitating learning—however, problems can occur when clients consistently fall on either emotional extreme. When this happens, problem solving will be needed to help clients achieve more optimal levels of emotional engagement.

Overengagement

OVERVIEW

Overengagement is defined as experiencing an extreme level of emotional arousal that interferes with corrective learning. To be clear, it is normal for clients to experience intense levels of distress during exposure (e.g., rate their SUDS as 100, physically shake, cry intensely), and in most cases this does not mean the client is overengaged. In fact, experiencing intense emotions is often a desired outcome of exposure as it indicates that clients are doing exposure fully and without avoidance. The critical factor in determining whether a client is overengaged is based on what, if anything, they are learning during and as a result of having these intense emotional reactions. If they are learning that they can tolerate very intense emotions without anything terrible happening, they are unlikely to be overengaged. Similarly, if they are able to attend to and retain information that is present while they are intensely distressed, this level of emotional activation is unlikely to be a problem.

In contrast, if the intensity of clients' emotions is reinforcing rather than disconfirming their PTSD-maintaining beliefs (e.g., they believe thinking about their trauma will cause prolonged and intense emotions that will make them unable to function for days and this is what is actually occurring), or they are unable to learn anything at all (e.g., they dissociate and cannot remember what happened during the exposure), then this means they are overengaged and intervention is needed to decrease emotional arousal to a more effective level. Foa and colleagues (2019) identify two types of overengagement—a dissociative type and an emotionally overwhelmed type—each of which is described below.

DISSOCIATIVE TYPE

Defining the Problem. Most clients who receive DBT PE struggle with dissociation at some point in treatment. However, the type and severity of dissociation, as well as the degree to which it may interfere with DBT PE, varies widely across clients. For some clients, dissociation is relatively mild and may not interfere significantly with treatment—for example, they may zone out momentarily and miss part of the conversation, briefly stop talking and stare off into space, or become so absorbed in telling the story of their trauma that they temporarily forget where they are. In other cases, dissociation is more severe and becomes significantly interfering—for example, clients may glaze over and become nonresponsive for many minutes, be unable to recall what occurred during imaginal exposure and processing, or feel completely disconnected from their body or their surroundings when engaged in exposure. In general, dissociation that occurs repeatedly or for extended periods of time during treatment is likely to result in poorer outcomes because it blocks emotional activation (e.g., by numbing and blunting emotions) and/or interferes with learning (e.g., by disrupting information processing and memory). Indeed, higher in-session dissociation has been shown to predict less improvement in PTSD during trauma-focused treatment (Kleindienst et al., 2016).

Potential Solutions. From a behavioral framework, dissociation is viewed as a behavior that is typically prompted by intense emotional arousal and is negatively reinforced by a reduction of aversive emotions and awareness of the cues that elicit them. In addition, dissociation is often reinforced by the external environment—for example, therapists and other people in clients' lives may respond to dissociation by reducing demands and/or increasing care, concern, and support. Dissociation is typically unintentional, meaning that it is a classically conditioned behavior that occurs automatically in response to certain stimuli. At times, however, dissociation can be done intentionally—for example, clients may purposefully make themselves space out or become numb to escape a particularly upsetting situation. It is important to validate that, for many clients, dissociation was learned in the context of chronic trauma from which there was no other means of escape and may have served an adaptive function in helping them to survive situations that were otherwise unbearable. In the context of DBT PE, however, dissociation that functions to reduce contact with trauma-related emotions and stimuli is viewed as a maladaptive behavior likely to interfere with treatment. When dissociation is maladaptive, you should maintain a clear expectation that it must be controlled even (and perhaps especially) if it feels uncontrollable or is not being done intentionally.

There are three main types of solutions for addressing problematic dissociation during DBT PE. The first involves using DBT skills to prevent and/or reduce the intensity and duration of dissociation. Ideally, clients will use mindfulness skills to recognize the warning signs that dissociation is imminent and move quickly to short-circuit this response. Typically, client-specific warning signs for dissociation (e.g., fogginess, stuttering, yawning, feeling cold, tunnel vision) and DBT skills that are effective in preventing or reducing dissociation when these warning signs are present (e.g., TIP, mindfulness, self-soothing) have already been identified in Stage 1. These skills should be applied and fine tuned as needed to prevent and manage dissociation during DBT PE, ideally without stopping or excessively disrupting the treatment procedures. For example, clients who struggle with dissociation during DBT PE may complete imaginal exposure while engaging in grounding strategies, such as holding an ice pack over their eyes, sucking on a sour candy, standing on a balance board, holding smelling salts under their nose, or doing wall squats. Importantly, if these types of skills are used to manage dissociation during exposure, the goal should be to use them only when needed (i.e., when dissociation is imminent or has already started) and not at other times, and generally to titrate their use as treatment progresses so that clients eventually complete exposure tasks without using skills that artificially decrease their level of distress.

The second type of solution to consider involves modifying the exposure task so that it is less distressing and therefore less likely to prompt dissociation. For imaginal exposure, it can be helpful to have clients keep their eyes open (rather than closed) and/or recount the trauma in the past tense (rather than the present tense). Both strategies are likely to decrease the vividness with which the trauma memory is recalled, and keeping eyes open can have the added benefit of helping clients to remain more aware of their present surroundings. The intensity of imaginal exposure can also be titrated by having clients focus on less distressing parts of the memory (e.g., not the hot spots) or write down the narrative rather than say it out loud. Similarly, *in vivo* exposure tasks can be modified to make them less distressing by changing the duration of the task, the number of feared stimuli that are present, the distance from the stimulus, and the context in which the situation is approached (e.g., time of day, location). As a last resort, safety behaviors (e.g., wearing a hooded sweatshirt, holding a pet) may be *temporarily* allowed during exposure to reduce distress and prevent dissociation, as long as there is an explicit plan to eliminate these safety behaviors as soon as possible. Finally, for clients who are still struggling to control dissociation at the beginning of DBT PE, it may be wise to start with less distressing exposure tasks, such as the second or third most distressing trauma memory and *in vivo* exposure tasks that elicit SUDS in the 20–40 range. This can provide clients with an opportunity to build mastery in managing dissociation during exposure before moving to more distressing tasks.

The third type of intervention involves using informal and formal contingency management to strategically reinforce clients' efforts to prevent and manage dissociation, and if needed, apply aversive consequences when problematic dissociation persists. Informal contingency management refers to the therapist's in-the-moment responses to the client that are intended to decrease the likelihood that problematic dissociation will continue. This primarily involves reinforcing nondissociative behaviors using whatever responses the client finds rewarding (e.g., praise, smiling, leaning forward, warm tone, open body posture). In contrast, when clients consistently dissociate in ways likely to interfere with treatment, you may respond in ways the client finds aversive (e.g., demanding that they stop dissociating, leaning back, closed body posture, withdrawing warmth). Typically, these types of informal contingency management strategies are implemented in combination with efforts to coach the client to use skills to reduce dissociation.

In cases where dissociation is severe, not responding sufficiently to other interventions, and proving to be a significant barrier in treatment, you may consider using formal contingency management strategies to address it. Clients must be oriented in advance to the rationale for using formal contingency management, which can be framed as a strategy that will help them gain control over problematic dissociation (which is typically something they want) by giving them more of the things they like when they do not dissociate and fewer of the things they like when they do dissociate. I often use the phrase "Contingencies create capabilities" to explain to clients that they may not be able to consistently prevent dissociation during exposure now, and if

TABLE 14.2. Designing Formal Contingency Management Plans for Maladaptive Dissociation

1. Orient the client to the rationale for using formal contingency management for dissociation and involve the client in collaboratively designing the plan.
2. Define the targets using behaviorally specific terms, including:
   a. Nondissociative behaviors to increase (e.g., using skills to prevent dissociation from lasting for longer than 2 minutes during exposure).
   b. Dissociative behaviors to decrease (e.g., engaging in impulsive sex after exposure when dissociated).
3. Identify specific rewards (reinforcers) for the nondissociative behaviors and determine when they will be provided.
   a. Reinforcers must be tailored to the specific client and possible to implement (e.g., affordable, accessible, within your own and others' limits).
   b. Provide small reinforcers immediately (e.g., praise, high-fives, stickers) and earn larger reinforcers over time (e.g., extra contact, a special gift, being excused from an unpleasant activity that is usually required).
4. Identify specific aversive consequences (punishers) for the dissociative behaviors and when they will be provided.
   a. Aversive consequences must be nonharmful, less frequent than reinforcement, and under the control of the client (i.e., they stop as soon as the client stops the problem behavior).
   b. Aversive consequences can involve the removal of something positive (e.g., a favorite video game is taken away, between-session contact is lost for 24 hours) or the addition of something negative (e.g., engaging in an activity that is disliked).
5. Consistently implement the agreed-upon plan and do not reinforce the targeted dissociative behaviors, including if/when an extinction burst occurs (i.e., a sudden and temporary increase in a behavior at the beginning of the extinction process).

we put effective contingencies in place, this will help them to develop these much-needed capabilities. Ideally, clients will then agree to participate in collaboratively designing and implementing a formal contingency management plan to address dissociation that is interfering with making progress in DBT PE. Guidelines for how to design a formal contingency management plan for maladaptive dissociation are provided in Table 14.2, although these are general behavioral principles that could be applied to change any problem behavior. It is important to note that in behavioral theory, the term *punisher* is used to refer to any consequence that is likely to reduce the occurrence of a problem behavior, and does not mean punishment in the colloquial sense (e.g., being punitive, harsh, or critical). To be most effective, formal contingency management must be implemented in a compassionate and nonjudgmental manner.

CLINICAL TIP

Using DBT PE with Clients with Dissociative Identity Disorder

There is a paucity of research on how to treat PTSD among people with dissociative identity disorder (DID). Treatment outcome studies for DID have not typically reported PTSD as an outcome (see Brand, Classen, McNary, & Zaveri, 2009, for a review) and the largest study of psychotherapy for DID to date found that PTSD symptoms decreased over time but remained at clinically significant levels after years of treatment (Brand, Classen, Lanius, et al., 2009). Although no studies have evaluated evidence-based PTSD treatments in the context of DID, a study of PE found that clients with high levels of trait dissociation were significantly less likely to remit from PTSD than those with low levels of trait dissociation (31% vs. 90%; Hagenaars, van Minnen, & Hoogduin, 2010). DBT PE has also not been evaluated specifically with people with DID—however, 46–74% of clients in DBT PE studies have been above a cutoff for dissociative disorders, and treatment resulted in large improvements in both PTSD and dissociation (Harned et al., 2012, 2014; Harned, Schmidt, et al., 2021). Given this, it seems reasonable to use DBT PE with clients with DID, although more research with this population is clearly needed.

Clients with DID are likely to pose significant challenges during DBT PE, including struggling to manage dissociation during exposure and having fragmented trauma memories that may be split across different personality states. In addition, the dissociative behavior of switching to alternate personality states may or may not interfere with DBT PE depending on its frequency, function, and the context in which it occurs. The following recommendations for using DBT PE with clients with DID are based on the principles underlying DBT, expert guidelines for treating PTSD in DID (International Society for the Study of Trauma and Dissociation, 2011), and recommendations for adapting DBT for DID (Foote & Van Orden, 2016).

Treatment Strategies to Consider

- Prepare clients for the possibility of an exacerbation of dissociation at the start of DBT PE and identify skills to prevent dissociation from interfering with treatment.

- When selecting trauma memories to target, assess the degree to which the client remembers the event in different personality states.

- As much as possible, plan to have the client complete treatment tasks without switching to another personality state.

- If other personality states "hold" the trauma memory or important details of it, discuss the pros and cons of doing imaginal exposure while in a different personality state and collaboratively decide how best to proceed.

- Ensure that switching between personality states is done only if/when it functions to promote trauma processing (e.g., by enabling more contact with trauma-related emotions and facilitating integration of trauma memories into a coherent narrative).

- Do not encourage or reinforce maladaptive dissociative behaviors (e.g., switching that disrupts exposure or functions to escape trauma-related emotions).

- Use shaping principles to reinforce progress toward the goal of being able to describe the trauma narrative in detail without engaging in any dissociative behavior.

- During processing, help clients to better understand the relationships between traumatic events and different personality states, and target trauma-related beliefs and emotions that may be contributing to the maintenance of these states.

- Monitor outcomes closely and make adjustments if DID-related behaviors are not improving, are worsening over time, and/or are interfering with resolving PTSD.

EMOTIONALLY OVERWHELMED TYPE

Defining the Problem. The second type of overengagement involves experiencing excessive levels of emotion that persist for extended periods of time and interfere with corrective learning. Examples may include overwhelming sadness with intense sobbing that makes the client unable to talk or complete imaginal exposure, extreme shame that causes the client's mind to shut down and stop processing information, and intense anger that leaves the client unable to focus on anything but the anger itself. This type of overengagement is similar to the concept of the skills breakdown point in DBT, which is when emotional distress is so extreme that the person is overloaded, cannot focus their attention on anything else, and is unable to process information. When emotions reach these extreme levels, particularly when they persist at this intensity for multiple sessions, they are likely to interfere with the person's ability to attend to and process corrective information. When this occurs, the emotions (whether justified or not) will need to be downregulated to levels that are more effective and will enable new learning to occur.

Potential Solutions. Similar to the dissociative subtype of overengagement, the overall goal is to reduce the intensity of clients' emotion—this is typically accomplished by using DBT skills during exposure. In DBT, when emotions are extreme and clients are at their skills breakdown point, the first step is to use crisis survival skills, such as TIP, distraction, and self-soothing to bring down arousal quickly. Whenever possible, it is preferable to have clients select crisis survival skills that can be applied while continuing to engage in exposure (e.g., holding ice) or that require only a brief break (e.g., to take a sip of a soothing drink) rather than strategies that will require an extended interruption of exposure (e.g., a 10-minute guided imagery practice). These types of crisis survival skills are general arousal reduction strategies that will help to decrease distress in the short term (during exposure) and should ideally be paired with emotion regulation skills (during processing) that will help to decrease the specific emotions that are leading to becoming overwhelmed in the long run.

The second type of solution is to modify the exposure task in a way that makes it less distressing. The previous section on managing dissociation includes a variety of suggestions for how to modify exposure tasks that can also be used for clients who experience the emotionally overwhelmed type of overengagement.

Potential Solutions for Overengagement

- Start with exposure tasks that elicit mild to moderate distress before gradually moving to more distressing tasks.
- Coach clients to use DBT skills that will help to decrease the intensity of emotions and prevent dissociation during exposure.
- Target maladaptive dissociation with informal and/or formal contingency management.
- Modify the exposure task to make it less distressing initially and work toward doing the exposure at its full intensity over time.

Underengagement

DEFINING THE PROBLEM

Underengagement is defined as experiencing low levels of emotional activation during exposure that interferes with corrective learning. While recounting their traumas, underengaged clients often exhibit flat affect, report feeling numb, and rate their SUDS as quite low. In addition, clients' trauma narratives may sound like they are reciting a script or reporting the news rather than describing a highly distressing event that they have personally experienced. Underengagement may be caused by intentional efforts to suppress emotions, but in some cases, clients are actively trying to experience emotions and are not able to access them. Underengaged clients may even report feeling frustrated by their inability to experience emotions and view their emotional numbness as an undesirable state that they want to change. Underengagement is likely to interfere with achieving improvement in PTSD because it blocks emotional activation and prevents a full test of clients' expectancies. For example, clients often have a variety of problematic beliefs about the likely consequences of experiencing intense emotions (e.g., that they will go crazy, be unable to function, be rejected, or kill themselves) and underengagement makes it impossible to disconfirm these beliefs.

POTENTIAL SOLUTIONS

The first step in addressing underengagement is to determine whether clients are doing anything, intentionally or unintentionally, to suppress or avoid their emotions. In other words, are they actively trying not to feel anything or are they open to allowing emotions to be present? If clients are not willing to experience emotions or are doing something to keep them blunted, you should start by validating clients' desire to suppress emotions before moving to reiterate the rationale for why avoidance of emotion will undermine the treatment. It may be helpful to assess clients' beliefs about the likely outcomes of emotional experiencing and encourage them to test the accuracy of these beliefs by doing exposure in an emotionally engaged way. In general, strategies to increase motivation and willingness to allow emotions to be experienced fully may be helpful, such as evaluating the pros and cons, linking experiencing emotions to achieving goals that are important to the client, obtaining and strengthening commitments, and setting rewards for emotional engagement.

A second set of solutions involves coaching clients to use a variety of acceptance-focused DBT skills to increase the intensity of emotions during exposure. If willfulness about allowing emotions is contributing to underengagement, clients can practice willingness instead by using half-smile and willing hands during exposure. Clients may also benefit from practicing radical acceptance, including acceptance of the need to experience emotions, acceptance of their own difficulty accessing emotions, and acceptance of the emotions themselves when they arise. Mindfulness of current emotion can be particularly helpful for the underengaged client—for example, low levels of emotional arousal may be amplified by having clients stay in the exposure situation and temporarily shift their attention to observing their emotion and experiencing their body sensations as fully as they can. Mindfulness skills can also help to increase engagement during exposure—for example, clients can be encouraged to closely observe the exposure cue, describe the trauma memory out loud in as much detail as possible, and fully participate in exposure without holding back.

Finally, underengagement can be addressed by modifying exposure tasks in ways that will make them more emotionally evocative. For imaginal exposure, clients can be coached to describe the trauma in greater detail, including internal details of their thoughts, emotions, and sensations during the trauma, as well as external details that are central to the trauma itself, such as the sights, sounds, and smells present in the most distressing moments. Additionally, imaginal exposure can be combined with *in vivo* exposure to cues that are related to the trauma memory. For example, while recounting the trauma clients may look at a photo of the perpetrator, smell the type of cologne that the perpetrator was wearing, or wear clothes similar to what they had on at the time. Common ways of modifying *in vivo* exposure tasks to make them more emotionally intense include increasing their duration, the number of feared stimuli present during the task, and/or proximity to the cue. In addition, you may consider having clients complete multiple *in vivo* exposure tasks at once, such as walking alone at night while wearing shorts or sharing personal information and asking for a favor in the same interaction. Finally, both imaginal and *in vivo* exposure can be combined with activities designed to generate physical sensations that resemble emotional reactions, such as briefly running in place or doing jumping jacks to get one's heart rate up. These types of sensation-inducing activities may help to activate emotions while engaged in exposure.

Potential Solutions for Underengagement

- Increase clients' motivation and willingness to allow emotions to be experienced fully.
- Coach clients to use DBT skills that will help to increase the intensity of emotions during exposure (e.g., mindfulness and reality acceptance skills).
- Ask clients to include more internal and external details in the imaginal exposure narrative to make the memory more vivid and likely to elicit emotion.
- Modify the exposure task to make it more challenging and emotionally intense.
- Engage in brief activities to induce physical sensations prior to or during exposure tasks.

Problems with Corrective Information

Defining the Problem

Once clients are doing exposure with an effective level of emotional activation, the next problem that can occur is that the information present during and/or after exposure is not sufficiently disconfirming the problematic beliefs that are maintaining their PTSD. For example, clients typically need to learn that approaching trauma-related memories and situations is not dangerous, that they are competent people who can cope effectively with difficult things, and that the traumas they have experienced were not their fault and do not mean they are bad, unlovable, or worthless people. If clients are not obtaining information during exposure and processing that facilitates this corrective learning, then their PTSD is unlikely to improve.

Potential Solutions

To determine whether there are problems with the amount or type of corrective information that is present, you must first be able to answer the question "What does my client need to learn?" More specifically, you must understand which problematic beliefs are activated by the situation or trauma memory so that you can determine what information is needed to disconfirm these beliefs. For example, if a client is afraid that thinking about their trauma will cause them to experience intense sadness that will never end, then imaginal exposure will need to elicit intense sadness so that they can discover how long this avoided emotion lasts. If a client is afraid that they will be harmed or rejected by others, then exposure tasks will need to put them in contact with people who treat them with care and respect. If a client believes that their actions during a traumatic event mean they are a coward, then they will need to be presented with information that helps them develop a more compassionate perspective about their own behavior, and so on. Once it is clear what clients need to learn, then you can evaluate the adequacy of the corrective information that is present. There are several solutions to consider when there are problems with the nature or intensity of the corrective information.

First, the exposure task may need to be redesigned to better match clients' fears and maximally violate their expectancies. For example, if a client who did not complete high school is afraid they will be kicked out of events, such as public lectures, due to their lack of education, then going to such an event, sitting quietly, and leaving without talking to anyone will likely provide them with some corrective information but not enough to fully disconfirm their beliefs. Instead, to increase the mismatch between what they expect and what actually occurs, it would be more effective to have the client tell one or more people at such an event that they dropped out of high school so that they can learn that they will not be kicked out even when others know about their lack of formal education.

During imaginal exposure, a common example that arises is that clients expect that we will reject them once we hear the details of their trauma. Typically, corrective information for this shame-related belief is provided by expressing warmth and care toward clients after imaginal exposure is complete. In some cases, this may not fully disconfirm clients' expectancies if, for example, they believe that you are only treating them positively because you are in a therapy office and that you would be unwilling to be associated with them in a less private setting. In such cases, to maximally violate clients' expectancies it may be useful to accompany clients into public places to demonstrate your willingness to be seen with them, such as by taking a walk outside together at the end of an exposure session. In general, to be most effective, exposure tasks need to be done in the conditions under which the feared outcomes are judged most likely to occur so that clients will obtain corrective information that maximally violates their expectancies.

Even if the task is effectively designed to activate and fully disconfirm clients' beliefs, problems may arise if avoidance or safety behaviors function to dilute or neutralize corrective information. Thus, a second potential solution is to ensure that clients are completing exposure tasks without engaging in behaviors likely to reduce the potency of the disconfirming information they encounter. In the prior example of the client who is afraid of being rejected due to their lack of formal education, this could occur if they take a benzodiazepine before attending a lecture and telling people they did not complete high school. In this case, even if people respond positively to their disclosure, they may attribute this to the fact that the medication enabled them to remain calm and appear confident, rather than to the fact that people are unlikely to reject them. Similarly, in the case of a client who believes you would be too embarrassed to be seen with them outside of the therapy office, if the client stares at the ground and does not look at you while you are walking together in public, then they would not be able to take in all of the available corrective information about your actual reactions.

A third potential solution to consider is to directly provide clients with corrective information if they are unable to generate it on their own. For example, a client may believe that their experience of being forced to have sex does not "count" as rape because they willingly chose to go to the perpetrator's apartment. After several sessions of imaginal exposure and processing, the client may continue to equate agreeing to go home with the perpetrator with consent for sex and be unable to generate alternative interpretations despite repeated efforts to help them do so. In such cases, it may be necessary to directly provide corrective information to clients by suggesting alternative interpretations, using self-disclosure to model more adaptive ways of thinking, and/or providing didactic information to counteract clients' inaccurate beliefs. For example, this might include providing the client with a legal definition of sexual consent and directly stating that their behavior does not qualify as consent. These types of more direct challenges to clients' problematic beliefs are often needed when the amount or intensity of corrective information that is otherwise available is insufficient to achieve change.

Finally, in some cases, the information present during and after exposure may reinforce rather than disconfirm clients' beliefs. For example, at times clients are rejected, have panic attacks, get in accidents, and engage in dysregulated behaviors as a result of completing exposure tasks. When clients' feared outcomes actually occur, the first step is to help them evaluate the severity of these outcomes. If the outcome is unpleasant but not severe (e.g., the client stuttered and turned red when talking to a stranger), then you can help clients reevaluate the perceived cost of the outcome. In contrast, if the outcome does have potentially serious consequences (e.g., the client is harmed by others or does something self-damaging), then you should help clients to cope effectively with the outcome and generate solutions to reduce the likelihood that it will happen again. If the negative outcome that occurred was both serious and a low-likelihood event (e.g., getting in a car accident), you can help clients to identify a wise mind path forward that includes a reasonable assessment of the potential for future risk and does not encourage excessive avoidance of the situation. However, if the negative outcome was serious and seems likely to occur again, then the wise decision may be to avoid the situation unless or until something changes that reduces the probability that it will be dangerous. For example, if a client is afraid they will physically attack people in public and they initiate a physical fight with a stranger during an *in vivo* exposure task, then this may suggest a need to avoid similar situations until the client is able to control physical aggression.

Potential Solutions for Corrective Information Problems

- Redesign the exposure task to maximally violate clients' expectancies. Conduct exposure in the conditions under which the feared outcome is believed to be most likely to occur.

- Assess for and eliminate avoidance or safety behaviors that may be diluting or neutralizing the corrective information that is present.

- Increase the amount or intensity of corrective information by providing additional information that directly counteracts clients' problematic beliefs.

- If feared outcomes occur, help clients to evaluate the probability and severity of the outcome. Make a wise mind decision about whether/how to continue approaching the cue versus avoiding it until risk is lower.

Problems with Information Processing

Defining the Problem

Sometimes information is present during exposure and processing that fully disconfirms clients' problematic beliefs, but something interferes with clients' ability to process and retain this new information. There are three steps in information processing that are necessary for new learning to occur: (1) the new information must be encoded, (2) the information must be stored in long-term memory, and (3) the information must be retrievable in other contexts in the future. Problems at any of these stages will lead to a failure in memory that interferes with corrective learning and impedes progress. For example, problems may occur if clients do not sufficiently pay attention to the information present during exposure (e.g., because they are distracted or selectively attending to only one aspect of the cue) so that it does not get encoded. Additionally, problems may occur if something interferes with consolidating and storing corrective information in memory, such as fatigue, intoxication, dissociation, or difficulty understanding the information. If this occurs, clients may be unable to retrieve information that was learned through exposure and processing when something activates their old problematic beliefs and associated emotions in the future.

Potential Solutions

As a basic starting point, clients should be instructed to do everything they can to optimize their ability to process information effectively, such as eating healthily, getting enough sleep, avoiding substances, controlling dissociation, and treating physical illnesses. These types of brain-boosting strategies are particularly important immediately before, during, and after exposure to ensure they are as clearheaded and able to learn as possible at the times when it is most needed. Additional strategies for addressing memory problems are described below.

ENHANCING MEMORY ENCODING

To get new information into short-term memory, you first need to consciously pay attention to it. Therefore, it is critical that clients utilize mindfulness skills while engaged in exposure to bring their full attention to the present moment. As with any mindfulness practice, this requires clients to notice when their attention has wandered and nonjudgmentally bring it back, often repeatedly, to focusing on the exposure task. Often clients find it harder to stay mindful after they have completed the same exposure multiple times and the cue is no longer novel. If this

---

Potential Solutions for Information Processing Problems

- Use PLEASE skills to maximize cognitive functioning (e.g., eat healthily, get enough sleep, avoid substances).
- Use mindfulness skills to pay close attention to the information that is present during exposure and processing.
- Vary the way in which exposure is completed to enhance attention and later retrieval.
- Minimize potential distractions and practice one-mindfulness while doing exposure.
- Review and consolidate newly learned information before and/or after exposure.
- Rehearse newly learned information out loud or in one's mind.
- Write down or make recordings of key new insights and review them regularly.
- Use retrieval cues to help remember previously learned information in new contexts.

occurs, it may be helpful to introduce some variability into the task so that it is not the same each time clients do it, such as by changing the context in which they complete the task or varying the specific behaviors they engage in. In addition, emotion tends to increase attention, so finding ways to increase or vary the intensity of clients' distress during and across exposure trials may help them remain attentive. Clients can also vary the exposure cues they are approaching by, for example, doing a different *in vivo* exposure task each day or changing the words they use in each repetition of the narrative. Conducting variable exposure not only helps to increase attention but has also been shown to have long-term benefits in enhancing later retrieval and reducing the likelihood of renewal effects after treatment (Craske et al., 2014).

Clients often report that they are more easily distracted when they do exposure on their own compared to during therapy sessions. To address this, you can coach clients to create an environment at home that minimizes distractions. For example, when listening to an imaginal exposure recording, clients may be instructed to sit still in a private location, silence their phone or other devices likely to make noise, and close their eyes to avoid being distracted by visual cues in their environment. Clients may also need to ask people with whom they live to not interrupt them and to help keep children, pets, or other potential distractions away from them while they are doing exposure homework. In addition, clients should be coached to use the skill of one-mindfulness during exposure: when doing exposure, only do exposure. Thus, when clients are listening to their imaginal exposure recording, they should not be engaged in other tasks like driving, exercising, cleaning the house, or watching TV at the same time.

ENHANCING MEMORY STORAGE

To increase the likelihood that encoded information will be stored in long-term memory, it is important to make the new learning that occurs during exposure explicit so that clients are aware they have learned something new. This process of consolidating newly learned information into clear facts that can be more readily retained is built into the Exposure Recording Form, which is designed to explicitly call clients' attention to what was learned as a result of the exposure (e.g., that feared outcomes did not occur). In addition, you can ask targeted questions focused on helping clients to notice and articulate new learning, such as "What did you learn during your *in vivo* exposure practice this week?" or "How did what happened during today's imaginal exposure differ from what you expected?" You may also explicitly draw clients' attention to corrective information that is present by saying things such as "Are you surprised to discover that thinking about your trauma in detail does not interfere with your ability to work?" When clients voice a more adaptive belief for the first time, you can highlight it as new, ask them to say it again, and then discuss what it is like to have that thought (e.g., "What does it feel like to say out loud that it wasn't your fault?"). In sum, repeatedly highlighting discrepancies between previously held beliefs and newly learned information helps to get this corrective learning more firmly anchored in memory.

ENHANCING MEMORY RETRIEVAL

Even if clients develop important new insights and perspectives during exposure and processing, it will do no good if they are unable to recall this new learning in other contexts. Indeed, for PTSD to improve, this newly learned information must become more powerful than the original learning. Prior learning does not get erased when something new is learned   rather, the goal is for new learning to override or inhibit the original learning, which requires that it be retrievable when it is needed, especially when old beliefs and associated emotions are activated. A key strategy for enhancing memory retrieval is to rehearse newly learned information. For example, at the end of a session you can ask clients to restate the new learning that occurred and assign homework to practice saying these things out loud to themselves. Clients can also be instructed to mentally rehearse new learning immediately before and/or after completing exposure tasks to ensure it will be recalled at times when old maladaptive beliefs are particularly likely to be activated. Important new insights can be written down or recorded to ensure clients can remember and review them at times when they would be helpful. Over the course of treatment, clients may benefit from keeping and regularly reviewing a running list of new beliefs that they develop. Finally, clients can use retrieval cues to help remember important facts during or after exposure, such as objects that remind them of the context in which prior new learning occurred (e.g., a photo, a bracelet).

CLINICAL TIP
Using DBT PE with Clients with Cognitive Challenges

There are a variety of conditions that may reduce clients' capacity to learn, such as intellectual disability and traumatic brain injury (TBI). These conditions can lead to cognitive challenges, such as difficulty thinking clearly, reasoning, concentrating, and remembering new information. While DBT PE has not been specifically researched in these populations, research on DBT and PE separately have shown that these treatments can be effective with people with cognitive challenges. In particular, DBT has been adapted for people with intellectual disabilities (Brown, 2015) and shown to result in large reductions in challenging behaviors in this population (Brown, Brown, & Dibiasio, 2013). In addition, multiple studies have found that PE (with no or minor modifications) is effective in reducing PTSD severity among veterans with mild to severe TBI (e.g., Ragsdale & Voss Horrell, 2016; Sripada et al., 2013; Wolf et al., 2015). Moreover, some research suggests that veterans with and without TBI demonstrate a comparable ability to learn in the process of PE as indicated by similar rates of within- and between-session habituation and extinction (Ragsdale et al., 2018). Given that DBT PE is intended to be tailored to the needs of individual clients, it would be appropriate to consider utilizing strategies derived from these studies of DBT and PE to support clients with cognitive difficulties to maintain focus, increase comprehension, and retain information as they engage in DBT PE.

Supportive Interventions to Consider

- Individualize and simplify forms for specific learning and processing needs.
- Provide support in completing forms or use other methods of self-monitoring (such as audio recording) for clients with difficulty reading or writing.
- Repeat information and regularly check comprehension.
- Limit the amount of material presented in a single session. For example, divide Session 2 of DBT PE into two sessions: Session 2A to complete psychoeducation and Session 2B to discuss the rationale for *in vivo* exposure and build the hierarchy.
- Extend sessions to compensate for slower processing speeds and concentration difficulties.

- Conduct joint sessions with family members or significant others to gain corroborating information (e.g., about avoided situations) and ask for support in completing assignments.
- Increase the use of memory-enhancing strategies, such as compensatory devices (e.g., smartphones) and detailed written instructions.
- Schedule between-session phone calls to assist with planning exposure activities and retaining rationales.

Problems with Changing Beliefs

Defining the Problem

Given that changing maladaptive trauma-related beliefs is a critical mechanism of action for reducing PTSD, clients with more rigid, extreme, and black-and-white thinking styles are likely to struggle more to make progress. Research has found that more rigid appraisal and interpretation processes and lack of cognitive flexibility are associated with a greater risk of developing PTSD (e.g., Schultebraucks et al., 2021), as well as greater PTSD severity and duration (e.g., Joseph & Gray, 2011; Steil & Ehlers, 2000). Clients who are cognitively rigid are often resistant to changing their beliefs, unable or unwilling to consider alternatives, and likely to ruminate and perseverate about their trauma in unhelpful ways. In addition, clients with more rigid thinking styles often have difficulty generating explanations for their traumas that are unique to the characteristics of the event and instead rely on global and stable attributions to explain how and why a trauma occurred. For example, a man who was raped may hold firmly to the global belief that he should be able to protect himself in any situation and struggle to consider how the characteristics of the situation in which he was raped limited his ability to fight off his assailant. If cognitive rigidity persists during treatment, it is likely to impede new learning and the development of novel perspectives, and clients will remain stuck in their old maladaptive ways of thinking.

Potential Solutions

There are a variety of factors that can contribute to cognitive rigidity and strategies to address each are discussed in detail below.

INCREASE WILLINGNESS TO CHANGE BELIEFS

For some clients, cognitive rigidity is caused by an unwillingness to let go of a specific belief or generally to consider alternative perspectives. Unwillingness to change unhelpful beliefs typically signals that the client feels that doing so would be threatening in some way. It is therefore important to search for and label the threat. What do clients assume will happen if they were to change the way they think about themselves, others, or the trauma? Is there something they think they will lose that is important to them? Or do they think they will gain something valuable by holding on to their unhelpful beliefs? At times, the perceived threat is linked to a specific belief or emotion that feels important to maintain, whereas at other times the perceived threat may be a more general fear of what might happen if they were to do things that would be likely to result in improvements in PTSD. Examples of common perceived threats are provided in Table 14.3.

TABLE 14.3. Common Perceived Threats to Changing Trauma-Related Beliefs

Loss of important relationships

Example: Blaming oneself for the trauma may enable the person to maintain a relationship with the perpetrator or others (e.g., family members), whereas blaming the perpetrator could lead to a loss of valued relationships.

Loss of identity

Example: "I am a veteran with PTSD" may provide a person with a strong sense of identity and connection to others who are similar to them, whereas allowing change to occur that could result in a loss of the PTSD diagnosis would threaten this identity.

Loss of control

Example: Hindsight bias (e.g., "I should have known it was going to happen") can increase the person's sense of control over future trauma, whereas viewing the situation as unpredictable can heighten a feeling of being unsafe or powerless.

Loss of benefits

Example: A person who receives financial assistance or other disability-related benefits due to PTSD may fear losing these benefits if PTSD is effectively treated.

Loss of valued characteristics of the self

Example: Letting go of unrealistic expectations about one's behavior (e.g., "I should always be able to protect myself") may threaten the person's sense that they possess this valued trait.

Loss of social support

Example: A person who receives care and attention from others due to being a rape survivor may fear that they will lose this social support if they no longer appear to be suffering as a result of the rape.

Loss of sense of validity

Example: Experiencing intense distress due to past trauma can function to validate the seriousness of what occurred, whereas no longer being seriously impacted by it may lead the person or others to invalidate or discount the significance of the trauma.

Loss of justice

Example: A person who frequently expresses judgments and anger about their past trauma may fear that they will never receive justice for what was done to them if they were to be less angry and more accepting.

Once the threat is identified, then the potential probability and/or cost of the threatening outcome can be evaluated. For example, if the client is afraid they will have to end their relationship with their parents if they acknowledge that their past behavior was abusive, how likely is this and how bad would it be? Are there other possible outcomes that could occur instead? Is it possible that they could choose to remain in a relationship with their parents and still acknowledge the problematic nature of their past behavior? Or if they do choose to distance themselves from their parents, is it possible this could be temporary until they feel less angry and more able to manage a relationship with them? Could it be the case that confronting their parents about their past behavior might lead them to apologize, perhaps even bringing them closer? Finally, clients should be encouraged to think through how they would cope if the threatening outcome were to occur. The DBT cope ahead skill can be used to plan and rehearse ways that clients would respond if their worst possible outcome did occur. For example, if the

---

Potential Solutions for Cognitive Rigidity

- Identify, problem-solve, and cope ahead for perceived threats to changing beliefs.
- Weigh the pros and cons of changing the way they think.
- Teach clients how to generate and consider different interpretations.
- Increase awareness that there are multiple ways to view any situation.
- Encourage dialectical thinking and look for ways to balance and synthesize extremes.
- Validate both old and new perspectives and allow for meaning to evolve over time.
- Observe and detach from distressing thoughts rather than trying to change them.
- Help clients to differentiate between thoughts and facts.
- Make decisions based on wise mind rather than on specific thoughts that arise.
- Use defusion strategies to reduce the impact of specific thoughts.

---

client became completely estranged from their parents, are there people from whom they could get support? If there are certain things that they rely on their parents for, how would they get those needs met in other ways? Additionally, clients should be encouraged to consider potential positive outcomes of changing the way they think. For example, letting go of self-blaming or self-critical beliefs often leads to reduced guilt and shame and an increased sense of self-respect and personal value. This process of considering multiple potential outcomes of changing one's belief, weighing the pros and cons of adopting a different point of view, and thinking through strategies to address the threatening outcome often helps to increase clients' willingness to let go of their belief and find out what actually occurs.

TEACH FLEXIBLE THINKING

If cognitive rigidity is due to a skills deficit (i.e., an inability to generate alternative interpretations), then clients can be taught how to think more flexibly. In DBT, the skill of check the facts is used to teach clients how to generate and consider different interpretations about a specific prompting event. This approach is similar to attribution retraining, which has been used to help people who have experienced a trauma learn to generate different causal explanations for the event and reduce cognitive rigidity (Joseph & Gray, 2014). The key element of these approaches is to teach brainstorming skills—namely, how to generate as many other possible interpretations as they can. To some extent, the content of these alternative interpretations may be less relevant than the experience of seeing that there is always more than one way to view a situation. To that end, clients should be encouraged not to censor themselves and to allow themselves to suggest interpretations that are extreme or highly improbable, as well as ones that may be more plausible. If clients struggle to identify alternatives, they can be asked to consider viewpoints they may have heard from other sources, such as movies, books, or people in their lives and/or to think about what they would say if someone they care about voiced the same belief. If needed, you can also help to generate alternative perspectives, perhaps taking turns with the client to create as long a list as possible.

Once multiple possible interpretations have been generated, clients can be asked to identify one or more that feel most likely and/or effective. To that end, it can be helpful to have them consider the likely outcomes of adopting a specific alternative perspective. For example, what emotion(s) would they experience? What action urges would they have and what might they do differently in their lives? How would they feel about themselves and other people? What predictions might they have for the future? Thinking through these potential outcomes can help clients to identify new interpretations that are likely to be most effective and then weigh the pros and cons of sticking with their old unhelpful belief versus allowing themselves to flexibly adopt an alternative one that seems both accurate and effective.

ENCOURAGE DIALECTICAL THINKING

In some cases, cognitive rigidity can be due to a lack of dialectical thinking. This can mean that clients think in rigid black-and-white terms. They are either weak or strong. The person who abused them is either good or bad. The world is either dangerous or safe. The trauma was either caused by their own behavior or the perpetrator's behavior. Often clients vacillate between these extremes because neither pole is entirely accurate, and each leaves out something important. Dialectical thinking encourages us to instead consider that two extremes that seem like opposites can both be true at the same time. Finding a way to synthesize and balance these opposites—using "and" instead of "or"—can lead to new and more flexible ways of thinking. Examples include:

- I can often protect myself from harm *and* I cannot keep myself safe all the time.
- The person who abused me has positive qualities *and* negative qualities.
- The world is usually safe *and* it can be dangerous at times.
- My behavior increased my risk of being victimized *and* the perpetrator is responsible for their actions.

Another version of nondialectical thinking can occur when clients find it difficult to allow for meaning and truth to evolve over time. For example, if they have always believed that being beaten by their parents was an acceptable form of discipline, allowing this perspective to change can feel destabilizing and cause clients to question their sense of reality. Clients may ask themselves, "How is it possible that I was so wrong?" or "How could things be so different from what I have always thought?" When this occurs, clients may feel pulled to rigidly hold to their original point of view since it feels familiar and comfortable, rather than allowing for the possibility that their understanding and perspective can change, often quite dramatically, over time. Dialectical thinking would involve being able to validate both their original and new perspectives—even if they are polar opposites—and accept that both have felt true at different times. Very often the old beliefs are a by-product of an invalidating environment, and these shifts in understanding can be explained by being out of those environments and getting exposed to new people and information.

CLINICAL TIP
Addressing Client and Therapist Polarization about What Is "Right"

Given the focus on helping clients to change their inaccurate beliefs to more accurate ways of thinking, it is not uncommon for therapists and clients to at times find themselves in a polarized debate about who or what is "right." You may be arguing for a point of view that you firmly believe is true and would be in the client's best interest to believe and the client may be holding firmly to their opposing point of view and arguing for why they believe it is accurate. As an example, I once treated a veteran who had PTSD related to witnessing traditional cultural practices involving the sexual abuse of boys during his deployments. Although he had tried several times to persuade local troops to change these abusive practices and had successfully intervened to stop one incident he witnessed, he firmly believed that he had not fought hard enough against these abuses. As a result, he had intense guilt and shame and viewed himself as a weak and morally compromised person who deserved to die. When I first heard this story, I was frankly incredulous that he would think it was his responsibility to change such an established and accepted (albeit abhorrent) cultural practice, particularly as a lone and distrusted American soldier who was there to conduct an entirely different wartime mission. I tried mightily to get him to recognize that he had done the best he could in a terrible situation, that nobody could have achieved what he was thinking he should have done, and that his decision not to push harder to change these abusive practices made sense and was likely wise in context. At times he agreed with some of the points I made, but no matter what I said, he held rigidly to his belief: "I should have fought harder against these abuses." We were polarized, and neither one of us was willing to give up our sense of being "right."

When this type of polarization occurs, it can be helpful to remember a key tenet of dialectics: There is no absolute truth, and therefore, there can be multiple "right" answers. As therapists, we must be willing to metaphorically drop the rope—that is, to stop the tug-of-war between our own and the client's point of view and instead look for what is being left out. What is valid on their side? Are there elements of my own side that are invalid or inaccurate? Is there a synthesis between our two opposing points of view that acknowledges the validity in both sides?

In the above case, we were eventually able to find several syntheses that included elements of both my own and the client's perspective: (1) "I could not have changed these cultural practices *and* I wish that I had tried harder to do so" and (2) "I am a person who usually fights hard for what I believe in *and* I did not fight hard in this situation." These more balanced thoughts enabled this client to begin to radically accept his own inaction, which led to sadness rather than guilt and shame about the fact that he had not been able to stop the abuse he had witnessed. As this example shows, it is important to remember that the goal is to help clients find new perspectives that work to decrease unjustified emotions, not to get them to adopt our point of view. Thus, as therapists we must be willing to let go of our own beliefs about what is "right," allow ourselves to think flexibly, and join with the client to search for a reasonable synthesis that will be effective in reducing suffering.

INCREASE MINDFULNESS OF THOUGHTS

At times, the most effective strategy to address particularly rigid beliefs is to teach clients to observe and detach from their distressing thoughts rather than try to change or control them. This can be a useful approach when clients recognize that an upsetting thought and their usual behavioral responses to it are not effective but continue to believe the thought is true. The goal of an acceptance-focused approach is to help clients change their relationship to their own thoughts and beliefs, viewing them as simple mental events and not concrete reality or facts. In DBT, this is done by teaching clients the skill of mindfulness of current thoughts, which involves learning how to observe their thoughts, beliefs, assumptions, and interpretations by noticing them come into their minds and letting them go without getting attached to them.

This type of mindfulness may lead to more flexible thinking by teaching clients to observe the changing nature of their thoughts without reacting to them as if they are facts that should govern their behavior. Instead, clients can be encouraged to choose to do what their wise mind says is effective even if they have a thought or belief that suggests otherwise. For example, a client who believes "I don't deserve to get better" can notice this thought without allowing it to stop them from choosing to engage effectively in DBT PE. Similarly, when clients voice thoughts that have already been identified as unhelpful, you can simply highlight that this has occurred and encourage them to respond effectively, rather than getting caught up in trying to change these thoughts (e.g., "Oh no, your 'why bother' thoughts have shown up today! What can you do when that thought comes up to make sure you stay effective?"). In this way, clients learn that thoughts are just a series of mental events, some of which are helpful and some of which are not, rather than beacons of truth that must be acted on.

Another way to practice the DBT skill of mindfulness of current thoughts is to play with thoughts using cognitive defusion strategies. Often this is done by repeating a particularly upsetting thought out loud over and over, perhaps using silly accents, saying it at different speeds, or singing it to the tune of a familiar song. Thoughts can also be imagined to take different shapes and forms, such as captions in a comic book, mythical creatures that battle one another, or balloons floating into the sky. The goal of these types of defusion strategies is to reduce the potency of specific thoughts and to see them as what they are (e.g., sounds, mental events), rather than as facts or literal meanings that must be taken seriously.

CLINICAL TIP

Using DBT PE with Clients with Psychotic Disorders

Although it was long believed that trauma-focused treatments should not be used with people with psychotic disorders, there is increasing evidence that these treatments can be effective in reducing PTSD in this population (Swan, Keen, Reynolds, & Onwumere, 2017) and may indirectly lead to decreases in psychotic symptoms, such as paranoid delusions (Brand, McEnery, Rossell, Bendall, & Thomas, 2018). Given these advancements, individuals with psychotic disorders, including those with active psychosis, were included in my most recent study of DBT PE (Harned, Schmidt, et al., 2021). In general, current recommendations are to not exclude individuals with psychotic disorders, such as schizophrenia or schizoaffective disorder, from PTSD treatments on the basis of these diagnoses, and instead to allow these individuals to receive trauma-focused treatment if/when they meet the standard readiness criteria for these treatments.

That said, individuals with psychotic disorders may pose particular challenges when delivering DBT PE, including being more likely to have entrenched delusional beliefs that may be especially resistant to change. When delivering DBT PE to individuals with psychotic symptoms, you are encouraged to utilize the following research-supported strategies from cognitive-behavioral therapy for psychosis (CBTp; Morrison, Renton, Dunn, Williams, & Bentall, 2004), as well as from expert guidelines and recommendations for using trauma-focused treatments with people with psychotic disorders (e.g., Brand, Hardy, Bendall, & Thomas, 2020; van den Berg, van der Vleugel, Staring, de Bont, & de Jongh, 2013).

Treatment Strategies to Consider

- Include family members or support persons in treatment (e.g., to obtain collateral information about the timing of traumatic events and the onset of psychotic symptoms).

- Address possible cognitive impairments, such as poor concentration and distractibility, using strategies such as repeating instructions and working slowly.

- Provide psychoeducation about the links between trauma and psychosis.

- Prioritize traumatic events that are most connected to the onset and content of hallucinations and delusions.

- Consider doing imaginal exposure to psychotic imagery (e.g., of feared catastrophes or hallucinations) and to events the person falsely believes occurred.

- Prepare in advance for the possibility of a temporary exacerbation of psychotic symptoms at the beginning of imaginal exposure sessions.

- Address delusions (e.g., paranoid beliefs about danger) using *in vivo* exposure and cognitive interventions focused on evaluating the helpfulness of the usual behavioral response rather than direct challenges of delusional content.

- Use acceptance-oriented strategies to reduce distress related to experiencing psychotic symptoms rather than trying to change their occurrence.

- If medications appear to be interfering with learning, consider not taking them prior to sessions if possible and safe.

Problems with Decreasing Emotional Intensity

Defining the Problem

In addition to belief change, the second critical mechanism of action for improving PTSD is to decrease the intensity of trauma-related emotions over time (i.e., between-session habituation or extinction), particularly those that are unjustified or ineffective. Although the troubleshooting strategies described so far have focused primarily on optimizing learning and subsequent belief change, in theory they should also help to reduce the intensity of trauma-related emotions. However, at times changing beliefs is not sufficient to change an emotion. For example, clients may no longer think from a logical perspective that they are repulsive, but they may still feel disgust toward themselves. Similarly, clients may recognize that there is no evidence to suggest that they are inherently bad, but they may continue to feel ashamed of themselves. When clients are not able to think their way out of feeling something, then emotions are likely to stay elevated and interfere with achieving improvement in PTSD.

Potential Solutions

When emotions are not decreasing in intensity even when clients recognize that they do not fit the facts, then behavioral (as opposed to cognitive) emotion regulation strategies are needed to change them.

REDUCE EMOTIONAL VULNERABILITY

In some cases, emotional vulnerability may be interfering with reducing the intensity of emotions. High emotional sensitivity and reactivity, general moodiness, and lack of energy can make it difficult to regulate emotions even when clients are trying to do so. To optimize their ability to regulate emotions, clients may need to use the ABC PLEASE skills from DBT, which focus on increasing pleasant events in the short- and long term, doing things that build a sense of mastery, coping ahead for upcoming stressors, and taking care of your body. By reducing emotional vulnerability, clients will be more able to access wise mind and use skills to effectively regulate emotions.

USE OPPOSITE ACTION

Often emotions are not changing because clients continue to act as if they are justified even when in wise mind they know that they are not. For example, as a result of imaginal exposure and processing, a client may now recognize that being sexually abused does not make them a worthless person. However, if they continue to act as if they are worthless by doing things such as putting others' needs ahead of their own, not asking to be treated with respect, and refusing to do kind things for themselves, then the emotion of shame is likely to persist. When knowing the facts does not sufficiently change an emotion, clients should be coached to use the DBT skill of opposite action to do the opposite of the emotion's action urge repeatedly and all the way (see Chapter 15 for specific examples). Opposite action can be done in a formal and structured way (e.g., using *in vivo* exposure) and/or informally by coaching clients to notice emotion-driven urges when they arise and choose to act opposite when they know the emotion is unjustified or ineffective. These types of opposite-to-emotion actions can help reduce stuck emotions by ensuring that their actions are not inadvertently maintaining the emotions they want to change.

USE PROBLEM SOLVING

It is also important to consider the possibility that an emotion may not be changing because it is justified (i.e., fits the facts of a situation that is prompting it) and that problem solving how to avoid or change the situation may be needed to get the emotion to decrease. For example, if someone in the client's current life (e.g., a partner or parent) is actively treating them as if they are incompetent and worthless, it is likely to be harder to get shame related to past events in which they were treated similarly to change. Or if a past abuser continues to do things in the present that block important goals (e.g., preventing the client from being able to spend time with other family members), then anger is likely to remain high. When present-day situations

---

Potential Solutions for Stuck Emotions

- Use ABC PLEASE skills to reduce emotional vulnerability and maximize the capacity to effectively regulate emotions.
- Act opposite to emotion urges repeatedly and all the way.
- Problem-solve present-day situations that are contributing to stuck emotions.

are contributing to and making it difficult to change painful emotions, then the DBT skill of problem solving can be used. This skill involves accurately describing the situation and what is problematic about it, identifying your goal in solving the problem, brainstorming as many possible solutions as you can, choosing a solution that matches your goal and seems likely to work, putting the solution into action, and evaluating the results. If one solution doesn't work, then additional solutions should be tried until the emotion that is being exacerbated by a current problem is reduced.

Deciding When to Pause the DBT PE Protocol

Although the goal is to complete DBT PE in one continuous course of treatment, there are times when DBT PE must be paused because a significant problem has occurred that makes it either unsafe or ineffective to continue. If this happens, DBT is used to target the problems that caused DBT PE to be stopped with the goal of resuming DBT PE as soon as these problems have been sufficiently resolved. As Marsha Linehan (1993) wrote in the DBT manual, "Because of its middle position in the three stages, the reduction of posttraumatic stress reactions is often started, stopped, and restarted" (p. 171). Therefore, you need to be prepared to make challenging clinical decisions about whether and when to pause and subsequently resume DBT PE when problems derail the treatment.

The core dilemma that is faced when deciding whether to pause DBT PE lies in finding an effective balance between pausing when it is not needed versus not pausing when it is needed. In my experience, clinicians tend to be more worried about the possibility of continuing DBT PE when this might be risky or ill-advised and therefore tend to err on the side of pausing rather than pushing forward when significant problems arise. Since there is no way to know in advance whether pausing versus continuing is likely to be most effective, the best we can do is make principle-driven (rather than emotion-driven) decisions in consultation with our DBT team and then closely monitor outcomes and adjust our course if needed.

The guidelines that are used to decide when to pause DBT PE are based on the same principles as the criteria for determining when a client is ready to start DBT PE. First, the principle of risk management specifies that reducing life-threatening behaviors must be prioritized over other targets—thus, decisions about whether to pause DBT PE must include consideration of potential safety issues. Second, in accord with the principle of contingency management, when making these decisions we must take into account whether pausing DBT PE would be likely to increase versus decrease a problem behavior. Third, the principle of outcome optimization emphasizes the importance of maximizing the likelihood that DBT PE will be effective in improving PTSD, which means that DBT PE may be paused if serious problems are making the treatment not work and efforts to solve these problems have not been effective. The principle-driven guidelines that are used to determine when to pause DBT PE are listed in Table 14.4. These guidelines are organized in terms of DBT's target hierarchy, with more stringent guidelines for stopping applied to life-threatening behaviors, and more flexible guidelines applied to therapy-interfering and/or quality-of-life-interfering behaviors.

Responding to Life-Threatening Behaviors

If clients engage in behaviors that lead you to believe they are at imminent risk of suicide, DBT PE should be paused. Indices of acute suicide risk vary between clients but often include

TABLE 14.4. Guidelines for When to Pause DBT PE

Pause DBT PE when life-threatening behavior occurs, including:

1. Behaviors indicative of imminent risk of suicide

2. Suicidal or nonsuicidal self-injurious behavior

Consider pausing DBT PE when therapy- or quality-of-life-interfering behavior occurs if:

3. Pausing would decrease the likelihood of the behavior, and/or

4. DBT PE is unlikely to be effective while the behavior is present, and/or

5. The problem must be treated now and cannot be effectively addressed while continuing DBT PE.

---

things like engaging in suicide preparation behaviors, communicating intent to kill oneself, or engaging in aborted or interrupted suicide attempts. Typically, increases in suicidal thoughts or urges that are not accompanied by intent to act or preparatory behaviors, and when the client remains firmly committed to staying alive, are not viewed as reasons to pause DBT PE. However, if clients are believed to be at imminent risk of suicide, meaning that they are likely to try to kill themselves within days, then reducing immediate threat to life must be prioritized over continuing DBT PE.

In addition, consistent with the rule that clients must be abstinent from both suicidal and nonsuicidal self-injury to be considered ready to start DBT PE, if these behaviors occur during DBT PE, they will automatically cause the treatment to be paused. This is true regardless of the intent or potential lethality of the behavior, meaning that low-risk forms of nonsuicidal self-injurious behavior will trigger DBT PE to be paused in the same way that a nearly lethal suicide attempt would. This contingency is primarily intended to motivate clients to maintain control over these behaviors, particularly because urges to engage in these behaviors may temporarily increase at the beginning of DBT PE. Indeed, many clients report that knowing that DBT PE will be paused if they attempt suicide or self-injure helps them to not act on urges to engage in these behaviors. Given this, it is critical that you clearly communicate this contingency to clients prior to starting DBT PE. Encouragingly, research has shown that relatively few clients engage in NSSI (0–20%) or attempt suicide (0–15%) during DBT PE (Harned et al., 2012, 2014; Harned, Ritschel, et al., 2021; Harned, Schmidt, et al., 2021; Meyers et al., 2017), and this contingency is often an important factor in reducing the risk that these behaviors will occur.

Requiring that DBT PE be paused if life-threatening behavior occurs also functions as a risk management strategy intended to mitigate against the possibility that these behaviors will be exacerbated by DBT PE. Indeed, given that self-injurious behaviors most often function to provide temporary relief from emotional distress, the occurrence of these behaviors during DBT PE suggests that clients may not yet have sufficient skills to safely tolerate and regulate the intense emotions elicited by exposure. If so, continuing to ask clients to do exposure tasks designed to elicit intense distress, without shoring up their skills first, may lead to additional instances of these behaviors. Finally, given concerns that DBT PE is likely to be less effective if clients are attempting suicide or self-injuring, particularly if these behaviors occur in close proximity to exposure and interfere with the corrective learning process, pausing DBT PE until these behaviors are resolved may also help to optimize the effectiveness of the treatment.

CLINICAL TIP

What If Pausing DBT PE Is Likely to Reinforce Life-Threatening Behaviors?

After reading the above, you may be concerned about the possibility that pausing DBT PE in response to suicide attempts and nonsuicidal self-injury may inadvertently reinforce these behaviors. This is a valid concern and may be a risk for some clients, particularly those who are highly ambivalent about doing DBT PE. Infrequently, clients who are ambivalent about DBT PE may engage in life-threatening behaviors to get the treatment to stop. In other cases, pausing DBT PE in response to these behaviors may be experienced as a positive outcome even if this was not the client's intention. Based on both clinical experience and data on clients' treatment preferences, it is a relatively small proportion of DBT clients who do not want DBT PE and an even smaller number who decide to initiate the treatment despite being very unsure they want to do it. If you are treating such an ambivalent client, it is recommended that you emphasize the voluntary nature of the treatment and maximize the client's sense of control over the decision about whether and for how long to do DBT PE. In addition, it can be helpful to troubleshoot in advance the possibility that clients may engage in life-threatening behavior in order to not have to continue DBT PE and obtain a commitment that they will directly communicate a desire to stop instead. If you end up in the unfortunate position of having to pause DBT PE due to life-threatening behavior with a client for whom this is reinforcing, other strategies can be implemented to make this pause as nonreinforcing as possible (e.g., applying other consequences the client finds to be aversive while DBT PE is paused).

Responding to Therapy-Interfering and Quality-of-Life-Interfering Behaviors

Whereas you are expected to pause DBT PE if life-threatening behaviors occur or are believed to be imminent, you may or may not choose to pause DBT PE if therapy-interfering or quality-of-life-interfering behaviors arise that are creating problems in treatment. These may include a wide variety of potential behaviors, such as inconsistent session attendance, suppressing emotions during exposure, dissociation, excessive substance use, increased psychotic symptoms, and homelessness. If these types of problems arise, the decision about whether to pause should be made after carefully considering the following three issues:

First, would pausing DBT PE be likely to decrease the likelihood of the behavior? As previously described, being able to receive effective treatment for PTSD is a desired outcome for many clients, and when this is the case, having to pause DBT PE is likely to be experienced as an aversive consequence that clients will work to avoid. Therefore, and perhaps somewhat paradoxically, we are usually more likely to pause DBT PE with clients who are motivated to continue the treatment and less likely to pause DBT PE with clients who might prefer to stop. For example, if a client who really wants to do DBT PE is completing imaginal exposure homework only once per week, you might choose to implement a contingency in which the client must do imaginal exposure at least three times per week to continue with DBT PE. Ideally, this contingency will motivate the client to do more homework, and if not, the experience of having to stop a desired treatment should help to decrease the likelihood that insufficient homework completion will be a problem again when DBT PE is resumed. In contrast, if a client who is not completing enough exposure homework is highly ambivalent about doing DBT PE, saying that you will pause the treatment or actually stopping it is unlikely to be effective in motivating them to do more homework and may instead be viewed as a welcome reprieve from a treatment they are unsure they want.

Second, will the behavior prevent DBT PE from being effective? As discussed in detail in this chapter, there are many possible behaviors that can make DBT PE not work. If progress in improving PTSD is slow or nonexistent, you should follow the troubleshooting steps previously described to identify the problem and try to solve it. If the interfering behavior persists despite repeated efforts to solve it, DBT PE may be paused because continuing is unlikely to lead to positive outcomes. Deciding to stop because the client is not improving can be a challenging decision, especially if you and/or the client are particularly tenacious and motivated to keep trying to make the treatment work. Although there is no rule about how long to persist in the face of nonresponse, one study of PE found that clients who do not experience at least a 10% reduction in PTSD symptoms by Session 8 (i.e., after six sessions of imaginal exposure) are unlikely to achieve meaningful change with additional sessions (Ready, Lamp, Rauch, Astin, & Norrholm, 2020). Although this should not be viewed as a definite cutoff point, if clients have achieved very minimal or no change in PTSD after eight or more sessions, then it may be wise to pause the treatment to focus on addressing whatever is interfering with making progress.

Third, does the behavior have to be treated now, and if so, can this be done while continuing DBT PE? Sometimes quality-of-life problems arise during DBT PE that are urgent and may be a higher priority than treating PTSD, such as serious medical illnesses, an abusive relationship, housing or financial problems that have reached a crisis level, criminal behavior that is likely to lead to arrest, or the sudden death of a loved one. When these types of acute problems are present that threaten to significantly disrupt the client's life, whenever possible the preferred option is to address the co-occurring problem during concurrent DBT while continuing to deliver DBT PE. However, there are times when it is simply not possible to treat both problems at once either because there is not enough DBT session time to adequately target the co-occurring problem or DBT PE may be contributing to or exacerbating the other problem. For example, if a client has received an eviction notice and will be forced to leave their apartment in 2 weeks, one or more entire sessions may be needed to help the client identify resources and mobilize to find a new place to live, rather than trying to figure this out in only 30 or 60 minutes. Alternatively, if an urgent problem—such as a significant increase in auditory hallucinations that has put the client at risk of losing their job—is being caused in whole or in part by DBT PE, then you may opt to pause the treatment so that the problem will resolve more quickly and/or a potential crisis will be averted. However, given that many clients' lives are characterized by unrelenting crises, you need to be careful not to fall into a pattern in which DBT PE is frequently paused or preempted by problems in the client's life, particularly when they are unrelated to DBT PE and/or being exacerbated by untreated PTSD.

Deciding When to Resume the DBT PE Protocol after Pausing

If DBT PE is paused, this should not be viewed as a failure. It is to be expected that clients' readiness for DBT PE may wax and wane over time and that stressors will sometimes arise in clients' lives that overwhelm their capacity to cope. Moreover, the decision about whether clients are ready to start DBT PE is a challenging and subjective one, and it may be the case that we discover once we begin DBT PE that we misjudged this and more preparatory work is needed. Therefore, rather than feeling ashamed, hopeless, or judgmental about whatever occurred that led DBT PE to be paused, it is infinitely more useful for therapists and clients to double down in their efforts to figure out what went wrong and work together to resolve it so that DBT PE can be resumed as soon as possible. This work is done during DBT individual therapy, which continues to be delivered while DBT PE is paused using whatever session structure is typical for your practice of DBT (e.g., one 1-hour session/week). Given that sessions are usually longer and/or more frequent when delivering both DBT and DBT PE, clients typically receive less individual therapy while DBT PE is paused. This reduction in session time can also function as a contingency that may reduce the likelihood that the problem behavior will recur.

Importantly, *there is no fixed length of time that clients must wait to resume DBT PE once it has been paused*. Instead, the length of time that DBT PE is paused depends on when clients demonstrate readiness to continue—this may be relatively brief (e.g., taking 1 week off before resuming) or require more time (e.g., several months). Overall, the goal is to resume DBT PE as soon as possible while also not returning too quickly to DBT PE if the problem has not been sufficiently resolved. The criteria that are used to decide when to resume DBT PE are listed in Table 14.5 and are based on the principles of risk management, contingency management, and outcome optimization. In addition, these criteria are described in *DBT PE Handout 21 (Preparing to Resume DBT PE)*, which is reviewed with clients and used to set specific goals for what they need to do to resume DBT PE.

If the Behavior Was Life-Threatening, It Is No Longer Occurring

Consistent with the expectation that clients must completely abstain from suicidal and nonsuicidal self-injury to start DBT PE, if these behaviors are what caused DBT PE to be paused, then they must be absent before DBT PE is resumed. However, unlike when first starting DBT PE, *there is no specific amount of time that clients must be abstinent from suicidal and self-injurious behaviors before DBT PE is resumed*. Instead, the decision about when to resume should be based on whether you and the client believe they can refrain from these behaviors if DBT PE is restarted. At times, the pause in DBT PE may be quite brief (e.g., 1 week) if the client quickly and effectively solves the problem that caused self-injury to occur and firmly commits to not self-injuring again. In other cases, it may take months to get the behavior back under control and feel confident that clients will be able to safely engage in DBT PE without serious self-injurious behaviors recurring.

TABLE 14.5. Guidelines for When to Resume DBT PE after Pausing

1. If the behavior was life-threatening, it is no longer occurring.
2. For other types of behavior, it is controlled enough that it will not interfere with DBT PE.
3. Problem solving has successfully addressed the factors that contributed to the behavior.
4. The client is committed to preventing the behavior from happening again.
5. When appropriate, the client has made repairs.

For Other Types of Behavior, It Is Controlled Enough That It Will Not Interfere with DBT PE

When the problem that caused DBT PE to be paused is a therapy-interfering or quality-of-life-interfering behavior, then it is up to you and the client to decide how much it must change before DBT PE can be resumed. In some cases, it may be important for the behavior to be completely absent. For example, if the problem is that the client hit their children, the therapist may require this high-priority behavior to be totally stopped before DBT PE is resumed. In other cases, a harm-reduction approach may be used in which the goal is to reduce the behavior to a level that ensures it will not interfere with treatment. This is often the case with behaviors like substance use, dissociation, and disordered eating for which the goal may be to ensure that clients can control these behaviors enough that they will not occur before, during, or for several hours after any exposure task, but they are not required to completely refrain from these behaviors to resume DBT PE. When the problem was the absence of an effective behavior, then therapists typically require clients to demonstrate the capacity to emit the effective behavior at a level consistent with what would be needed during DBT PE. For example, if the client was not doing imaginal exposure homework because they did not like the sound of their voice in the recording, then you may require them to record their DBT session and listen to it four times per week before resuming DBT PE. Whatever change in behavior is desired, it is important that the goal be specifically and behaviorally defined (e.g., in terms of frequency, severity, duration, and topography) so that it is clear exactly what clients need to do to demonstrate readiness to resume DBT PE.

Problem Solving Has Successfully Addressed the Factors That Contributed to the Behavior

While DBT PE is paused, you and the client should engage in standard DBT problem-solving procedures (e.g., chain and solution analyses), and before DBT PE is resumed, solutions should be in place that have effectively addressed the factors that contributed to the behavior occurring. There are innumerable factors that can contribute to problem behaviors, including things that preceded the behavior (e.g., interpersonal conflict, intense shame, intoxication, finding a sharp object) and/or occurred after the behavior (e.g., increased support from a family member, getting to skip school). Whatever the critical controlling variables may be, it is important that the client has implemented solutions that have worked to change or reduce the impact of these factors.

The Client Is Committed to Preventing the Behavior from Happening Again

In addition to engaging in active problem solving to address the past behavior, clients must also be fully committed to preventing the behavior from occurring again in the future. This often means that clients are committed to continuing to use the solutions that have been generated to ensure that a similar chain of events does not happen again, as well as to implementing other solutions as needed (e.g., if urges to engage in the same problem behavior arise in a different and unplanned-for context). DBT strategies for obtaining and strengthening commitments should be used and thorough troubleshooting of factors that might interfere with following through on this commitment should be conducted. If clients are unwilling to commit to preventing the behavior, their level of commitment is weak or fluctuates over time, or significant barriers exist that make it unlikely that they will keep this commitment, then additional work to strengthen their commitment will be needed before DBT PE is resumed.

When Appropriate, the Client Has Made Repairs

In DBT, when clients engage in behaviors that negatively impact others, they are typically expected to make repairs. Therefore, when clients engage in behaviors that cause DBT PE to be paused, it is important to consider whether these behaviors caused harm to others. In some cases, actual physical harm may have occurred to a person (e.g., hitting a partner) or to property (e.g., punching a hole in your office wall). More often the harm is emotional (e.g., causing a parent to worry that they are dead) or something that damages a relationship (e.g., repeated verbal attacks). When the behavior that led DBT PE to be paused negatively impacted you or other people, then clients should make appropriate repairs before DBT PE is resumed.

This can be done using the "correction–overcorrection" contingency management strategy from DBT, which includes (1) withdrawing something positive or adding an aversive consequence after a problem behavior occurs, (2) requiring the client to engage in a new behavior that corrects the effects of the problem behavior and goes past these negative effects to overcorrect the harm that was done, and (3) stopping the aversive consequence as soon as the overcorrection occurs. For example, if a client overdoses during DBT PE on a stash of old medications they told you they had disposed of, then this is likely to negatively impact the therapy relationship by causing you to be unsure of whether you can trust them to be honest in the future. You may immediately provide a negative consequence by stopping DBT PE and withdrawing warmth. The correction–overcorrection procedures might include having the client repair the direct effects of the behavior by addressing the problems that led them to lie about getting rid of lethal means and go beyond these effects by explicitly sharing information with you each week that they have urges to lie about to demonstrate their willingness to be forthright. Once these overcorrections have occurred, then DBT PE may be resumed.

Concluding Comments

Encountering problems during DBT PE is the norm rather than the exception. What varies is the nature of the problems and the degree to which they interfere with achieving positive outcomes. When problems arise, a principle-driven approach is used to determine what the problem is and how to address it, as well as whether and when to pause and resume the treatment. Typically, clients complete DBT PE with only minor to moderate problems arising that do not seriously interfere with treatment. At times, however, more serious problems are encountered that may require DBT PE to be paused and restarted, perhaps even repeatedly. Ultimately, most clients succeed in achieving significant improvements in PTSD, which is a testament to their own and their therapists' determination to overcome the challenges that arise during treatment.

CHAPTER 15

Targeting Specific
Trauma-Related Emotions

PTSD can be conceptualized as a disorder of emotional avoidance. Traumatic events naturally evoke intense emotions that often feel overwhelming and unmanageable. When these emotions and the trauma cues that elicit them are consistently avoided, PTSD is likely to develop and become chronic. During DBT PE, our task is to break this cycle that is maintaining PTSD by helping clients to experience their trauma-related emotions without avoiding and apply strategies to regulate them effectively in the long term. Depending on the emotion and the degree to which it is justified or unjustified, different interventions are needed to regulate it to a level that is effective and appropriate to the situation. These interventions may include a variety of DBT strategies that aim to change the beliefs, actions, and expressions associated with the emotion.

In this chapter, I discuss how to select and implement tailored interventions to regulate six specific trauma-related emotions: fear, guilt, anger, shame, disgust, and sadness. These interventions are primarily implemented during the processing portion of sessions to target the emotions that have been activated by imaginal exposure but may be used at other times as well (e.g., during homework review). In addition, clients are often asked to practice the strategies discussed in session in their lives outside of therapy.

Fear

Fear is commonly viewed as the core emotion in PTSD as it is a hardwired response to trauma. Fear is likely to be particularly intense for clients who experienced an event that was life-threatening or in which they or someone they care about were physically harmed or seriously threatened. For these types of danger-focused traumas, fear is often the primary emotional response that occurred at the time of the traumatic event and continues to arise in the present in response to a wide range of internal and external cues that are perceived to be dangerous. Fearful clients tend to overestimate the likelihood of danger, feel as if they are constantly under threat, and live in a chronic state of hyperarousal. Although fear at the time of a past traumatic event is both natural and justified, fear in response to present-day cues that pose little to no risk of harm is unjustified and requires down-regulation. Table 15.1 describes the typical action urges, experience, and beliefs associated with fear, as well as strategies for decreasing unjustified fear. (Justified fear is rarely targeted during DBT PE except to encourage clients to adaptively avoid dangerous situations.)

Targeting Unjustified Fear

In DBT PE, unjustified fear is primarily reduced by repeatedly approaching feared but safe situations and trauma memories via *in vivo* and imaginal exposure, respectively. During exposure, clients may also be coached to act opposite to fear, such as by changing their facial expressions and body language to appear calm and confident rather than tense and afraid. As a direct result of exposure, clients learn that the anticipated harms either do not occur or are not as bad as expected, and fear naturally dissipates. Thus, therapists often do not need to spend much, if any, time actively working to change fear-based beliefs during processing and instead may focus on strengthening and generalizing the fear-related learning that occurs during exposure. For example, you may draw the client's attention to the fact that the feared outcomes of exposure, such as being attacked, losing behavioral control, or experiencing intense emotions, either did not occur or were coped with effectively, and then extend this learning to other contexts in which they are likely to encounter similar trauma reminders.

TABLE 15.1. Regulating Unjustified Fear

Characteristics of fear	Strategies to decrease unjustified fear
	Action urges
To freeze, escape, hide, or fight back	*Act opposite by:* Approaching the feared cue repeatedly without freezing or fighting back
	Expressions
Darting eyes, tensing muscles, rapid breathing, jittery, jumpy, trembling, shrinking away	*Change the experience by:* Keeping eyes and head up, relaxing muscles, breathing slowly, acting calm and confident
	Common beliefs and interpretations
• The world is dangerous and I am likely to be harmed. • People are likely to hurt me and can't be trusted. • I am powerless and can't keep myself safe from harm. • I have to be on guard all the time. • Trauma memories are dangerous. • It is not safe to feel emotions.	*Change beliefs to:* • The world is generally a safe place and I am unlikely to be harmed. • People are unlikely to hurt me and can often be trusted. • I can keep myself safe in most situations. • I can let down my guard and still be safe. • Thinking and talking about my trauma is not dangerous. • I can experience intense emotions without anything harmful happening.

Guilt

Guilt is pervasive among individuals receiving DBT PE and is typically the first emotion targeted for regulation during processing. This is because clients' initial reactions to imaginal exposure almost always include judging their behavior at the time of the trauma and blaming themselves for the event, both of which are likely to elicit intense guilt. Importantly, guilt is an event-specific emotion—that is, guilt is tied to interpretations of a specific traumatic event as being their fault because of the way they did or did not behave at the time. Clients can typically cite a litany of reasons why they believe they are to blame for the specific traumas they have experienced. These often include beliefs that they should have known the event was going to happen and been able to prevent it, they should have acted differently or made different choices during the event that would have stopped it sooner or reduced the harm it caused, and/or they should have responded differently after the event was over. Overall, guilt occurs when clients attempt to answer the question of "why" a specific trauma happened and reach the conclusion that it is due to their own actions or inactions.

To determine the degree to which guilt is justified or unjustified, it is first necessary to specifically define the behaviors about which the client feels guilty. Next, it must be decided whether the guilt-inducing behaviors violate the client's personal values or a generally accepted moral code. In most cases, you can readily determine that guilt is unjustified because the client's behaviors were normative and values consistent, such as being friendly to a stranger, wearing makeup, drinking alcohol, or walking outside alone. This determination can be more difficult in cases where the client's behavior was consistent with their values and/or the moral code of their environment at the time of the event but is inconsistent with their present-day values and/or environment (e.g., initiating sexual behavior with an abuser). When clients' behavior was contextually appropriate at the time and did not cause harm to others, then guilt is unjustified even if they no longer ascribe to those values or live in that environment. In some cases, there may have been competing moral codes at play at the time of the trauma, such as a veteran whose religious beliefs conflicted with military values related to killing others, and it may have been impossible to adhere to both simultaneously. When the client's behavior was consistent with one important moral code but not another, guilt is typically also unjustified.

In contrast, guilt is justified if the client engaged in behavior that violates their personal values and the moral code of their environment, such as breaking laws, lying, or behaving in offensive ways. In addition, some level of guilt or regret is justified when the person is responsible for causing harm to others even if unintentionally (e.g., accidentally hitting a pedestrian while driving). At its extreme, guilt is justified when clients have intentionally perpetrated crimes or violent acts toward others that violate clear moral codes (e.g., murder, sexual assault, war atrocities).

Targeting Unjustified Guilt

When guilt is unjustified, the task is to down-regulate guilt to a level that fits the facts of the traumatic event. This factual information is typically obtained by paying close attention to the client's description of the trauma during imaginal exposure, as well as by asking clarifying questions during processing to understand exactly what occurred. Many clients exhibit a hindsight bias, believing that they should have known the event was going to happen and been able to prevent it from occurring. In these cases, it is often useful to help clients think through the facts of what they did know—and when they knew them—as the event was unfolding. Often there was no indication that the situation was likely to be dangerous until it was too late to avoid it. For example, a veteran may believe he should have known a bomb was present even though he was actively scanning the road and did not see anything suspicious before it detonated and killed his friend. For events for which there was little to no advanced indication of danger, the goal is to help clients realistically evaluate the predictability of the event, as well as their own ability to control its occurrence.

In other cases, clients may have chosen to enter a risky situation (e.g., engaging in sex work in an alley) or to ignore potential signs of danger (e.g., choosing to go home with a date who had made repeated unwanted sexual advances throughout the evening). When the risk was at least somewhat foreseeable, it is important to help clients nonjudgmentally understand and accept why they made the choices they did at the time even though they may have been risky. In addition, it is rare that anyone could have known with 100% certainty that an event was going to happen, and it can be helpful to draw clients' attention to the fact that the event was at least somewhat unpredictable. Perhaps most importantly, putting oneself in a risky situation is not the same as being to blame for the traumatic event, particularly when it was perpetrated by someone else. For example, choosing to get in a car with a stranger may be risky, but it does not give the person permission to rape you. Instead, clients should be helped to develop a dialectical perspective that acknowledges (without judgment) that they may have done something that increased their risk of victimization while also holding the perpetrator responsible for harming them.

Most clients also feel guilty about the ways in which they responded (or didn't respond) during or after the traumatic event. Clients often hold themselves to unrealistic standards in terms of how they think they should have behaved as the event was unfolding. For example, they may think they should have been able to fight off a person who was larger and stronger than them or that their own behavior somehow justified the harm that was done to them. When clients' expectations for themselves are unrealistic, it can be useful to ask them if they would hold a friend or family member to the same standard if they were in the situation. Most clients will react as if it is preposterous and irrational to assume, for example, that their own child should be able to fight off a much larger adult or that their sister would deserve to be beaten for not immediately obeying her husband's request to make him dinner. Furthermore, clients often assume that if their behavior had been different the event would have had a more positive outcome when in fact it is impossible to know this. Indeed, it is possible that behaving differently (e.g., fighting back) could have made the outcome worse rather than better. In general, it is important to help clients contextualize their behavior at the time of the trauma by thinking through why they responded the way they did given the reality of the situation they were in and the options that were available to them at the time. In essence, how is it understandable that clients did exactly what they did and didn't do whatever it is that they now think they should have done? Rather than judging their own behavior, the goal is to help clients see that they did the best they could in a terrible situation, validate how their behavior makes sense in context, and shift responsibility to the person(s) who were actually culpable.

In addition to implementing cognitive interventions aimed at changing guilt-inducing beliefs, clients can also be coached to use the DBT skill of opposite action to reduce guilt. As shown in Table 15.2, this could include things such as acting proud while describing their actions at the time of the trauma, engaging in the behavior that causes guilt over and over without apologizing, and doing kind things for themselves. These types of opposite actions for guilt can be done during imaginal exposure, in daily life when the opportunity arises, and/or as formal *in vivo* exposure exercises. The following dialogue provides an example of addressing unjustified guilt during processing with a client who had been gang raped by her boyfriend and several of his friends.

TABLE 15.2. Regulating Unjustified Guilt

Characteristics of guilt	Strategies to decrease unjustified guilt
Action urges	
To repair the harm, apologize, appease, make amends, self-punish, and stop engaging in the behavior that elicits guilt	*Act opposite by:* Not apologizing or making repairs, telling supportive people about the behavior, repeatedly engaging in the behavior
Expressions	
Flushed red face, head bowed, mumbling or quiet voice	*Change the experience by:* Looking innocent and proud, putting shoulders back and head up, maintaining eye contact, and speaking clearly
Common beliefs and interpretations	
• The trauma was my fault. • I should have known the event was going to happen. • My actions (or inactions) caused the trauma to occur. • I should have done more to stop the event from happening. • I did something bad or wrong during or after the event.	*Change beliefs to:* • The person who harmed me is responsible for this event. • I could not have known this was going to happen. • My actions did not justify the harm that was done to me. • I did the best I could in the situation. • The decisions I made at the time of the event are understandable in context.

THERAPIST: During imaginal exposure you said, "I should have known this was going to happen." What did you mean by that?

CLIENT: I should have known this was going to be a dangerous situation. If I had just left the party earlier with my friend, I wouldn't have been raped.

THERAPIST: And what emotion do you feel when you think about the rape as something you could have prevented?

CLIENT: I feel guilty and like it was my fault.

THERAPIST: Yes, self-blame usually causes guilt. So why exactly do you think you should have known this was going to be a dangerous situation?

CLIENT: Because they were drunk, and I should have known that it wouldn't be safe for me to be alone with drunk men.

THERAPIST: Had you ever been alone with your boyfriend and his friends before when they were drunk?

CLIENT: Yes, I spent the night at his apartment a lot and he often had friends over and they would drink while we all hung out.

THERAPIST: Had you ever been raped before when you hung out with him and his friends while they were drinking?

CLIENT: No.

THERAPIST: So how were you supposed to know that it was a dangerous situation on this particular night when it never had been before?

CLIENT: One of the guys who raped me was someone I had never met before. He was the cousin of my boyfriend's friend and he was visiting from out of town.

THERAPIST: Was this the first time someone had shown up at a party or been at your boyfriend's apartment that you hadn't met before?

CLIENT: No, he had a lot of friends and I didn't know any of them before I met him.

THERAPIST: So, having guys around that you didn't know was not an unusual thing and had never been dangerous to you before, right?

CLIENT: True.

THERAPIST: Was there anything else about this particular night that would have indicated that it was a dangerous situation to you?

CLIENT: Well, look what happened! I mean, obviously it was dangerous.

THERAPIST: There's no doubt that it turned out to be dangerous, but it's not clear to me how you should have known that in advance. It sounds like it was a situation you had been in many times before without anything bad happening. When was the first time you felt afraid or in danger that night?

CLIENT: When I came out of the bathroom and they were all standing there, and the one guy grabbed my arm and started pulling me into the bedroom.

THERAPIST: If I were you, I would have felt totally blindsided in that moment. Was there any sign before then that they were about to rape you?

CLIENT: No, they were just playing video games and drinking before I got up to go to the bathroom.

THERAPIST: So, it's not fair to look back and say, "I should have seen it coming." It sounds like there just weren't any signs of danger until they ambushed you as you were coming out of the bathroom, and then it was too late to get away.

CLIENT: If I think about it that way, it makes me want to stay away from men completely. Because if you can't predict when men will rape you, then you're never safe.

THERAPIST: I think there is an important balance to find between taking excessive precautions, which is how you've been living your life since the rape—avoiding lots of situations that you think could be dangerous even though they are generally safe—and taking excessive risks, which would mean ignoring clear signs of danger and behaving recklessly. In the middle is wise-minded action where you pay attention to both emotion and logic to make decisions about which situations are or are not likely to be risky to you.

CLIENT: I just wish there was a way to always keep myself safe.

THERAPIST: I do too! And the facts are that we can't, and if we structure our lives to try to minimize any potential danger, then our lives will get very small and limited. For example, driving a car can be a dangerous thing to do. Lots of people get seriously injured or die in car accidents every day. If we wanted to be absolutely sure that we won't get hurt in a car accident, what would we need to do?

CLIENT: Never get in a car.

THERAPIST: Exactly. And how would that affect our life if we never got in a car?

CLIENT: It would be hard to go places, so it would be hard to travel or see friends or go to work.

THERAPIST: So, what would be a wise-minded action a person could take when driving that takes into account that it can be dangerous?

CLIENT: Making sure that you always wear your seat belt.

THERAPIST: Right, so we want you to wear a seat belt in your life, but we don't want you to refuse to ever get in a car. At the time of the rape, were you wearing your seat belt?

CLIENT: I guess you could say I was. I was with my boyfriend who I trusted, and I had had some drinks but I wasn't drunk. And I wasn't flirting or doing anything provocative around those guys.

THERAPIST: I agree, it doesn't sound to me like you took any excessive risks. This was just a normal situation, like driving a car, and on that night it ended in a terrible tragedy. So, what does your wise mind say about your guilt now?

CLIENT: That I didn't do anything risky and I couldn't have known they were going to rape me.

THERAPIST: Great! Let's have you write down that thought so you can remind yourself of it this week.

Regulating Justified Guilt

When guilt is justified, the goal is to ensure that it is at a level that both fits the facts of the situation and is effective for the client. The intensity of guilt that is justified depends on the situation, with less intense guilt (e.g., regret) being reasonable for mild transgressions (e.g., lying about one's age) or when clients did not intend to cause harm to others (e.g., accidents), and more intense guilt (e.g., remorse) being appropriate for more serious wrongdoings (e.g., bullying a peer) or when clients intended to harm others (e.g., physical assaults). Thus, the first task is often to determine the level of guilt that is justified by considering the context of the situation, the person's values and knowledge at the time the event occurred, the degree to which they intended to cause harm to others, and their role in the event (e.g., direct perpetrator, collaborator, bystander). In this process, it is important that you do not minimize clients' harmful behavior or provide false reassurances when clients have truly done something problematic. This is not done to judge or "shame" the client, but rather to validate their sense of reality that they have done something harmful and join with them to figure out how to effectively resolve their justified guilt.

> **CLINICAL TIP**
> ### Working with Perpetrators
>
> Historically, exposure therapy was viewed as inappropriate for treating PTSD caused by perpetration of acts of violence or other serious harmful behavior. This was due to concerns that repeatedly exposing a perpetrator to a memory of an event in which they inflicted harm on others would desensitize them to its severity and increase their risk of reoffending. However, exposure therapy is now viewed as appropriate for perpetration-induced PTSD *when the person has remorse for their behavior*. Perpetrators who feel remorse are often wracked with guilt and shame about their behavior, view it as abhorrent and repulsive, and are fully committed to not reengaging in the behavior. In these cases, it is appropriate to proceed with DBT PE to reduce PTSD symptoms caused by acts of perpetration, which may also pave the way for the client to make effective repairs.

When guilt is justified, it can be ineffective if it is so intense that it seriously interferes with the client's ability to function or causes extreme misery. This can occur, for example, if clients believe that their harmful actions make them entirely bad people who deserve to suffer eternally. When justified guilt is ineffectively extreme, it can be down-regulated by helping clients to problem-solve the behavior that is causing guilt, including making repairs, committing to avoiding the behavior in the future, and seeking forgiveness. Repairs can be made directly to the person(s) who were harmed, or if that is not possible, clients can find ways to repair the harm in a more general sense by working to prevent or repair similar harms to others. For example, a client who forced her younger brother to engage in sexual behavior when they were children may directly apologize to him as an adult and attempt to make things better for him now. Or the repair may be more indirect, such as donating to organizations that provide services to abused children or volunteering with children who are in need.

In addition to direct problem solving, it is also critical to help clients with justified guilt develop more dialectical and balanced ways of thinking about themselves and their behavior. Similar to unjustified guilt, it is important to contextualize clients' behavior by helping them to think through how the values-inconsistent or immoral behavior was possible in the context of the situation. This is not intended to minimize or reduce their responsibility for it, but rather to help them understand how it occurred in a less judgmental way, which may also facilitate more effective problem solving about how to avoid a recurrence. Clients' harmful acts should also be considered in the context of their life as a whole. Often clients who have engaged in behavior that justifies guilt will discount or minimize the positive things they have done in their lives and instead view themselves as entirely bad people. Instead, clients should be helped to adopt a "both–and" approach that acknowledges both their positive and negative behaviors. Overall, the goal is to help clients let go of extremes and work toward dialectical balances that acknowledge the truth in both sides. Examples include "I did a harmful thing that hurt someone *and* I do not deserve to suffer forever" and "I have done things I regret *and* I have done things I am proud of."

Ultimately, clients who have engaged in acts that justify guilt must be helped to radically accept their own past behavior and work toward self-forgiveness. Radical acceptance is not the same as approval, but rather involves accepting that they did what they did, even though they wish they hadn't, rather than constantly trying to "undo" this painful reality or staying stuck in thinking it should not have happened. Importantly, radical acceptance involves accepting just the facts of the situation. For example, a client who got in an accident while driving drunk might have to accept "My decision to drive while intoxicated resulted in another person's death" but should not accept "I'm a terrible person who can't be trusted to make good decisions." This focus on acceptance of their past behavior without judgment can help clients to build self-compassion, let go of self-loathing, and begin to shift toward forgiveness.

Anger

At the beginning of treatment, anger is often low to moderate and may be directed at the self and/or others. As unjustified guilt and self-blame decrease, anger typically becomes more intense and is directed solely toward the perpetrator or others who played a role in the trauma. This increase in anger typically occurs in the middle portion of treatment and, for many clients, is the first time they have experienced significant anger toward the people who are to blame for causing them harm. Anger is often accompanied by thoughts about having been treated unfairly, questions about why the perpetrator chose to harm them and others failed to protect them, and a desire for justice to be served to those who were responsible. Thus, the presence of anger often reflects a momentous and positive shift toward appropriately holding others, rather than themselves, responsible for the traumas they have suffered.

Anger is justified when you or someone you care about is harmed, threatened, or insulted by others, an important goal is blocked, or an injustice has been committed. Thus, anger directed toward perpetrators of trauma, others who could have intervened but did not (e.g., witnesses), and people or organizations that put the client in a dangerous situation (e.g., military leadership) is justified. On the other hand, anger is unjustified if it is directed toward people who were not actually in a position to intervene or could not reasonably have been expected to know the trauma was occurring. For example, a client who was sexually abused by a neighbor may feel angry toward their parents for not protecting them from this abuse. However, if the client hid the abuse from their parents and they did not know it was occurring, then anger is understandable but not justified. Some clients also experience unjustified self-directed anger that can take the form of intense self-hatred or self-invalidation.

Targeting Unjustified Anger

When anger is unjustified and self-directed, the interventions are similar to those for unjustified guilt. This is because clients who are angry at themselves are often judging their own behavior at the time of the trauma (e.g., "I was stupid to get so drunk") or the way it has impacted them (e.g., "I'm mad at myself for not being able to better control my emotions"). When anger is fueled by self-judgment about their own actions, then helping clients to contextualize their behavior, generate compassionate reasons for why they responded as they did, and shift responsibility to those who were culpable will also help to reduce self-directed anger. When unjustified anger is directed toward others, it is important to help clients check the facts about the role the people with whom they are angry actually played in the event. Clients may feel angry toward people, such as parents, other family members, or authority figures, who they believe should have known the trauma was occurring and protected them, when in fact there is no evidence that the people did know or were in a position to intervene. In these cases, helping clients shift from thinking "these people should have done something" to instead accepting that they could not, often moves clients from feeling angry to feeling sad.

Targeting Justified Anger

When anger is justified and other-directed, it must first be determined whether the intensity of the anger is effective for the client. Justified anger is typically effective when it is focused on the people who have caused the client harm, can be regulated when needed, is not causing the person to be pervasively or chronically angry, and may even be motivating the client to engage in self-protective or value-consistent behaviors. When this is the case, you will primarily validate clients' anger, reinforce and strengthen the adaptive beliefs that are prompting justified anger (e.g., "I did not deserve to be abused"), and encourage clients to allow themselves to experience anger effectively. This acceptance-focused approach typically leads to a natural reduction in anger over time as clients process, accept, and come to peace with what was done to them. In some cases, clients may wish to seek justice for the harms that were done to them, and you can help them think through the pros and cons of options for seeking legal or other types of recourse. For clients whose trauma was perpetrated by a family member, there are often difficult decisions to be made about whether and how to confront the perpetrator, tell others in the family about the trauma, and maintain relationships with those who were involved. Often clients begin to wrestle with these issues during DBT PE but may not reach a wise-minded decision about how to move forward until after DBT PE is complete.

For some clients, justified anger can become ineffective when it interferes with successful emotional processing of trauma and limits their progress in treatment. Several studies of PE have found that high levels of pretreatment anger predict less improvement in PTSD and a greater likelihood of dropout (e.g., Foa, Riggs, Massie, & Yarczower, 1995; Rizvi, Vogt, & Resick, 2009). In a study of DBT PE, clients who did not achieve remission from PTSD were more likely to show increases in anger across imaginal exposure trials, whereas clients who remitted from PTSD exhibited a slight decrease in anger from the first to last imaginal exposure trial (Harned et al., 2015). These studies suggest that interventions designed to reduce justified anger may be needed to improve outcomes for clients whose anger interferes with exposure (e.g., by blocking the activation of other emotions, such as fear or sadness) and/or is not naturally decreasing across the course of treatment. In addition, justified anger may be targeted for down-regulation when it causes problems in clients' lives more broadly, such as chronic irritability, intense bitterness or resentment, or verbal or physical aggression. When anger is justified and ineffective, you need to balance the acceptance strategies described above, particularly validating the reasons that clients are angry, with change strategies for reducing the intensity of anger to a level that is more effective for the client.

An important first step in changing justified anger is to ensure that this is the client's goal—it is likely to be impossible to decrease anger in a client who wants to remain angry. Some clients are reluctant to reduce anger because it feels like they would be letting the people who harmed them off the hook for what they did. However, as the common saying goes, holding on to anger is like drinking poison and hoping that it will kill someone else. Thus, the goal of reducing anger is for the client to suffer less, not to exonerate the people who caused them harm: The perpetrator(s) will remain to blame for their harmful actions even if the client is less angry about what they did. Once clients agree to the goal of reducing anger, the way to do so is by using the skill of opposite action. As shown in Table 15.3, this may be done by acting opposite to angry urges, such as by gently avoiding or being kind to the person with whom they are angry and speaking at a normal volume rather than yelling. Clients can also be coached to change judgmental language that fuels anger (e.g., "My dad was an asshole") to factual descriptions (e.g., "My dad was often critical of me").

Perhaps the most challenging, and often transformative, way to practice opposite action to anger is to help clients build understanding and acceptance for the people who have harmed them. Understandably, therapists often feel reluctant to suggest that clients might try to increase compassion toward a perpetrator or another person who played a role in their trauma. To be clear, clients would be 100% justified to remain angry for the rest of their lives at the people who caused them so much harm. At the same time, holding on to this type of bitterness and resentment is likely to be toxic for clients (and to have no impact on the people who harmed them). Therefore, encouraging clients to find ways to understand and accept the other person—while continuing to hold them responsible for what they did—is often critical to helping clients achieve freedom from their suffering. This approach to opposite action to anger is typically implemented in mid- to late treatment after clients have had an opportunity to sufficiently experience, express, and be validated for justified anger, and are now recognizing the need to reduce the intensity of their anger. To achieve this, you need to help clients identify the understandable reasons the other person did what they did. Does the context of the situation help to

TABLE 15.3. Regulating Ineffective Anger

Characteristics of anger	Strategies to decrease anger
Action urges	
To physically or verbally attack someone, make aggressive gestures, swear, blow up, criticize and judge people	*Act opposite by:* Gently avoiding or doing something kind for the person with whom you are angry, looking for nonjudgmental reasons for the person's behavior
Expressions	
Pacing, clenching fists, pointing fingers, raising voice, hitting or breaking things	*Change the experience by:* Unclenching fists, holding hands open (willing hands), relaxing muscles, half-smiling, talking at normal volume, sitting or standing still
Common beliefs and interpretations	
• The people who harmed me are bad and evil. • They should not have done what they did to me. • People who are similar to those who harmed me are bad and evil (e.g., all men, police).	*Change beliefs to:* • My perpetrator harmed me and is not an entirely bad person. • My perpetrator's behavior was harmful and can be understood in context. • The other person was doing the best that they could do (and needed to do better). • Just because someone is similar to the person who harmed me does not mean they do the same bad things.

explain their actions? Did the person's learning history make them more likely to engage in the behavior? Did the person lack the skills to behave more effectively? Below is an example of a therapist working to help a client reduce his anger during processing by building compassion for his physically abusive mother.

CLIENT: (*with raised voice*) What kind of mother would beat her child for practicing the piano? I mean, what was I supposed to do? I had a concert that week and needed to practice. She's a useless fucking excuse for a mother! People like her should not even be allowed to have children if they are just going to abuse them!

THERAPIST: I agree that your mother's abusive behavior was incredibly problematic and caused you a lot of pain and suffering. At the same time, I'm worried that continuing to feel this angry toward her is only going to cause you to suffer more. What do you notice about how you are feeling as you talk about her in this way?

CLIENT: I feel like I want to scream and yell and hit something.

THERAPIST: Right, that's what anger makes us want to do. I've noticed that your anger has been getting more and more intense over the past several weeks. Do you think it's causing problems for you to be this angry?

CLIENT: Yeah, I feel angry most of the time now and I can't control it. I yelled at my wife and my kids a few times this week over minor things. I hate it when I do that! It makes me feel like my mother.

THERAPIST: Would you like to work on reducing your anger toward your mother? I think that will help you to be less angry in general.

CLIENT: But she deserves for me to be angry at her—she was a terrible mother!

THERAPIST: There is no doubt that your anger toward her is justified. She caused you a lot of harm. However, it seems like your anger has reached a level that is not effective for you—it's making you feel miserable most of the time and causing you to be irritable toward the people you love, right?

CLIENT: That's true.

THERAPIST: So, the reason to work on reducing your anger is to make *you* less miserable, not to somehow suggest that you don't deserve to be angry or that your mother didn't do anything wrong. Your mother abused you and being less angry with her is not going to change that reality, but it will make you happier.

CLIENT: OK, I see your point. I would like to be less angry.

THERAPIST: Good, I appreciate your willingness to give this a shot! One way for you to feel less angry toward your mother is to act opposite to your urges to judge her by instead trying to understand her behavior in a nonjudgmental way. That means really putting yourself in her shoes and trying to see things from her perspective. So, why do you think she physically abused you? How is it understandable even though we of course wish she hadn't done it?

CLIENT: I don't know. How is any of her behavior understandable? She was abused by her parents when she was a kid, and she knew how painful it was. Why would she do the same thing to her own kids?

THERAPIST: That's a good question. Why do you think she did?

CLIENT: I guess if your own parents hit you, that you might think this was normal or somehow OK.

THERAPIST: Yes, that can definitely happen. People often parent in ways that are similar to how they were raised as children. And it sounds like she was raised to believe that physically punishing children was a reasonable parenting strategy.

CLIENT: Her parents were even worse to her than she was to me. She used to say things to me like "You should be glad I'm not whipping you with a belt like my mom did to me." So maybe she thought that she was actually going easy on me.

THERAPIST: That could be. It's possible she even thought she was somehow being kind to you by not punishing you as severely as her own mother had punished her.

CLIENT: That would be ironic, since hitting kids is never kind. But I could see how she could think that.

THERAPIST: Are there other reasons you think she may have physically abused you?

CLIENT: She was generally unhappy. My dad abandoned us when I was little, and she had been left alone to raise me and my sister without any help. She was always stressed out about money and she barely got any sleep because she had to work two jobs.

THERAPIST: It sounds like she may have been quite emotionally vulnerable. We are all more likely to get angry when we are stressed out and tired, and it sounds like that was true for her most of the time.

CLIENT: Yeah, I don't know how she did it really. She often only got 2 or 3 hours of sleep at night. In the event we have been talking about, she had fallen asleep on the couch and I didn't realize it. So, when I started playing the piano, it woke her up. I can understand why that would make her angry, but I didn't deserve to be hit for it.

THERAPIST: It sounds like there are several understandable reasons for her behavior. She had been raised to believe that physical punishment was a reasonable parenting strategy, and she may have even thought that she was being easy on you by using less severe forms of punishment than her own parents had. It also sounds like she was chronically tired and stressed out, and that having her sleep disrupted was particularly upsetting to her given how little sleep she got.

CLIENT: Yeah, all those things are true.

THERAPIST: So how do you feel when you think about your mother in this way?

CLIENT: I feel some empathy for her. I can see that she was probably doing the best she could. I just wish she had been able to do better.

THERAPIST: Me too. Does this change your anger at all?

CLIENT: Yes, I feel less angry now. Instead, I feel sad for both of us.

Shame

Shame is often the most painful and pernicious emotion that our clients experience: It is frequently at the core of their desire to be dead and a critical link in the chain to self-injurious behaviors. Unlike guilt, which is event specific and focused on one's behavior ("I did something bad"), shame is global and about oneself as a person ("I am bad"). Shame is often associated with general negative beliefs about the self as being inadequate, unworthy, incompetent, and unlovable that influence how clients perceive themselves in all aspects of their lives. For many clients in DBT PE, these types of self-critical beliefs developed early in life and represent an internalization of the invalidating environment in which they were raised. For example, a client may have developed the belief "I don't matter" as a result of having been neglected by their parents as a child. These early self-invalidating beliefs are often then reinforced by traumas and experiences of mistreatment that occur later in life. For example, when clients who were abused as children experience intimate partner violence as adults, they are likely to interpret this later trauma as further proof that the negative beliefs they developed about themselves as children are true. As a result, individuals who have experienced repeated traumas often have particularly intense shame and extreme negative views about themselves that are quite entrenched and difficult to change.

Shame is considered to fit the facts (i.e., be justified) if a person's behavior or characteristics would cause them to be rejected by a person or group they care about if they were made public. This might include specific behaviors, such as failing a test or crying, or more general characteristics, such as one's sexual orientation or political beliefs. Importantly, the determination of whether shame is justified or unjustified depends on the interpersonal context within which the shame-inducing information is shared—it is not inherent in the behavior or characteristic itself. For example, most clients believe that people will reject and judge them if they were to learn about the traumas they have experienced. In the context of therapy, this shame is typically unjustified: Therapists are not going to reject clients when they share the details of their trauma. However, with some people, such as family members who have previously responded to clients' trauma disclosures with blame and criticism, shame may be justified. Similarly, clients who identify as sexual minorities may be rejected by some people due to their sexual orientation (e.g., members of certain religions) and accepted by others (e.g., other sexual minority people and their heterosexual allies).

Targeting Unjustified Shame

When shame is unjustified, the goal is to decrease it to a level that fits the facts (see Table 15.4). Because shame is often particularly intractable, this typically requires a two-pronged approach: (1) helping clients to develop new perspectives about the shame-eliciting details of past traumas and (2) creating new experiences in the client's present-day life that disconfirm their negative beliefs about themselves. The first intervention typically occurs during processing and involves addressing shame-related beliefs that are activated by imaginal exposure. Often shame can be reduced by working to generalize learning about a specific traumatic event to clients' global beliefs about themselves as people. For example, if a client has the belief "I always make bad decisions," then helping them to recognize that they made reasonable decisions at the time of a specific traumatic event may provide evidence that can be used to disconfirm the general belief about their poor decision-making abilities. In this way, efforts to reduce unjustified guilt and self-blame related to specific traumatic events can often have downstream effects in helping to change more global shame-related beliefs.

To maximize reductions in shame, you also need to extend the processing discussion beyond the specific traumatic event(s) that are being targeted via imaginal exposure to include other experiences in the client's life that have contributed to this style of self-critical thinking. As part of this process, it is often useful to help clients understand how these beliefs developed and have been maintained as a result of cumulative traumatic or invalidating experiences. For example, when did they start thinking about themselves as being bad or inferior? What events contributed to the development of this belief? Once formed, how did this preexisting belief get applied to understanding later traumas or other events in their life more broadly? These discussions often help clients begin to recognize that these long-standing beliefs are not necessarily

TABLE 15.4. Regulating Unjustified Shame

Characteristics of shame	Strategies to decrease shame
Action urges	
Hide, keep information secret, withdraw from people, criticize and punish self	*Act opposite by:* Share information about yourself and your behavior with others who won't reject you, repeat the behavior, validate and do something kind for yourself
Expressions	
Curl up, shrink, cover face or body, no eye contact, blushing, speak quietly and with frequent pauses	*Change the experience by:* Sit up straight, face forward, hold head high, make eye contact, reveal face and body, talk at normal volume without pausing
Common beliefs and interpretations	
• I am bad and unlovable. • I am stupid, incompetent, and weak. • I am worthless and don't deserve to be treated well. • There is something wrong with me as a person. • I have to be perfect all the time.	*Change beliefs to:* • There are things about myself that I like and things I wish that were different. • I do not deserve mistreatment. • I am likable, especially to people I care about. • I can do hard things. • There is nothing inherently wrong with me. • It is OK to make mistakes.

facts but rather were caused by specific events and then became a lens through which they interpreted their later experiences.

For most clients, these global negative beliefs about the self are long-standing and habitual ways of thinking that have typically gone unquestioned and been repeatedly reinforced by people in their lives. As a result, clients often have few if any prior experiences that would provide them with models for how to think about themselves in a more positive way. Thus, if you ask clients to generate more self-validating interpretations of themselves and their behaviors, many simply will not be able to do so effectively. If this occurs, you may need to be more directive when targeting shame-related beliefs, including directly challenging these beliefs and suggesting more adaptive ways for clients to think about themselves. You may also need to be particularly emphatic and irreverent when addressing these entrenched self-critical beliefs, calling "bullshit" on clients' beliefs about themselves, saying unexpected or humorous things that make them think about themselves differently, and demanding that they give up self-critical beliefs because they are ineffective.

Although we are often initially the ones generating more validating and accurate ways for clients to think about themselves, over the course of treatment this responsibility should fall more and more to clients. For example, through a process of shaping, we may initially provide clients with new, more validating perspectives, then increase our demand that they rehearse and generate self-validating statements while actively blocking them from repeating self-invalidation and judgment. Ideally, by the end of DBT PE, clients will be readily able to self-generate validating ways of thinking about themselves and their behaviors in both past and present situations. The following is an example of targeting unjustified shame during processing with a client who believes that there is something inherently wrong with her that makes her unlikable. This belief developed due to pervasive experiences of traumatic invalidation in her family and peer groups throughout her life, and imaginal exposure was focusing on a specific invalidating event in which she had been rejected and excluded by peers in middle school.

THERAPIST: What is feeling particularly painful about this event now?

CLIENT: The part about not having friends. The feeling separate and alone and like it's always been that way and it's always going to be that way and there's nothing I can do about it.

THERAPIST: That is painful. So, let's start with the not having friends part. That was a fact, right? You actually did not have any friends at this point in eighth grade.

CLIENT: Right.

THERAPIST: So, what does that mean to you that you did not have any friends?

CLIENT: That there must have been something wrong with me. I was hardly ever able to make friends and the few times I did, I always messed things up in some way. When I think about this particular event, and standing there all alone and watching everyone else have fun, I just think that it was meant to be like that. It has something to do with who I am, like it's in my nature.

THERAPIST: And what emotion do you feel when you think that the reason you had no friends is because there was something wrong with you?

CLIENT: I feel ashamed, and I hate myself.

THERAPIST: Yes, judging your entire self as bad or wrong typically makes people feel shame.

Thinking back on that event now, do you think that's true? That there was something wrong with you and that's why you didn't have friends?

CLIENT: Are we talking objectively?

THERAPIST: We're talking about what you think in wise mind.

CLIENT: I guess I don't even know what it actually means to have something wrong with me.

THERAPIST: Interesting. Say more.

CLIENT: Well, now I'm questioning what that even means, to have something wrong with oneself.

THERAPIST: OK, well what are the possibilities of what it could mean?

CLIENT: It's something beyond what you say or do.

THERAPIST: Like it's something more innate. Part of your cells in some way.

CLIENT: Yeah, but what does that mean?

THERAPIST: It's the difference between shame and guilt. When people feel guilty it is about something they said or did, like a specific behavior. Which is painful, but often not as painful as shame. Shame is about your entire being, like who you are in the world is flawed in some way. Is that the distinction you're getting at?

CLIENT: Yeah, that's what I was trying to get to.

THERAPIST: So, from wise mind, do you think that the answer to why you didn't have friends is because of something that was inherently wrong with you? Or something you said or did? Or something else?

CLIENT: I don't think it's about what I said or did. Because it was year after year after year, and I've thought a lot about it and I genuinely can't figure out what I could have done that would have made so many people not want to be my friend.

THERAPIST: OK, so what would explain it?

CLIENT: I don't know. I know last week we talked about how I was different than the other kids in my school, like I was Puerto Rican and they were White, which meant that I looked different and ate different foods and things like that. And maybe that made them not like me. But I still feel like it was deeper than that, that something else is wrong with me.

THERAPIST: If there was something wrong with you, what could it be?

CLIENT: I don't even know. Like if I stop thinking about myself, what sort of examples are there of things that are wrong with people? I don't even know if that really exists.

THERAPIST: I agree.

CLIENT: So, if that doesn't really exist for other people, then why would it exist for me?

THERAPIST: Excellent question.

CLIENT: Unless I'm the exception to the rule, but I know that's not wise mind.

THERAPIST: That's totally true.

CLIENT: So no, there's nothing wrong with me.

THERAPIST: Oh my god, I feel like jumping up and down!

CLIENT: But I got there just logically. It doesn't actually feel true.

THERAPIST: I know, that's straight logic. I think you are now actually in reasonable mind, and you've closed the door on emotions completely. Because your emotions are still going to pull you back into thinking that it just feels true that there's something wrong with you, right?

CLIENT: Yes.

THERAPIST: So, what we've got to do is grab on to the logic side. Because you're completely correct, and we've got to get those facts to feel more true than they currently do. That might just happen through repetition, by walking yourself through those logical steps over and over. So, tell me again how you got to the point of thinking there was nothing wrong with you. And while you do it, I want you to practice opposite action for shame. So, uncurl yourself, sit up straight, make eye contact with me, and say it like you mean it.

CLIENT: OK. (*sits up, makes eye contact*) It couldn't have been true that I said or did some terrible thing year after year, situation after situation, without me being able to say what it was.

THERAPIST: Great, keep going and increase your volume.

CLIENT: (*louder*) So it would have had to be something that was just inherently bad or wrong about me. But what would that be? I don't think those things exist in other people, so how could they exist in me? So that must mean there's nothing wrong with me.

THERAPIST: It makes me so happy to hear you say that! And I completely agree, there is nothing wrong with you. How do you feel when you say it?

CLIENT: I feel less ashamed. And like maybe there's some hope that things can be different for me in the future.

THERAPIST: Yes, I feel very hopeful. From my perspective, the most plausible explanation for why you did not have friends at that age is because you were different than the kids you grew up with. You were the only non-White kid in your school, you were devoutly Catholic and others were not, and you were incredibly smart. All of those things made you different—not in a bad way—just different. And the fact that you were different likely made other kids not include you, which is what got this whole belief system started.

CLIENT: I can see that.

THERAPIST: So, the solution is not to judge yourself—you're perfectly likable—but instead to find people who are similar to you. That is something you are already starting to do, and we will keep working on it, because it is completely possible for you to have friends.

CLIENT: Well, now you've screwed up my whole belief system!

THERAPIST: Good, I'm glad to hear it!

As this example illustrates, the therapist is often a powerful source of corrective learning for clients about whether they are in fact the terrible people they believe themselves to be. Therapists not only help clients to reappraise their past traumatic experiences in more self-validating ways but they also fundamentally do not reject the client. This experience of being cared for and accepted—particularly by someone who knows about one's most shame-inducing experiences—is often both a foreign and incredibly meaningful one for clients. At the same time, discovering that a single person is not rejecting is unlikely to be sufficient to generalize learning about one's self-worth to other contexts. Thus, it is almost always necessary to identify ways in which clients can get even more corrective feedback that will help to disconfirm their negative beliefs about themselves. In DBT PE, this is done by using *in vivo* exposure to target unjustified shame (see Chapter 9). For example, if the client in the above example believes "If people really knew me, they wouldn't like me," then *in vivo* exposures might involve sharing personal information with other people who are unlikely to reject her.

Targeting Justified Shame

If shame is justified (i.e., they are likely to be rejected), and the shame-eliciting behavior does not violate the client's values (i.e., guilt is unjustified), then clients are coached to validate their behavior and seek out people and environments that are more accepting. Clients also have a choice to make about whether they wish to keep the shame-eliciting information hidden from people who are likely to reject them or reveal it and tolerate others' judgment. In addition, some clients may choose to try to change others' beliefs to be more accepting and/or engage in activism or advocacy efforts that aim to shift cultural values to be more accepting of people like themselves (e.g., people with mental illness). In contrast, if shame is justified and the shame-eliciting behavior violates the client's values (i.e., guilt is also justified), then the effective course of action is to change the behavior to be consistent with their own values, as well as those of important others in their life.

Disgust

Disgust involves a visceral sense of revulsion toward something that is believed to be potentially contagious. This can include physical disgust that is prompted by exposure to objects that are viewed as toxic or contaminated, such as bodily fluids, spoiled food, and disease-carrying animals. Disgust can also be social in nature and elicited by people who are considered offensive, distasteful, or morally abhorrent. In the context of trauma, disgust is often self-directed and related to beliefs about being physically contaminated by one's traumatic experiences. (See Table 15.5.) For example, a woman who was raped may feel disgusted by herself because she feels as if her body has been made dirty by the rapist. At the start of treatment, disgust is often primarily self-directed, and over the course of treatment shifts to being directed toward others, such as perpetrators who are viewed as foul and revolting people due to their behavior. This transition to disgust toward perpetrators typically occurs around the same time that clients begin to feel other-directed anger—however, disgust toward others often remains moderate to high at the end of treatment, whereas anger tends to decrease.

TABLE 15.5. Regulating Unjustified Self-Directed Disgust

Characteristics of self-directed disgust	Strategies to decrease self-directed disgust
Action urges	
Sequester oneself, stay away from people to avoid contaminating them, wash, conceal body	*Act opposite by:* Move close to others, initiate physical contact, do not wash, take in one's body
Expressions	
Shuddering, curling upper lip, wrinkling the nose, closing eyes, holding breath, turning away	*Change the experience by:* Turning toward, half-smiling, relaxing face muscles, opening eyes, breathing normally
Common beliefs and interpretations	
• I am dirty and gross. • My body is repulsive. • I am permanently contaminated because of what happened. • If other people get close to me, they will be infected by me.	*Change beliefs to:* • My body is clean and free from physical contaminants that were present at the time of the trauma. • Other people do not find me to be disgusting. • Touching or being near other people does not infect them.

Disgust is justified when there is an actual danger of physical or social contamination. In the case of physical disgust, this would mean that there is a risk of infection or illness if one were to come into contact with the disgust-eliciting object. Physical disgust at the time of the trauma is justified when the event involved being near or touching potential contaminants, such as sexual fluids, feces, blood, or dead bodies. However, continuing to feel disgust when those substances or objects are no longer present is not. Social disgust toward people who engaged in immoral or damaging behavior at the time of the trauma is also justified, whereas disgust toward people whose behavior did not violate social or moral norms is not.

Targeting Unjustified Disgust

When disgust is unjustified and self-directed, it is typically prompted by beliefs about oneself as being dirty, contaminated, and physically repulsive. Clients who believe they are disgusting often avoid people and isolate themselves. Whereas fear and shame lead to avoidance of others as a way to protect oneself from perceived physical or social danger, self-directed disgust motivates avoidance of others as a way to protect other people from feeling sickened or repulsed. Therefore, the corrective learning that is typically needed is to discover that you are not physically contaminated and other people are not disgusted by you. Below is an example of targeting disgust-related beliefs during processing with a client who had been sexually abused by her brother throughout her childhood.

THERAPIST: I see that you are having really intense disgust. You rated it as 100. What are you feeling disgusted about?

CLIENT: I feel disgusted by myself.

THERAPIST: How so? What do you think is disgusting about you?

CLIENT: I just feel dirty.

THERAPIST: Do you feel like your body is somehow physically contaminated? Like there is something about it that is actually dirty?

CLIENT: Yeah, I feel like my brother's semen is still inside me. Like it's in my cells now or something and it's just always going to be there.

THERAPIST: That's really common. A lot of people who were sexually abused feel as if their body has been permanently contaminated by their abuser.

CLIENT: I just hate that feeling, like he's still inside me. It just makes me feel gross. (*makes an "ugh" noise and shudders her shoulders*)

THERAPIST: Well, if you are thinking that your brother's semen is still in your body, it makes sense that you would feel disgust.

CLIENT: I agree.

THERAPIST: But you're not thinking that his semen is somehow indestructible, are you? Like the fact that it was on your body 10 years ago means it is still there now?

CLIENT: It feels that way.

THERAPIST: How many times do you estimate you have showered since your brother's semen last came into contact with your body?

CLIENT: I don't know, a lot. I usually shower every day.

THERAPIST: Well, you must be really terrible at washing yourself if you haven't managed to get his semen off your skin in the thousands of showers you have taken since the abuse stopped!

CLIENT: (*laughs*) No, I wash really thoroughly.

THERAPIST: So, think for a minute from wise mind. Where do you think your brother's semen is now that was on your body 10 years ago?

CLIENT: Well, the semen that was on my skin probably washed off and went down the drain in the shower. But I also had to swallow his semen sometimes, and you can't wash that away.

THERAPIST: Are you thinking about this like that old wives' tale about bubblegum? Like that if you swallow gum it stays in your stomach for a really long time before it can be digested?

CLIENT: Maybe.

THERAPIST: Well, here's a fact for you to consider: After you eat it takes around 24–72 hours for your food to be digested. So, the same would be true if you swallow semen.

CLIENT: OK.

THERAPIST: And once your food has been fully digested, what happens to it?

CLIENT: (*grinning*) I shit him out!

THERAPIST: Yes, you did! If you ask me, I think you got the last word in this whole scenario, because one way or another his semen is now living in the sewer system.

CLIENT: Ha! That's right!

THERAPIST: So, when you think about it this way and acknowledge the fact that his semen can no longer be on your skin or in your body, how does that make you feel?

CLIENT: It makes me feel less disgusted with myself, and like I'm not somehow carrying him around in me still. It makes me feel like I may finally be able to be rid of him.

In addition to addressing beliefs about the trauma that are fueling unjustified disgust during processing, you should also assess for disgust-related avoidance that is occurring outside of session. For example, are clients washing excessively or avoiding physical contact with people due to feeling dirty and contaminated? If so, it will be important to change these avoidance behaviors through informal opposite action or planned *in vivo* exposure. For example, clients may be instructed to notice and block urges to shower when it is not needed or to intentionally do things that they think may disgust others, such as making appropriate physical contact. In addition, if clients are disgusted by their own body, they can work on fully taking in their body by smelling, looking at, and touching themselves without acting disgusted. In general, opposite action for disgust is often a helpful strategy for reducing unjustified self-directed disgust that arises both in and outside of therapy.

Targeting Justified Disgust

When disgust is justified and directed toward others, acceptance-oriented interventions are typically used, such as validating clients' disgust and reinforcing adaptive beliefs about the disgusting nature of others' behavior. You may also self-disclose your own feelings of disgust toward the people who caused the client harm. In most cases, other-directed disgust, even when intense, is both justified and effective: Disgust does not tend to interfere in client's lives or cause them to feel miserable in the same way that intense anger toward others does. Whereas intense anger is typically a sign that clients are judging rather than radically accepting another person's behavior, clients can reach a place of radical acceptance of another person and still feel disgusted by them. Radical acceptance requires clients to accept the facts of what happened, but it does not mean that they have to approve of those facts. Disgust toward perpetrators and others responsible for one's trauma is a sign of nonapproval of their behavior, which is typically an effective and valid stance for clients to maintain in perpetuity. Thus, justified other-directed disgust often remains moderate to high at the end of treatment.

Sadness

Once other emotions have been reduced to levels that fit the facts of the situation and/or are effective, what is typically left to process is sadness. Often clients have spent a lifetime avoiding feeling sad about the traumas and losses they have suffered due to fears that they would not be able to tolerate this grief and it would literally kill them. In DBT, inhibited grieving, or the tendency to avoid feeling sadness or grief about past losses, is an important secondary target that often contributes to clients' behavioral dyscontrol and general misery. For clients with a history of trauma, there is much to be grieved about the tragic events they have experienced and the suffering they caused. Thus, when clients are finally able to radically accept these traumas, rather than judging themselves or others or denying or minimizing the reality of what occurred, they often feel intense sadness. Admittedly, this is not a very reinforcing outcome for having worked so hard to gain a new perspective on and accept one's traumas, and at the same time it is a necessary, and temporary, stage of recovery. Therefore, you should encourage clients to view this stage of acute mourning as a sign of immense progress and reassure them that this too will pass if they allow themselves to experience rather than inhibit their grief. As sadness is felt and naturally subsides, clients typically reach a place of resolution, peace, and freedom from a past that has long been holding them hostage.

Sadness is justified if you have lost someone or something important to you, or your life is not the way you would like it to be. Losses caused by trauma may be concrete (e.g., the death of a friend or the loss of one's physical functioning) and psychological (e.g., the loss of one's sense of personal validity). In addition, the lives of people who have experienced trauma are often far removed from what they would like them to be. For clients in need of DBT PE, trauma has often made it difficult for them to form close relationships, engage in their communities, work or go to school, experience happiness, and generally have lives that feel as if they are worth living. Therefore, sadness about trauma-related losses and the ways in which their lives have been negatively impacted by trauma in the past and present is completely justified. On the other hand, sadness is not justified if it is about anticipated future losses unless there is a realistic limitation on the future that makes it reasonable to assume that the loss will actually occur. For example, it would be justified for a childless woman in her 60s to grieve the fact that she will never have her own biological children, whereas this future-oriented sadness would not be justified for a healthy woman in her 30s.

Targeting Unjustified Sadness

When sadness is unjustified, the goal is to reduce it to a level that fits the facts of the situation. Typically, unjustified sadness is prompted by inaccurate interpretations about the impact of past traumas (e.g., "I am permanently damaged by my abuse"), overgeneralizations about one's past (e.g., "I have never experienced anything positive in my life"), and/or unrealistic predictions about the future (e.g., "I will never be loved"). When this occurs, helping clients to check the facts about these interpretations and develop more accurate ways of thinking often helps to reduce sadness to a level that is appropriate to the actual losses they have experienced. In addition, helping clients to describe just the facts about the past (e.g., "I often felt as if my mother did not love me") rather than adding judgments (e.g., "I was unlovable") can also help to decrease the intensity of sadness to a level that fits the facts. Sadness also has a way of snowballing such that when it arises in the context of a specific loss, people tend to feel sad not only about that one event but also about other perceived or actual losses they have experienced. Helping clients to stay focused on the specific loss they have experienced, rather than their entire history of losses and/or anticipated future losses, will also help to reduce sadness to a level that is justified to the event. Finally, when sadness is unjustified, opposite action can be used to decrease its intensity (see below).

Targeting Justified Sadness

When sadness is justified, it is important to consider whether the intensity of the sadness is effective for the client. Justified sadness is typically effective when it is not pervasive and overwhelming, can be regulated when needed, and does not make it impossible to experience pleasure. Essentially, we want clients to find an effective balance between inhibited grieving in which sadness is constantly avoided and unrelenting grieving in which sadness is constantly experienced—in this middle ground lies effective sadness. When justified sadness is effective, clients are encouraged to grieve their losses in whatever ways they find helpful. At the same time, these efforts to grieve must be balanced with efforts to ensure that sadness does not become all-consuming. Helping clients figure out when to shift from allowing to changing sadness, which skills to use to make each end of this dialectic possible, and how to monitor whether they have gone too far to one end or the other is often at the crux of the coaching that therapists provide during this phase. For example, you may encourage clients to balance time spent allowing sadness by crying and journaling about past losses with time spent engaging in activities that will bring pleasure, meaning, and a sense of connection into their lives.

When justified sadness is ineffectively intense and may even have reached the level of a major depressive episode, clients need to increase their use of emotion regulation strategies designed to reduce the frequency and intensity of sadness. (See Table 15.6.) This may include opposite action for sadness, which typically involves activating behavior and increasing connection with others rather than being inactive or isolating. In addition, clients can be encouraged to increase their participation in pleasurable events, as well as activities that function to build mastery and a sense of competence. The following excerpt provides an example of helping a client whose son died by suicide to regulate his sadness to a level that is effective.

CLIENT: I spent so long feeling like it was my fault that he killed himself or angry at him for doing it, that I think I never really grieved his death. And now that I have accepted that he killed himself, without judging myself or him for it, I just feel incredibly sad all the time.

THERAPIST: That's because it is incredibly sad. You lost your son in a tragic way and you miss him terribly every day. Sadness is a completely natural reaction to such a massive loss, and it makes sense that it's gotten particularly intense now that you have let go of your judgments and have radically accepted his death.

TABLE 15.6. Regulating Sadness When It Is Not Effective

Characteristics of sadness	Strategies to decrease sadness
Action urges	
Withdraw, isolate, be inactive, ruminate about past sad events	*Act opposite by:* Spend time with people, get active, build mastery, focus on the present moment
Expressions	
Moving slowly, talking little or not at all, shuffling feet, crying or sobbing, moping, slumping	*Change the experience by:* Moving quickly, talking frequently in an upbeat tone, picking feet up, stopping tears, sitting or standing up straight, perking up, (half) smiling
Common beliefs and interpretations	
• My life will never be what I want it to be. • Life is meaningless without [person they have lost]. • My life has been nothing but trauma and suffering.	*Change beliefs to:* • My life is not what I want it to be right now and it can be different in the future. • I will always miss [person] and it is possible to find purpose and meaning without them. • I have experienced a lot of sad things in my life and I have also experienced positive things.

CLIENT: *(crying)* I still wish I could get him back. I wish I could go back and change things somehow so that he would still be alive, but I know I can't.

THERAPIST: I wish that were possible too, and it's really painful to accept that it's not.

CLIENT: I don't know if I'll survive this sadness—it feels like it's taking over my life. Yesterday when I was at the store I just started crying out of nowhere. People were looking at me and probably thought I was crazy, but I just couldn't stop it. That's been happening a lot and I can't seem to control it.

THERAPIST: Does it feel like you're sad most of the time now?

CLIENT: I feel sad all the time now and I'm worried I'm starting to get depressed. I don't feel like doing anything anymore and I'm exhausted all the time.

THERAPIST: It sounds like it might be helpful for us to think about ways to find a balance between feeling sad, which we need you to do some of the time, and getting a break from sadness so that it doesn't take over your life and turn into depression.

CLIENT: I agree.

THERAPIST: Are there things you're doing on purpose to feel sad or grieve your son?

CLIENT: No, it just comes up without me doing anything and often it's at inconvenient times.

THERAPIST: Sadness is like a barrel of rainwater that collects over time. If we never open the spigot and let some of the water out, it will eventually overflow. However, if we make sure that we regularly take water out of the barrel, it will stay at a level that is effective and won't spill out everywhere. In your case, you have a lot of sadness that has built up since your son's death because you have rarely opened the spigot and let it come out. And now it has reached the point of overflowing and is leaking out at times when you don't want it to.

CLIENT: That makes sense.

THERAPIST: So, I think what we need you to do is intentionally open the spigot some of the time to get your sadness to a level that is more effective.

CLIENT: How would I do that?

THERAPIST: I'm not sure exactly, but often doing things like looking at reminders of your son, talking about him with people, or thinking about things you did with him will bring up sadness.

CLIENT: Yes, those things would definitely make me feel sad.

THERAPIST: Is there something you could imagine doing every day that would bring up sadness at a time and place where it would be reasonable to allow yourself to just cry and grieve without trying to make it stop?

CLIENT: I could go into his bedroom and look at his things.

THERAPIST: That sounds like it would work. So, let's plan to have you stay in his bedroom and allow yourself to feel sad, including crying if you feel like crying, until the sadness naturally subsides. If you really focus on your sadness and don't try to block it, it should come like a wave, increasing for a bit before it decreases again. Usually this lasts no more than 10 or 15 minutes if you make sure that you stay focused on just the facts. So, what are the facts that need to be grieved?

CLIENT: (*crying*) My son is dead because he killed himself. And I am never going to see him again or be able to watch him grow up.

THERAPIST: Yes, those are the facts and they are incredibly sad. So, if you go in his bedroom and focus on those facts your sadness will come up and then it should come back down. I'd say you should do that for no longer than 30 minutes each day, but it may take less time than that for the sadness to naturally decrease. Are you willing to do that every day this week?

CLIENT: Sure, I'll try it.

THERAPIST: Great! My hope is that if you build in time every day where you are intentionally opening the spigot and allowing yourself to feel sad, that this will help it to stop overflowing at other times. However, if sadness comes up at other times when it is reasonable to allow yourself to cry until it naturally subsides, then that would also make sense to do.

CLIENT: OK.

THERAPIST: So, let's think about the other side of this dialectic, which is strategies to reduce sadness when needed. This is where we think about using opposite action for sadness. What do you have urges to do when you feel sad?

CLIENT: I just want to be alone and not do anything.

THERAPIST: Right, that's typically what happens when we feel sad. So, to reduce sadness you would need to do the opposite of those things, which would mean being around people and staying active. Ideally, you would find activities to do that are things you typically enjoy or that make you feel competent. Do you have any ideas about what those things could be?

CLIENT: I could spend more time with my wife and friends. My wife and I used to do things together a lot like go out to dinner, take walks, or watch movies together. My buddies and I like to watch sports together or do active things like mountain biking.

THERAPIST: Those all sound great! What about things that make you feel good about yourself and give you a sense of mastery or competence?

CLIENT: When I fix things around the house, I usually feel good about that. We have a couple of things that I've been needing to fix for a while.

THERAPIST: Perfect! So, I'd suggest that you also do at least one pleasurable activity or an activity that makes you feel competent every day. These could be activities that involve spending time with your wife and friends, but they don't all have to be social activities. You may even want to schedule those activities for after you have done your intentional grieving each day, as they could help you to switch your focus away from the sadness to other things.

CLIENT: OK.

THERAPIST: The last thing that is really critical is that you need to work on staying mindful of the present moment when you are engaging in those activities. It's not going to do any good if you are watching a movie with your wife and thinking about your son the entire time. So, instead, work on being one-mindful and focusing your attention on the activity you are doing so that you can fully participate in it.

CLIENT: OK, I'll give it a shot.

THERAPIST: I appreciate your willingness, and I feel hopeful that this approach will help to get your sadness to a level that feels more effective for you.

Concluding Comments

Although DBT PE is first and foremost a treatment for PTSD, it also has a significant secondary benefit: It helps clients strengthen and generalize the emotion regulation skills they learn in DBT. DBT PE provides clients with the opportunity to repeatedly practice and hone these skills under particularly challenging conditions. Indeed, DBT PE could reasonably be described as an emotion regulation bootcamp as it requires clients to purposefully activate painful trauma-related emotions every day for months and then cope effectively with them. As a result of DBT PE, clients are therefore likely to learn a variety of important lessons about emotions and their ability to manage them, including:

- Emotions can be labeled and understood.
- Emotions can be tolerated even when they are extremely intense.
- Emotions do not last forever.
- Avoidance makes emotions last longer and get more intense in the long run.
- Experiencing emotions without avoiding causes them to decrease over time.
- Emotions can be experienced without engaging in maladaptive behaviors.
- It is possible to engage in wise-minded behavior even when emotional.
- Emotion regulation strategies can be used to change emotions to a level that is appropriate to the situation and effective.

As clients progress through DBT PE, you should actively work to highlight and strengthen this critical learning about emotions and emotion regulation. Ideally, by the end of DBT PE, clients will no longer view emotions as intolerable or feel the need to chronically avoid them—a shift in perspective that has far-reaching effects in terms of improving their quality of life.

CHAPTER 16

Working with Different Trauma Types

DBT PE can be used to treat PTSD related to any trauma type. Although the structure and core procedures of DBT PE remain the same regardless of the type of trauma being treated, you need to tailor your delivery of the treatment to address the specific characteristics of the traumas that clients have experienced. Therefore, it is important to be familiar with common issues that arise when working with different trauma types. In this chapter, I focus on the types of trauma that are most prevalent among clients receiving DBT PE, including child sexual abuse, child physical abuse, traumatic invalidation, sexual assault and rape, and intimate partner violence (IPV). Although it is not unusual for clients to have experienced other types of trauma, such as accidents or traumatic losses, these are less often the focus of treatment. That said, if a specific type of trauma is not included in this chapter, it is not meant to imply that it may not be important to target for some clients. Additionally, many of the trauma types reviewed here are likely to co-occur, making their separation into distinct types somewhat artificial. My intent is to provide an overview of the most common types of trauma that are treated during DBT PE and to suggest strategies for picking index events and addressing the themes that often arise when processing these traumas in treatment.

Child Sexual Abuse

Definition and Common Experiences

Child sexual abuse is the most common index trauma reported by clients who receive DBT PE and is generally defined as an adult or older adolescent using a minor for sexual stimulation. Child sexual abuse can include a range of behaviors, such as engaging the child in sexual activity (e.g., fondling, oral sex, vaginal or anal penetration), exposing a child to sexual body parts or sexual acts, and child sexual exploitation (e.g., being forced to engage in sex work or in the production of child pornography). Most perpetrators of sexual abuse are known to the child and often include family members or friends, neighbors, babysitters, or other adults with regular access to the child (e.g., teachers, priests, coaches). Child sexual abuse often begins with a grooming process during which the perpetrator gains the child's trust and affection by doing things such as buying them gifts, playing games with them, and giving them special attention before beginning to engage in inappropriate sexual behaviors with them. The child may be asked, pressured, threatened, or physically forced to engage in the sexual behaviors. In addition, perpetrators often use secrecy, blame, and threats to maintain control and keep the child from disclosing the abuse to others.

Children may have a wide variety of emotional reactions to the sexual abuse while it is occurring. For many sexual abuse survivors, the primary emotions present during the sexual abuse may have been positive ones, such as happiness and excitement. This is often the case when the perpetrator made the child feel special and loved, rewarded the child for the sexual behavior, and/or sexually stimulated the child so that the abuse was physically pleasurable. In other cases, the sexual abuse may have elicited negative emotions, such as fear, shame, and sadness. This is more likely to be the case when the abuse was perpetrated by someone the child did not like; was done in a violent or physically painful way; or included threats, insults, or humiliation. At times, sexual abuse may have been experienced as neither positive nor negative, but rather as a behavior that the child did not understand and had no particular reaction to at the time. Children's emotional reactions to sexual abuse typically change as they age, with younger children more often experiencing it as something positive or neutral, whereas older children and adolescents typically experience it as something unwanted and clearly negative as their awareness that it is inappropriate grows.

Picking an Index Event

Child sexual abuse is typically chronic and may occur repeatedly with the same perpetrator over months or years, which makes it challenging to pick a single incident to focus on for imaginal exposure. Moreover, because chronic sexual abuse often occurs in more or less the same way each time it happens, it is often hard for clients to clearly distinguish between events. Additionally, many clients have experienced sexual abuse from more than one perpetrator and decisions need to be made about whether to target both in treatment, and if so, which perpetrator to address first. When selecting a single event to target via imaginal exposure from a chronic trauma type, you should try to balance the goal of picking a highly distressing event (ideally the most distressing one) with the goal of picking an event that is reasonably representative of the larger pattern of sexual abuse. At times, these goals can be somewhat at odds because the most memorable and distressing event(s) are often ones that deviated in some way from how the sexual abuse typically occurred. For example, the sexual abuse may have happened in an unusual location, there may have been a witness when this was not usually the case, the sexually abusive behavior may have been done in an atypical way, or the perpetrator may have had an unexpected response. At the same time, these events typically include many elements that are representative of the sexual abuse more broadly and may therefore be useful events to select. It is also important to consider the primary problematic beliefs the client has about the sexual abuse and to select events that are clearly linked to those beliefs whenever possible. For example, if the client believes that their own flirtatiousness caused the abuse to occur, it would be useful to select an event that they view as evidence that this is true so that this belief can be more directly targeted.

It is also important to remember that no matter which event is picked for imaginal exposure, the larger pattern of sexual abuse, including details of other specific times it occurred, must be discussed during processing in order to generalize learning across events. Therefore, the single incident that is picked for imaginal exposure can be viewed more as a jumping-off point for discussing the broader experiences and dynamics of the sexual abuse that occurred, which may relieve some pressure in terms of needing to pick the "right" event. In addition, it may be the case that more than one event will need to be targeted to fully resolve the distress associated with chronic sexual abuse. For example, in cases where the sexual abuse occurred in significantly different ways (e.g., the sexual behavior was sometimes initiated by the perpetrator and sometimes by the client), there may be distinct beliefs and emotions tied to each form of the sexual abuse that cannot be adequately targeted with only one event. When this occurs, a second event can be selected for targeting either during the Trauma Interview in Session 1 or later in treatment after the first memory is complete.

Common Themes to Be Processed

Not Realizing It Was Wrong

Many clients who were sexually abused as children did not recognize the behavior as a problem at the time it was occurring. As adults or adolescents looking back on their experiences, they often struggle to understand how this could be true and believe they should have known immediately (or sooner than they did) that the sexual behavior was wrong. To address these types of beliefs, it is helpful to have clients think through what they understood about sex at the age at which the abuse began, when and how they first learned about normative sexual behavior (if at all), and what exactly led them to first recognize the behavior as problematic. In addition, clients can be encouraged to consider what the perpetrator taught them, directly or indirectly, about the acceptability of the sexual behavior and how this influenced their perceptions of it at the time. When the sexual abuse was done in a seemingly caring manner or in the context of a generally positive relationship, this may have made it difficult for clients to identify it as abusive. This can also occur in situations in which the client was an adolescent and believed they were in a consensual, real relationship with the perpetrator even though the person was an adult. In general, it is important to help clients nonjudgmentally understand why they did not view the behavior as problematic until whatever point they did begin to perceive it that way, and to normalize this as being both age appropriate and reasonable given the specific context in which their abuse occurred.

Self-Blame

Nearly all clients blame themselves in whole or in part for the sexual abuse they experienced. Clients often believe that they provoked or encouraged the abuse in some way and/or that they should have done something different to stop it from happening. Self-blame can be particularly pronounced for clients who at times initiated sexual behavior with their abuser and may even have sought the person out. When the perpetrator is someone with whom clients have an ongoing relationship, the pull to blame themselves for the abuse can be particularly strong because the alternative—blaming the perpetrator—is likely to have significant negative consequences. For example, clients may be reluctant to hold the perpetrator accountable for their behavior because they wish to maintain a relationship with the person, avoid causing tension in their family, or preserve their own sense of the person as a caring and positive presence in their life. This can lead to a difficult dialectical dilemma in which clients want to view themselves more positively (e.g., by not blaming themselves for their own abuse) while also not wanting to view their abuser negatively (e.g., by holding them responsible for what occurred). This can be particularly challenging to reconcile for clients who believed (or believe) that their abuser loved them, as it can be painful to accept that the person would knowingly do something so painful and damaging to them.

As with self-blaming beliefs more broadly, you should help clients nonjudgmentally understand how the behaviors they engaged in and the decisions they made at the time of the sexual abuse make sense given the context in which the abuse occurred. If at times clients initiated sexual behavior with their abuser, it is important to help them understand how this behavior is understandable (e.g., they were taught or expected to do so, they found the attention or touch of the abuser to be pleasurable, they did not understand that the sexual behavior was inappropriate) and does not make them responsible for what occurred. In addition, when clients lack relevant knowledge, didactic strategies can be useful to educate them about things such as legal definitions of sexual abuse, the age at which people are considered capable of consenting to sex, the grooming process, and other common dynamics of sexual abuse. When the sexual abuse was perpetrated by an adult, clients must be helped to recognize that sexual behavior between adults and children is never acceptable and is always the fault of the adult. This is because adults are in a position of power over children and possess the knowledge to understand that the behavior is inappropriate, whereas children can neither consent to nor fully comprehend the implications of engaging in sexual behaviors. In cases where the perpetrator was also a minor, consideration can be given to how much that person may or may not have recognized the sexual behaviors as problematic given their age and history, while also holding the person responsible for having caused harm to the client even if they may not have intended to do so or been fully aware of the seriousness of their behavior.

Experiencing Sexual Abuse as Positive and Pleasurable

It is quite common for clients to report that they liked, looked forward to, or wanted some aspects of the sexual abuse they experienced. This awareness can be particularly upsetting once clients reach an age when they recognize the sexual abuse as having clearly been problematic and harmful. Clients often struggle to understand how something so wrong could have felt good at the time, and frequently decide that it must mean they are perverted, disgusting, or morally reprehensible. When this occurs, it is important to help clients understand what exactly was positive about the experience and how this makes sense. Often clients enjoyed that the perpetrator expressed interest in them, spent time with them, gave them gifts, and/or appeared to love and care for them. These are, of course, completely normal things to enjoy, and this is even more true if children were not receiving adequate love and attention from other people in their lives at the time. Indeed, children who appear to not be getting their emotional needs met by others are often targeted by perpetrators of sexual abuse because of this vulnerability. In addition, it can be helpful to educate clients that abusers often intentionally make the experience enjoyable for the child so that they will be interested and willing to engage in the sexual behavior and less likely to complain about it to others.

It is also common for clients to have experienced sexual arousal or orgasm during the abuse, which usually causes intense shame, as well as disgust toward their body. They may interpret their experience of arousal as meaning they wanted the abuse to occur or consented to it, and they may have been told this was true by the perpetrator. When the perpetrator was of the same sex, this may also lead clients to question their sexual orientation and wonder whether they are gay because they were aroused by the behavior. It is important to both normalize sexual arousal during sexual abuse and educate clients about how and why this can occur, including when the abuse was done in a violent way, they disliked the perpetrator, and/or the experience was unwanted. The main point to convey is that sexual arousal is a natural physiological reaction to being touched in certain areas of the body and it cannot be controlled, just like we cannot control other reflexive responses, such as sweating. Thus, experiencing arousal or orgasm during sexual abuse does not indicate the person consented to or wanted the stimulation, nor does it necessarily mean that they found it to be pleasurable. In the field of sex research this is referred to as arousal nonconcordance, which occurs when there is a mismatch between genital arousal and subjective wanting or desire (Nagoski, 2021).

It can be helpful to use the analogy of tickling to explain this concept to clients. Often people laugh and smile while they are being tickled, because this is the body's natural response to tickling. However, when someone is tickled against their wishes or the tickler won't stop when they are asked, the person being tickled will likely continue to laugh and smile even though they are not enjoying the experience. The same is true for sexual arousal and orgasm: Our bodies are programmed to respond to touch in certain areas with physical arousal and we cannot prevent this even when it is unwanted. It is also important to acknowledge that at times the client may have experienced the sexual arousal as pleasurable or desired, which is also completely understandable and does not negate the fact that the behavior was nonetheless abusive.

Initiating Sexual Behavior with Others

A common behavioral warning sign that a child has been sexually abused is that they attempt to play sexual games or ask others to engage in sexual behavior with them, including other children as well as adults. Therefore, it is not unusual that clients report that they initiated or even forced sexual behaviors on others when they were children. These events often cause clients to experience overwhelming guilt and shame and to view themselves as sexual predators or pedophiles. This can be a challenging issue to process because guilt and shame are typically neither entirely unjustified nor entirely justified. On the one hand, guilt is unjustified because the client usually did not understand the behavior was considered inappropriate and it therefore did not violate their values (or the moral code of their abusive environment) at the time. On the other hand, guilt is justified to the extent that their behavior may have caused harm to others even if this was unintentional. Similarly, shame about these behaviors is likely to be unjustified in some contexts where rejection is unlikely (e.g., in therapy) and justified in others (e.g., with family members). You should educate clients that this type of sexualized behavior is a common consequence and sign of sexual abuse and help them to down-regulate guilt and shame to levels that fit the facts of the situation by using strategies described in Chapter 15 (e.g., increasing self-compassion, radically accepting their past behavior, and making repairs if appropriate).

To Tell or Not to Tell

Whether or not clients told others about their sexual abuse, they are likely to judge themselves for the disclosure choices they made. If they did not tell anyone, they may blame themselves for keeping it hidden. If they did tell someone, they may think they should have disclosed sooner, in a different way, to a different person, or not at all. Regardless, it is important to help clients understand in a nonjudgmental way the complex factors that influenced their disclosure choices. Most children who experience sexual abuse delay or never disclose their abuse to family, friends, or the authorities, and there are many potential reasons for this. Often the abuser makes the child promise to keep it secret and may threaten to hurt them or people they care about if they tell. If the child cares about the abuser, they may feel motivated to keep the abuse hidden to protect the person from getting in trouble. Sometimes children stay quiet because they are afraid they will not be believed or they will get in trouble if someone finds out what has been going on. If clients did tell someone about the abuse, they may hold themselves responsible for the perpetrator getting in trouble or for the stress it caused the people they told. In addition, if the people to whom they disclosed responded in ways that were unhelpful, dismissive, or even punitive, clients may judge themselves for having brought this added layer of suffering on themselves by disclosing.

In the present moment, there are often still challenging decisions to be made about whether and to whom to disclose sexual abuse, particularly when the perpetrator is a family member. For example, if the perpetrator is a stepfather who is still married to the client's mother or a brother who has a close relationship with the client's parents, choosing to tell other members of the family about the person's past abusive behavior is likely to have significant implications for the family system as a whole. As with any challenging interpersonal situation, clients should consider and weigh their priorities in the situation, which may include getting an objective met (e.g., ensuring that the person will be prevented from having contact with them), maintaining a relationship (e.g., with the perpetrator or someone close to them), and/or increasing one's self-respect (e.g., by telling the truth about their abuse). There are no easy or correct answers in situations like this, and clients should be encouraged to give themselves time and grace to reach a decision about how to move forward that feels most effective for them, while also allowing for the possibility that what feels wise may change over time as their beliefs and emotions continue to shift.

Understanding the Perpetrator's Motives

Many survivors of child sexual abuse struggle to understand their perpetrator's motives and ask questions, such as "I thought he loved me—how could he have done this to me?" and "Why would a parent do this to their own child?" Often clients will question the psychological makeup of the perpetrator and may wonder, for example, whether the person is sadistic, depraved, or evil. When clients felt particularly attached to the perpetrator, they may struggle to accept that the person abused them intentionally and instead hold on to the hope that they acted without awareness or understanding that the sexual behavior was wrong or likely to cause damage. When the perpetrator was a caregiver, it can be particularly painful to come to terms with the fact that the person who was supposed to protect them from harm had in fact done quite the opposite. Regardless of their relationship to the perpetrator, clients often struggle with intense feelings of betrayal as they come to terms with the fact that someone they trusted and may have loved took advantage of them for their own sexual gratification.

In this process, clients often become intensely angry at the perpetrator, which is both completely justified and an important part of the typical course of processing trauma. However, remaining intensely angry toward one's perpetrator in the long run is likely to lead to bitterness and resentment that impedes the client's recovery. When this occurs, and in general, it can be useful to help clients consider a range of possible reasons why their perpetrator chose to sexually abuse them that are not solely focused on the person's inherent badness and do not minimize their culpability. Starting from the fundamental DBT assumption that all behavior is caused, clients might consider factors such as the perpetrator's own history of abuse, their difficulty controlling sexual urges, the disinhibiting effects of substances, the person's need to feel loved and cared for, and so on. This process of finding nonjudgmental explanations for why the perpetrator may have sexually abused them is often an important strategy for helping clients to reach a place of full radical acceptance of what happened, which includes acceptance—but not approval—of the perpetrator and their harmful actions.

Seeking Justice

As clients' guilt and self-blame decreases and/or anger toward the perpetrator increases, many will raise issues related to wanting justice for the sexual abuse that was inflicted upon them. Unfortunately, the vast majority of child sexual abuse incidents are never reported to authorities. (See Chapter 7 for a discussion of the role of the therapist as a mandated reporter.) This may be because the child did not disclose their abuse at all or disclosed it only to a close friend rather than an adult. Even when children disclose their abuse to a parent or other adult, it is often not reported to authorities and instead a decision is made to manage it informally or within the family. If a formal report is made to child protective services, these agencies typically only investigate about half of the child sexual abuse incidents that are reported to them and even those that are investigated are unlikely to result in meaningful interventions. In addition, statutes of limitations often prevent adult survivors of sexual abuse who have delayed reporting from bringing a perpetrator to justice. Taken together, this means that very few clients are likely to experience any sort of legal justice for the sexual abuse they suffered. Even if it is possible to take legal action against a perpetrator, many clients do not want to pursue this. Reasons for not pursuing legal action often overlap with the reasons for not disclosing abuse, but also include fear (often justified) that the legal process itself will be traumatizing and may not result in conviction.

Thus, it is often necessary to help clients consider nonlegal avenues for seeking justice, which could potentially include things such as confronting the perpetrator, telling others about the person's abusive behavior, asking the perpetrator to acknowledge their behavior, seeking some type of restitution (e.g., an apology, money) from the perpetrator, or demanding that they seek treatment. When these types of direct methods of seeking justice are not desired or possible, clients may opt to achieve justice in a broader sense, such as by aiming to lead a happier, more fulfilling, and values-consistent life than their abuser. All too often, clients end up having to accept that the perpetrator is unlikely to be punished in a legal, social, or moral sense, and they must work to let go of bitterness and resentment about this injustice in order to reduce their own suffering.

Child Physical Abuse

Definition and Common Experiences

Child physical abuse is generally defined as the nonaccidental injury of a child. This includes acts such as hitting with a body part or object, kicking, shoving, shaking, choking, burning, and poisoning that result in physical injury. Physical injuries can range from red marks, welts, cuts, and bruises to muscle sprains, broken bones, and head trauma. Physical abuse can also include inactions that result in physical injury to a child, as well as threats of potential harm. In nearly all cases, physical abuse is perpetrated by a parent, caregiver, or other adult or older adolescent with authority over the child. In addition, it is more likely to occur in cultures, religions, or family systems in which corporal punishment of children is viewed as an acceptable form of discipline. Unlike child sexual abuse, child physical abuse frequently occurs openly within a family and the perpetrator may be physically violent toward other family members as well. However, children are typically expected to keep the physical abuse secret and hide or lie about their injuries to people outside the family. In addition, it is not uncommon for perpetrators of physical abuse to engage in sexually abusive and severely invalidating behaviors toward the child that may occur during and/or separate from incidents of physical violence.

Given that physical abuse by definition involves actual or threatened physical injury, it is almost uniformly a negative experience for the child. In addition to being physically painful, it is often highly emotionally distressing. Children who are physically abused frequently live in a state of heightened fear in which they are constantly looking for signs that the perpetrator is likely to lash out at them again, trying not to anger the person, and attempting to placate or make them happy instead. At times, the violence may be quite predictable and at other times it may occur unexpectedly. Often perpetrators of physical abuse use an authoritarian parenting style in which they have very high expectations of their children, lay out strict rules that they expect to be followed at all times, and require immediate and unquestioning obedience to their demands. When children break an explicit or unwritten rule, make a mistake, misbehave, or question an order, they are often swiftly and harshly punished. In these types of authoritarian households, children are often taught to believe that the use of physical violence is an acceptable and necessary parenting strategy to keep children in line. When the physically abusive person is consistently harsh and uncaring, children often strongly dislike the person, although they usually keep these feelings hidden to avoid punishment. In contrast, if the perpetrator is sometimes warm and nurturing toward the child, this can result in mixed feelings toward the person that fluctuate depending on how they are behaving.

Picking an Index Event

As with child sexual abuse, child physical abuse is typically chronic and often occurs across multiple years if not the person's entire childhood and adolescence. In addition, it is not uncommon for both parents to have been physically abusive if this was a generally accepted practice within the home, although one may have used physical punishment more frequently or severely than the other. When there are many potential incidents to select from, you should help clients identify an event that is highly distressing, emblematic of the larger pattern of abuse, and clearly remembered. Often clients select an event that involved a higher than usual degree of physical injury and/or in which they believed they were going to die. Other relevant factors to consider may include the prompting event (if any) for the violence, whether other people were present or injured, the client's in-the-moment response, and/or the reactions of family members or others who knew about the incident. Additionally, when the perpetrator engaged in multiple types of abusive behavior (e.g., physical and sexual abuse, as well as severe invalidation) and/or there were multiple perpetrators of physical abuse, you should consider selecting an event in which all of these types of abusive behaviors occurred to maximize efficiency and generalization.

Common Themes to Be Processed

Defining It as Abuse

As with child sexual abuse, many survivors of child physical abuse did not view the behavior as abuse at the time it was happening because they were taught to believe it was normal and acceptable. Unlike child sexual abuse, however, it is not uncommon for adult survivors of child physical abuse to continue to question whether the behaviors they experienced constitute abuse.

Whereas sexual behavior between adults and children is widely viewed as unacceptable, using physical violence to discipline children is still accepted as an appropriate parenting strategy in some cultures and families. As a result, clients who were physically abused as children may view themselves as having experienced harsh or strict parenting rather than physical abuse. In addition, whereas any sexual contact between an adult and child is considered to cross a clear, black-and-white line of being inappropriate, the boundary between perhaps tolerable forms of physical punishment (e.g., a single slap to the buttocks) versus unacceptable forms of physical punishment (e.g., repeatedly punching a child in the face) can be gray and harder to clearly define. Therapists often serve as educators in this process, providing clients with legal or other widely accepted definitions of child physical abuse to consider and allowing them to come to their own wise mind decision about how to define their experiences. Often clients do eventually choose to label their experiences as physical abuse, while also recognizing the dialectical truths in both sides (e.g., "The behavior was abusive and harmful to me *and* my mother believed it was an appropriate parenting strategy").

Believing the Abuse Was Deserved

In nearly all cases, perpetrators of physical abuse communicate to the child that they deserve to be physically punished. The reasons they are told they deserve to be hit, threatened, and hurt often include things such as having been bad, disrespectful, ungrateful, demanding, lazy, or incompetent. During treatment, clients often still believe that they deserved to be abused for whatever reasons the perpetrator told them this was true (e.g., "I was a bad child"). When processing specific incidents of physical abuse, clients will often point to things they did or failed to do at the time that they view as evidence these general beliefs are true. Even if an episode of physical violence was prompted by something the client did, it is important to help them recognize that their behavior may have prompted the violence but did not justify it. When their alleged misbehavior was minor or even benign, such as getting their clothes dirty or asking for a birthday gift, it is often easier to help clients recognize that the punishment did not fit the crime; indeed, in many families these behaviors would not be viewed as something that needed to be punished at all. However, when clients knowingly broke a clear rule or did something objectively problematic, such as skipping school or using drugs, clients may hold more firmly to the belief that they deserved to be beaten. Regardless, it is important to help clients recognize that intentionally injuring children is never an acceptable form of punishment and that there are many other nonviolent ways to punish a child if they have truly misbehaved. Moreover, it can be helpful to highlight that many of the "bad" behaviors that clients engaged in (e.g., drinking alcohol, not coming home, getting in a fight at school) may have been a response to the abuse they were experiencing.

Being Protected and Protecting Others

Because child physical abuse often occurs openly within families and the perpetrator may be violent toward multiple family members, there are frequently emotions and beliefs to be processed related to whether and how family members attempted to protect one another from the abuser. Many clients harbor feelings of anger and resentment toward family members, particularly parents or other adults, who may have witnessed or known about the physical abuse and did not intervene on their behalf to try to stop it. Anger about not having been protected by people who were in a position to do so is a completely justified response, and at the same time it may be necessary to help clients decrease this anger if it becomes ineffective. This is often done by asking clients to put themselves in the shoes of the other person and generate understandable reasons for their failure to intervene, such as that the other person was scared, less powerful than the abusive person, financially dependent on them, or otherwise under the abuser's control. Clients often end up embracing a dialectical stance that acknowledges both that others were responsible for protecting them from harm and it is understandable why they did not. Clients may also face difficult decisions about whether and how to address issues from the past with family members in the present, such as whether to confront a parent about their failure to intervene or limit contact with a parent who still lives with the abuser.

On the other side, clients may also feel guilty about their own perceived failure to intervene to protect family members, such as their mother and siblings, who were also being abused by the person. In many cases, clients attempted to directly intervene during one or more episodes of violence (e.g., by yelling at the abuser to stop). Clients may also have engaged in more indirect attempts to intervene, such as by strategizing with siblings about how to keep the abuser calm or trying to convince the other parent to leave the abusive relationship. In families in which multiple people were being abused by the same person, it is common for family members to have joined forces to try to prevent the person from becoming violent. This can often contribute to clients feeling as if it was their responsibility to protect others, including adults, from harm. In such cases, it is important to help clients recognize that the abuser was responsible for their own violent behavior and that children cannot be expected to intervene to stop a violent adult from harming others.

Actual or Perceived Threats to Life

In cases of more extreme physical abuse, the perpetrator may have threatened or actually attempted to kill the child. This may include things such as threatening a child with a weapon, poisoning a child with a toxic chemical, choking a child, or hitting a child with an object likely to cause serious injury. In some cases, the perpetrator may have explicitly communicated intent to kill the child and in other cases homicidal intent may have been implied or assumed. The experience of being trapped in a home with a person who threatens or attempts to kill you is an extraordinarily painful one. Not only does it leave the child in a constant state of fear for their life, but it is also likely to make them feel as if their life does not matter at all and is dispensable. Clients may ask particularly anguished questions, such as "How could she want to kill me?" When trying to understand the motives of an extremely violent parent or caregiver, it may be useful to have clients consider the other person's potential skill deficits, history of violence, substance use problems, mental illnesses, and values that may help to provide an explanation for the violent behavior that is not about the client's own perceived flaws. In addition, clients often have a lot of inhibited grief to process about the fact that their parent(s) were so poorly equipped to care for children, and need to grieve the tremendous damage they suffered as a result.

Breaking the Cycle of Violence

Many clients who were physically abused as children express concerns that they are or will become angry and violent people just like their abuser. Clients may compare themselves to their abuser, finding apparent similarities in their mannerisms, behavior, and reactions that they dislike and that make them afraid "I am just like them." When this occurs, it is important to ensure that clients are accurately observing their own behavior, as they are often prone to exaggerating the severity of their behavior (e.g., viewing expressing any anger at all as being highly problematic). If clients have a history of aggression toward others, they can be encouraged to think dialectically about these past transgressions by acknowledging the problematic nature of their aggressive behavior, committing to not repeat it, and making repairs when possible while also understanding with compassion how it occurred, particularly given their own history of abuse. For all clients, skills training focused on how to effectively experience and express anger without becoming verbally or physically aggressive is often needed to address real skills deficits, as well as to help clients gain confidence that they will be able to manage anger effectively when it does arise. In addition, if clients are afraid they will become aggressive toward others and there is no evidence to suggest this is true, *in vivo* exposure tasks that are designed to help them learn that this is unlikely to happen may be useful.

Although clients are often focused on being afraid they will harm others, it is also important to help them recognize that harming themselves is another way in which they may be continuing the cycle of abuse they experienced as a child. For many clients who were physically abused as children, self-injury can function as a way to physically punish themselves for their own perceived misdeeds. In some cases, clients physically harm themselves in the same ways they were harmed as children (e.g., hitting themselves in the face) and in response to the same types of behaviors they were punished for as a child (e.g., making a mistake). Clients may also engage in other behaviors that function as self-punishment, such as denying themselves pleasurable experiences or nice things, pushing themselves to work excessively, or not fulfilling their own basic needs (e.g., for sleep or food). In these cases, it is often an important goal of treatment for clients to stop treating themselves in the same harmful ways they were treated as children and instead to learn to treat themselves with kindness, respect, and compassion. For many clients, this is a very hard thing to do given their beliefs that they deserve to be punished, in which case activities related to doing nice things for themselves can be assigned as formal *in vivo* exposure tasks. In addition, clients can be taught how to use reinforcement and shaping to motivate and reward themselves, rather than relying on punishment to try to change their behavior.

Traumatic Invalidation

Definition and Common Experiences

Traumatic invalidation was first defined by Marsha Linehan (2015) as "extreme or repetitive invalidation of individuals' significant private experiences, characteristics identified as important aspects of themselves, or reactions to themselves or to the world" (p. 304). Invalidating behaviors can take many forms, such as being criticized, excluded, emotionally neglected, ignored, misinterpreted, treated unequally, blamed, and controlled (see Chapter 2 and *General Handout 2, What Is Traumatic Invalidation?* in Appendix A). Often these experiences of invalidation are also invalidated—for example, the invalidating person(s) may discount or minimize the harmfulness of their behavior, criticize the person's reactions to it, and/or deny that it occurred altogether (e.g., gaslighting). Together these invalidating behaviors strike at the core of the person's sense of self by communicating that they are unacceptable, unlovable, unimportant, incompetent, inferior, and don't belong. Traumatic invalidation is often done by parents or caregivers starting early in childhood and can include a wide range of experiences. At one extreme, it may involve overt and blatant mistreatment by parents who display constant contempt and disdain for the child, frequently tell the child they are hated and unwanted, and abuse the child physically and/or sexually. At the other end, traumatic invalidation may be ambiguous and unintentional, such as when well-meaning parents regularly convey disapproval and disappointment toward their child in an effort to help them improve and succeed, and these frequent slights are experienced as deeply emotionally painful.

Although traumatic invalidation often occurs in the family of origin, it can occur at any age and may be perpetrated by any important person, group, or organization. This may include experiences such as bullying by peers in school; regularly having one's character attacked by a boss; or being frequently criticized, controlled, and threatened by an intimate partner. Traumatic invalidation may also include societal or cultural invalidation related to repeated experiences of being criticized, excluded, or discriminated against because of one's race, sexual orientation, gender identity, religion, national origin, disability, or other personal characteristic. Although traumatic invalidation is typically repeated, it may also occur only once in a particularly extreme or life-changing way, such as when a person is given up for adoption as a child, suddenly and unexpectedly rejected by a spouse, excommunicated from one's church after coming out as gay, disbelieved and punished by a parent after disclosing sexual abuse, wrongfully searched and arrested by the police due to racial profiling, or fired from a job due to false allegations of misconduct. Experiences of traumatic invalidation can not only cause PTSD symptoms but can also have profound and long-lasting negative impacts on the person's self-concept, as well as their relationships with others (see *General Handout 3, The Impact of Traumatic Invalidation*).

CLINICAL TIP
What If Traumatic Invalidation Is Ongoing?

A complicating factor that can occur when treating traumatic invalidation is that it may still be happening. For example, it is not unusual for adult clients to report that their relationships with one or both parents continue to be characterized by frequent and painful invalidation that is consistent with how they were treated as a child. When the client is an adolescent or the perpetrator is an intimate partner, the client may still be living with and dependent on the invalidating person. If the client is a member of a marginalized group, they may regularly experience invalidation and discrimination in their day-to-day lives. When traumatic invalidation is ongoing, it is still possible to effectively treat the PTSD symptoms it has caused, but this is likely to require particularly strong corrective feedback to override the invalidating messages that the client continues to receive. In addition, treatment needs to include problem solving how to effectively manage and respond to present-day invalidation.

In such cases, the goal of DBT PE is both to process specific past invalidating events that are contributing to PTSD and help clients develop a more self-validating perspective about ongoing invalidation. In particular, processing past traumatic invalidation can help to reduce clients' unjustified emotions (e.g., shame, guilt, disgust at themselves) and associated negative self-directed beliefs so that they will be less likely to personalize or believe invalidation when it occurs. This, in turn, can help to reduce clients' reactivity to ongoing invalidation and enable them to cope with it effectively (e.g., without engaging in self-destructive behaviors). Additionally, if clients no longer buy in to the invalidating messages that are being directed at them, they may be better able to implement effective interpersonal strategies that may change the dynamics of specific invalidating relationships, such as asserting limits or reducing contact with invalidating people, asking to be treated with respect, not apologizing for their own valid behavior, and ending destructive relationships.

Picking an Index Event

Therapists often find it particularly challenging to identify a single episode of traumatic invalidation to target via imaginal exposure. As a starting point, it is important to remember that the primary goal of DBT PE is to treat PTSD, which means that any invalidating event that is selected for targeting should be clearly linked to symptoms of PTSD that are causing significant distress. Because traumatic invalidation is typically repeated over many years and the negative impact of these experiences may be cumulative (rather than linked to any particularly extreme episodes of invalidation), it can be challenging to identify one event to focus on. When targeting chronic traumatic invalidation, it is recommended that you select an event that is highly distressing to recall and is linked to the client's primary negative core belief(s). The goal is to find an event that the client views as strong evidence that their most distressing or impairing self-invalidating beliefs are true and involves the key invalidating person(s) who made them believe these things about themselves. If these criteria are met, then the event will likely be an effective choice to help the person process the broader pattern of invalidation they experienced and reduce the believability of their negative beliefs about themselves.

Common Themes to Be Processed

Defining It as Traumatic

It is quite common for clients to describe experiences that would be considered traumatic invalidation (e.g., "My mother was really critical and blamed me for all her problems" or "The kids in my school constantly bullied me because I was gender nonconforming"), but question whether these experiences "count" as trauma. This tendency to minimize or discount the traumatic nature of severe or repetitive invalidation comes up frequently during processing and clients often assume their reactions to these experiences are exaggerated and a sign of their own personal weakness or oversensitivity. You can help clients to broaden their view of trauma to include highly stressful events that cause physical, emotional, or psychological harm, while also highlighting that the fact that they have PTSD symptoms related to these events clearly indicates they were traumatic. In addition, it can be helpful to normalize clients' reactions as being common responses to these types of invalidating experiences. For example, research has found that childhood emotional and psychological maltreatment (e.g., bullying, controlling, insulting, excluding, isolating) causes comparably severe PTSD symptoms as sexual and physical abuse, as well as equally or more severe problems in other areas (e.g., self-injurious behaviors, substance use, skipping school, generalized anxiety, depression, attachment problems; Spinazzola et al., 2014). Overall, it is important to help clients stop minimizing the seriousness of the invalidation they experienced and the harm that it caused, while also accepting that their reactions are valid responses to this type of maltreatment.

Unlearning Self-Invalidation

One of the most damaging outcomes of traumatic invalidation is that it teaches the person to invalidate and criticize themselves in ways similar to how they have been invalidated by others. Clients often reflexively assume that their point of view, emotions, preferences, and behavior are wrong and likely to be off-putting, and that they are generally unacceptable people. This can include a wide variety of specific beliefs about their perceived negative qualities (e.g., that they are stupid, lazy, arrogant, ugly, rude, selfish, or manipulative), as well as contempt and hatred of themselves more globally. At its extreme, clients may question their own humanity, viewing themselves as so completely lacking in the qualities that make us human that they instead feel as if they are aliens, robots, or monsters. Imaginal exposure and processing directly target the origins of these self-invalidating beliefs with the goal of helping clients learn that their behaviors and responses at the time of the traumatic invalidation were understandable, and that the criticism and rejection they experienced from others was invalid in important ways. Just as critically, this discussion about the past occurs within an interpersonal context in which shame is not reinforced (i.e., you do not reject or criticize them), which provides another layer of learning about their personal validity and acceptability in the present. *In vivo* exposure offers another avenue to correct self-invalidating beliefs, particularly by conducting exposure to situations that cause unjustified shame because clients incorrectly assume they will be rejected. In addition, other skills from DBT can be utilized to directly target self-invalidation, such as check the facts, loving-kindness meditation directed at the self, and practicing self-encouragement and self-validation.

Developing Realistic Standards

Severely invalidating environments often teach clients to believe that they must be perfect at all times to avoid criticism and, as a result, they come to expect themselves to never make mistakes. Clients often hold themselves to strict rules of behavior, such as expecting themselves to never be late, to always be well groomed, to get straight A's, and to never lose their temper. If they break these rules, they believe they deserve to be harshly criticized or punished. Processing past experiences of traumatic invalidation can help clients reconsider whether the strict standards they were held to by their environment were reasonable or even desirable. You can also provide clients with didactic information about normative expectations (e.g., that children should not be expected to never cry) and self-disclose your opinions about the appropriateness of the standards clients were expected to meet.

In addition to processing these past experiences, clients need to learn how to set reasonable expectations for themselves in the present and to treat themselves with compassion when they do not meet these expectations. This is often done through *in vivo* exposure by having clients intentionally violate their own excessively strict rules to find out how the environment responds, which also creates opportunities to practice accepting and validating themselves when they are imperfect. Through this trial-and-error process, clients will ideally be able to identify new standards that match their own values rather than those of their invalidating environment while also being effective (e.g., help them to achieve important goals, do not cause them to be rejected by people they care about, reduce stress) and realistic (i.e., are generally achievable).

Trusting One's Inner Wisdom

Another painful outcome of traumatic invalidation is that it teaches clients to believe they cannot be trusted to make wise choices, often because others have told them their instincts or perceptions of reality are wrong. In many cases, clients also come to believe that they must be constantly monitored and told what to do by others to ensure they don't do things incorrectly. During imaginal exposure and processing, clients can be helped to see the ways in which their past behavior was effective and wise even if it was invalidated by others. In past situations in which clients made choices that were clearly unwise or ineffective, it is usually the case that they had some intuition or awareness about what would have been a more effective choice even if they did not follow it, or other factors contributed to their decision in ways that are understandable. In general, the goal is to help clients see that they did possess wisdom in the past even if their environment treated them as if they did not and/or their behavior did not always reflect it.

At the same time, it is important to help clients increasingly find and act on their wise mind in the present, rather than constantly distrusting their own instincts and looking to others for guidance. This can be done by designing *in vivo* exposure tasks that will enable clients to learn that they are more competent than they think by having them make decisions and solve problems independently. It may be useful to conceptualize this in terms of the dialectical dilemma between active passivity and apparent competence, with the goal being to help clients find an effective balance between the extremes of constantly asking others to do things they are capable of doing for themselves and acting as if they are more capable than they are such that they do not get the help they need.

Grieving the Pain of Not Being Accepted

The overarching experience of a person who is severely invalidated is that they are made to feel like an outsider who does not belong. Clients often describe feeling as if they were not loved, their presence was unwanted, and they were frequently shunned by people around them. Often clients were taught to believe that their personal qualities made them undesirable and they needed to change who they were to be accepted. However, even when they tried to mold themselves into more acceptable people, they were often still excluded from valued groups and abandoned by people who were important to them. These experiences of not being accepted are extraordinarily painful, leading to intense feelings of sadness and loneliness. Often clients coped by suppressing these emotions and acting as if they were not bothered by their exclusion or that they preferred being alone. Therefore, an important part of healing from traumatic invalidation is to face the intense sadness and pain of not having felt loved or accepted by important people in one's life despite desperately wanting to belong. Rather than inhibiting this grief, clients must be helped to acknowledge, experience, and radically accept the painful reality of these past experiences of being an outsider.

To that end, it is often helpful to frame their experiences as having been the result of a mismatch between their own personal qualities and those of their environment. Marsha Linehan describes this experience as being like a tulip in a rose garden: The tulip is not invalid or problematic, it is just different from the roses around it. In the case of our clients, many of the qualities they possess that were considered unacceptable by their invalidating environment, such as being outspoken, artistic, sensitive, inquisitive, or adventurous, as well as other key aspects of their identities, such as their sexuality, gender, and race, would be viewed as acceptable and even desirable in other contexts. More generally, our clients have often spent much of their lives in environments that were not well matched to their needs—for example, their need for attention and care may have exceeded the capabilities of their parents, or their progressive values may have been different from those of their conservative community. In this no-fault framework, clients can be helped to both validate their own needs and personal qualities and grieve the fact that they were not a good match for the people around them

Finding Validating Environments

As Linehan has often advised, if you are a tulip, don't try to be a rose. Instead, find yourself a tulip garden. This is often a critical part of recovering from traumatic invalidation—namely, to help clients find validating environments in which they are accepted and valued for who they are. To start, clients first have to stop trying to be someone they are not in order to gain approval. This may require them to spend time identifying and clarifying their own personal values, priorities, and goals. Clients may also need to practice, via *in vivo* exposure, how to say no to requests to do things they do not want to do, disagree with others who express opinions inconsistent with their own, and generally to act confidently about their own personal preferences and values. In this process, they often become clearer about what matters to them and who they want to be, as well as which people in their environment respond positively versus negatively to these qualities. If they find that people in their lives respond to them with disapproval and invalidation or seem to have values and interests that do not match their own, then they will need to actively work to find new relationships and communities to join that are a better match for them. When clients lack the interpersonal skills necessary to build new relationships, these can be taught and rehearsed in and out of session (e.g., how to find people who share similar interests, participate in conversations effectively, and join groups). This work to find more validating relationships and environments often begins during DBT PE and continues into Stage 3 and beyond.

Sexual Assault and Rape

Definition and Common Experiences

Sexual assault refers to sexual contact or behavior between adults that occurs without the consent of the victim, such as attempted rape, unwanted sexual touching, and forcing the person to perform sexual acts, such as touching the perpetrator's genitals. Rape is a form of sexual assault that involves sexual penetration without consent, including vaginal or anal penetration with any body part or object and oral penetration by a sex organ. Although the legal definitions of sexual assault and rape vary across states and countries, most definitions include some element focused on the victim's lack of consent. Consent to engage in sexual acts involves overt actions or words indicating agreement for specific sexual acts that was freely given by a person who had the capacity to consent. In contrast, sexual assault and rape involves the use of physical force, threats, emotional coercion, and/or manipulation to force the person into nonconsensual sexual activity and/or is done to a person who lacks the capacity to consent (e.g., due to intoxication or unconsciousness). In most cases of sexual assault and rape, the perpetrators are acquaintances of the victim, such as an intimate partner, friend, classmate, or neighbor, and the assault happens in a private location. Although the vast majority of sexual assaults and rapes are perpetrated by men against women, perpetrators and victims can be any gender.

Picking an Index Event

In many cases, sexual assault or rape is a single event, making the process of identifying an index event straightforward. Some clients, however, have experienced multiple sexual assaults or rapes by the same and/or different perpetrators. In the case of repeated sexual assaults by the same perpetrator, the same principles as previously discussed for other forms of chronic trauma apply. However, when the client has experienced multiple one-time sexual assaults by different perpetrators, then these should be prioritized in terms of the level of distress and impairment they currently cause. If clients report that multiple sexual assaults are comparably distressing, then it may be useful to select the one that occurred first, as this may provide a useful foundation for understanding how this original sexual assault may have contributed to the client's vulnerability and reactions to subsequent sexual assaults. Ideally, the learning from imaginal exposure and processing of one sexual assault may generalize to other assaults so that they do not need to be formally targeted. It is not unusual, however, to target more than one sexual assault, and when this is needed, processing of subsequent assaults typically goes more quickly because the client can draw on the learning that already occurred related to the previously targeted assault (e.g., regarding self-blame).

Common Themes to Be Processed

Defining It as Sexual Assault or Rape

Common harmful stereotypes about what constitutes "real" rape or sexual assault lead many clients to question whether their own experiences "count." These stereotypes often inaccurately suggest that sexual assault is restricted to incidents involving physical violence, injury, and/or penetration, which can cause clients to minimize their own traumatic sexual experiences if they do not meet these excessively narrow definitions. Other damaging stereotypes focus on who can perpetrate sexual assault and rape, such as faulty beliefs that rape only happens by strangers, which can lead clients to question whether their experiences of sexual assault and rape by acquaintances, dating partners, spouses, and past sexual partners "count." Problematic stereotypes also exist about who can be sexually assaulted or raped—for example, that only young, attractive females are raped, that males can't be raped (in general and by women in particular), or that certain types of people can't be raped (e.g., sex workers, spouses). These common myths may lead clients who do not fit stereotypical victim categories to discount the reality of their own experiences.

In general, clients often express problematic beliefs consistent with these types of damaging rape myths that cause them to minimize, discount, or invalidate their own experiences as not being "real" rape or sexual assault. When this occurs, you must help to debunk these myths by providing psychoeducation about definitions of sexual assault and rape (e.g., that physical force or penetration are not required), characteristics of perpetrators (e.g., that sexual assault and rape can occur in any type of relationship), and characteristics of victims (e.g., that people of all ages, genders, appearances, and sexual orientations can be sexually assaulted and raped). Ultimately, it is up to clients to decide how they wish to define and label their unwanted sexual experiences. Our role is to provide them with didactic information to correct harmful stereotypes and then allow them to reach their own wise-minded decision.

Issues of Consent

Given that determinations of nonconsent play a central role in distinguishing sexual assault and rape from nonvictimizing sexual behaviors, issues related to consent commonly arise in processing. Very often clients believe that they did not sufficiently express nonconsent. For example, they may say that they did not say "no" at all, or enough, or in the right way, and that this makes the experience their own fault and "not rape." Many clients believe they should have expressed nonconsent by fighting back or physically resisting, and if they did not, that it can't be rape. At times, clients may have consented to some sexual activity (e.g., fondling) and believe that this negated their ability to not consent to other types of sexual activity (e.g., intercourse), or that having consensual sex with the perpetrator once gave them the right to force sex the next time. Each of these beliefs represent common misunderstandings about how sexual consent is defined that you should help clients correct.

In general, sexual consent means actively agreeing to participate in a sexual activity so that the other person knows that the sexual activity is wanted. There are four key elements of consent that are often helpful to review with clients. First, consent must be *affirmative*. This means that the person must clearly express agreement in words (e.g., saying "yes" to sexual requests) or behavior (e.g., enthusiastically initiating sexual contact). The absence of a "no," a lack of physical resistance, or experiencing genital arousal does not indicate consent. Unless the person actively agreed to the sexual activity, they did not consent. Second, consent must be *freely given*. If perpetrators used overwhelming verbal pressure to get clients to give in to their advances, used emotional manipulation to make them feel guilty or inadequate for being sexually unwilling, or coerced them into saying "yes" by threatening them with negative consequences if they did not, then consent was not freely given. Similarly, if the client was incapacitated at the time of the sexual activity (e.g., due to being very drunk or asleep), then they were not able to give consent freely. Third, consent is *reversible*. This means that a person can change their mind at any time and retract their previous consent. For example, if the client consented to sex earlier in an encounter (e.g., while making out), they can still withdraw their consent as the encounter progresses (e.g., while naked in bed). Fourth, consent is *specific*. A person can consent to one sexual act (e.g., oral sex), but not another (e.g., vaginal sex). Therefore, if the client said "yes" to one type of sexual activity, this did not give the perpetrator permission to engage in other types of sexual activity without obtaining additional consent. If any of these key elements of consent were missing or violated, then the client did not consent to the sexual activity: Sexual activity without consent is sexual assault or rape.

Causal Attributions

Nearly all clients who have been sexually assaulted or raped view it as having been caused by their own behavior and therefore hold themselves responsible for what occurred. Often this is because they believe they put themselves in a risky situation (e.g., by going to the perpetrator's home), made "bad" or "stupid" decisions (e.g., drank too much alcohol), or generally "should have known better" (e.g., that men cannot be trusted), and that these errors in judgment make them complicit in their own assault. In addition, victims of sexual assault and rape often blame themselves because they think they were "asking for it." This typically includes ways in which they think they sexually provoked the perpetrator, such as by wearing revealing clothing, flirting, or willingly engaging in some sexual activity. Like when working to reduce unjustified guilt and self-blame more broadly, it can be helpful to encourage clients to think through why they made the decisions they made at the time, what information they had available to them as the incident was unfolding, and whether there was reason to believe they were putting themselves at risk. You should also take a firm stance that whatever decisions clients made or behaviors they engaged in—risky or not—did not give the perpetrator free license to sexually assault or rape them. Choosing to use drugs, walk home alone, get in a car with a stranger, wear a short skirt, or flirt is not the same as consenting to sexual activity. Moreover, even if the client may have been selected based on their behavior (e.g., being intoxicated), it does not make them responsible for the perpetrator's decision to sexually assault or rape them.

The flip side of viewing themselves as having caused their own sexual assault or rape is that clients typically do not hold the perpetrator responsible for their actions. This is consistent with sexist rape myths suggesting that women cause or provoke rape and men don't mean to perpetrate it. Often female clients absolve male perpetrators of responsibility because they believe he didn't understand what he was doing, didn't realize they were not interested in the sexual activity, or didn't mean to pressure them. Moreover, common stereotypes about male sexuality may interfere with holding men responsible for rape, such as beliefs about acceptable male sexual behavior (e.g., that men are supposed to try to pressure women into sex) and male sex drive (e.g., that once men are sexually aroused, they can't stop themselves from having sex). Other common reasons for not holding perpetrators accountable for sexual assault and rape may include attributing their behavior to being intoxicated at the time, or if the perpetrator was an intimate partner, believing that the person loved them and wouldn't have intentionally hurt or violated them.

Often as clients begin to stop viewing themselves as to blame for what happened they will naturally start to shift responsibility for the sexual assault to the perpetrator. You can help to facilitate this relocating of responsibility by highlighting the ways in which the perpetrator did not seek or obtain consent for the sexual activity or generally forced the client to engage in sexual activity that was unwanted. In addition, you can use didactic strategies to provide corrective information about rape myths that may be contributing to these faulty causal attributions, such as by emphasizing that men are responsible for controlling their sexual urges even when sexually aroused or intoxicated. In some cases, it may be useful to help clients separate the perpetrator's intentions from whether or not they were responsible for the assault by finding dialectical balances, such as "He may not have realized I did not want to have sex with him *and* it was his responsibility to obtain consent before acting" and "He may not have intended to harm me *and* he is still responsible for having caused me harm."

Patterns of Sexual Revictimization

Many clients have suffered repeated experiences of sexual abuse and assault across their lives by different perpetrators in a variety of contexts. As a result of this pattern of revictimization, clients often wonder what they have done or what it is about them that has caused them to be repeatedly targeted by sexual predators. Not surprisingly, they generally tend to blame themselves and to view their repeated experiences of sexual victimization as being due to their own poor decisions and incompetence. Helping clients to unravel the multiple factors that may have contributed to their sexual revictimization can be a delicate discussion that requires you and your client to acknowledge the painful reality that they may have done things that increased their risk of being repeatedly assaulted while at the same time holding firmly to the fact that this does not make these experiences their fault. No matter what, the person to blame for sexual assault and rape is the person who perpetrated it.

In these discussions, you can both normalize the experience of sexual revictimization and educate clients about it. For example, it is a well-established fact that individuals who are sexually abused in childhood or adolescence are at much greater risk of being sexually assaulted as adults than others. One of the most common explanations for this link is that early experiences of sexual victimization result in shame and a variety of negative self-directed beliefs that lead people to believe they are "damaged goods" and don't deserve to be treated with respect. These beliefs may have led clients to be more tolerant of being mistreated, including being subjected to unwanted sexual behaviors, and to have difficulty standing up for themselves or observing limits with people who were sexually aggressive. In addition, avoidant coping may have increased the likelihood that clients would deny or minimize warning signs that they may be in danger rather than acting quickly to escape a risky situation. Repeated victimization may also have led to habituation, such that signs of danger may not have been noticed or perceived as dangerous. Even in situations that were accurately perceived as dangerous, clients' difficulty trusting their own instincts may have led them to ignore rather than follow their wise mind.

Often the consequences of earlier sexual traumas, such as substance use, dissociation, and oversexualized behaviors, may have contributed to clients being in high-risk situations, impaired their judgment, and/or reduced their ability to defend themselves during a sexual assault. Moreover, these types of behaviors may have led them to be targeted by sexual predators because they were perceived as vulnerable. Overall, you must help clients to develop a self-compassionate understanding of their experiences of sexual revictimization, including not judging behaviors that may have increased their risk of repeated assaults, and move from self-blame and guilt to regret and sadness. In addition, it can be helpful to talk about how clients can decrease their risk of experiencing future sexual assaults while ensuring that the precautions they take do not become excessive in ways that overly restrict their lives.

Disclosure Experiences

Sexual assault has been described as a hidden epidemic because it is often not recognized and rarely reported. Many survivors suffer in silence because the stigma, shame, and self-blame associated with sexual assault deters them from either informally or formally disclosing their experiences. In addition, fears of being disbelieved, having to defend themselves in "she said, he said" situations, and being retaliated against by the perpetrator or others may cause survivors to stay quiet and not report their assault. When survivors of sexual assault do disclose their experience, it may be right away or years later and is often to one or more people they feel closest to, such as family, friends, or a romantic partner. If they receive a positive response, this can help to improve psychological well-being by reaffirming their self-worth, reducing self-blame, and increasing social support. However, negative responses to disclosures are likely to lead to additional psychological trauma and can increase feelings of shame, isolation, and PTSD symptoms.

Unfortunately, many clients have suffered not only the trauma of being sexually assaulted but also the trauma of having been blamed, disbelieved, ridiculed, or retaliated against when they disclosed their experience to others. In cases in which the perpetrator was a powerful or well-liked person (e.g., the leader of their church or military unit), clients may have been ridiculed and shunned by an entire community after reporting their assault. In many cases, the experience of having a therapist believe them, tell them it wasn't their fault, and provide support is the first positive response they have ever received and is likely to be a significant corrective learning experience in and of itself. In addition, helping clients process their past negative disclosure experiences and learn to view them as both undeserved and uncalled for is often an important part of recovering from the traumatic experience as a whole. In cases where the negative disclosure experience is as or more distressing than the sexual assault itself—perhaps reaching the level of traumatic invalidation—it will be important to address the disclosure experience in processing and, possibly, target it via imaginal exposure.

Intimate Partner Violence

Definition and Common Experiences

IPV refers to several types of abusive behavior by a current or former romantic partner or spouse, including physical violence, sexual assault, traumatic invalidation (commonly referred to as emotional or psychological abuse in the IPV literature), and/or stalking. The severity of these behaviors can vary widely with some perpetrators of IPV using violence in a single episode, whereas others engage in all four forms of abuse repeatedly over many years. Although IPV is committed most often by males toward female partners, it can be perpetrated and experienced by all genders. Additionally, IPV can occur in heterosexual and same-sex relationships, in adolescent and adult relationships, and whether or not sexual intimacy has occurred in the relationship. In relationships in which IPV is repeated, it often (but not always) follows a cycle that starts with a tension-building phase in which the abuser becomes increasingly irritable and hostile and the victim feels as if they are walking on eggshells and constantly trying not to upset their partner. This tension builds until an abusive incident involving physical or sexual violence occurs, after which the perpetrator often enters a "honeymoon phase" in which they may apologize, express guilt and remorse, attempt to win their partner back by buying them gifts or being particularly affectionate, and promise not to engage in the abusive behavior again. This eventually ends as tension begins to build again before the next abusive incident occurs.

Although episodes of acute violence may occur cyclically, in between these episodes perpetrators of IPV typically use numerous strategies to instill fear and maintain power and control over their partner. This may include using intimidation to make the person afraid (e.g., by making menacing looks or gestures, breaking objects, or displaying weapons) or making threats (e.g., to harm the person, kill themselves, or end the relationship). Perpetrators of IPV often use emotional or psychological abuse to erode their partner's self-esteem by calling them names, insulting them, making them feel guilty or inadequate, and humiliating them. In heterosexual relationships, male abusers often attempt to assert male privilege by treating their female partner like a servant, excluding her from decisions, and demanding strict obedience. In same-sex relationships, abusers may threaten to "out" the victim to their family, friends, or coworkers. Perpetrators often use economic abuse to make their partners financially dependent on them by preventing them from getting a job, taking their money, or not allowing them to have access to bank accounts. When the couple has children, the abuser may threaten to take the children away, harm them, or use visitations to abuse a former partner. Most abusers attempt to isolate their partners from friends and family, often refusing to allow them to spend time with other people and closely monitoring their activities and communications. When the victim attempts to confront the abuser about their behavior, they often respond by minimizing it, saying it was the victim's fault, or claiming that it didn't occur. Collectively, these abusive strategies often work to keep the victim in a chronic state of fear and shame, cut off from other sources of support, and dependent on the abuser, such that they are less likely to end the relationship or leave.

Before initiating DBT PE with a client who has suffered IPV, it is important to first establish that they are currently safe from serious harm. If clients are still in a relationship with the abuser, treating PTSD is typically discouraged if they are still actively being physically or sexually victimized, as priority should be given to ensuring their safety. In all cases where there is still a threat of violence from a current or former partner, it is recommended that clients create a safety plan that clearly defines what they will do and who they will contact if they feel they are in danger of being harmed by the person. Once safety is confirmed and/or sufficient precautionary measures are in place, clients can proceed with DBT PE assuming other readiness criteria have been met.

Picking an Index Event

Given that IPV is typically repeated, there are often multiple episodes of abuse to pick from when selecting an index event. Clients are encouraged to select the event that is currently most distressing, which is often one in which they sustained particularly serious injuries or felt as if their own or their children's lives were in danger. When clients experienced multiple types of abusive behavior from their partner (e.g., physical and sexual abuse as well as traumatic invalidation), picking an event in which all of these types of behaviors occurred is likely to increase the efficiency and effectiveness of treatment. Other factors to consider may include the overall representativeness of the abusive episode, such as the location, precipitating events, and the perpetrator's words and actions, as well as how clearly the client can remember it. In cases where the client suffered a head injury or lost consciousness and cannot remember some portion of the event, it can still be targeted as long as they can describe some elements of what occurred (e.g., what led up to the abusive incident and the first things they can remember after regaining consciousness).

Common Themes to Be Processed

Given that IPV includes multiple types of abusive behavior, including physical abuse, sexual assault, and traumatic invalidation, many of the themes already discussed in regard to these individual trauma types are likely to be relevant when working with clients who have suffered IPV. In addition, there are several common themes that are specific to IPV that are important to consider.

Choosing to Stay

As with other types of trauma, nearly all clients who have experienced IPV blame themselves for their own abuse. In IPV, this self-blame often focuses on the client's belief that they should have left their abusive partner sooner and is accompanied by self-judgment for having chosen to stay with the person for however long the abuse lasted. Often people in the clients' lives have expressed similar judgments and wondered why they didn't "just leave" the abusive relationship. However, very few victims of IPV leave immediately after the first incident of abuse and most stay in the relationship for months or years. In addition, leaving is often not a one-time event and instead typically involves multiple attempts to leave before the relationship is fully over. Therefore, it is important to both normalize clients' decisions to stay in and/or return to the abusive relationship and help them to identify the understandable reasons why they did not leave their partner sooner.

One crucial factor to consider is that leaving is often the most dangerous time for a victim of IPV and many abusers threaten to kill or seriously harm their partners if they leave. In addition, self-blame for their partner's violence and shame about being in an abusive relationship often reduce the likelihood that people will leave. Many victims of IPV continue to love their abusive partner and to hope and believe that they will change so that the relationship can be salvaged. If the couple had children, the victim may have wanted to keep the family together or been afraid of losing custody if they left. Cultural and religious values that support traditional gender roles and oppose divorce frequently contribute to women choosing to stay with abusive men. When the person was dependent on their abusive partner due to factors such as lack of money or resources, physical disability, or immigrant status, this can make it seem impossible to leave the relationship. Whatever the reasons, the goal is to help clients develop self-compassion for their decision to stay in an abusive relationship and recognize the ways in which the abuser's controlling and threatening behaviors led them to feel trapped and unable to leave.

Not Protecting Children from Harm

When the client's children were involved in the IPV either as witnesses or direct targets of the violence, this can contribute to intense feelings of guilt and self-recrimination for not having done enough to protect them from harm. It is not unusual for clients to hold a black-and-white view about this—for example, stating that they completely failed as parents and did nothing to protect their children. To assess the accuracy of these beliefs, it is necessary to clarify the facts about what exactly was done to or in the presence of children, and what, if anything, the client did to try to shield them from this harm. It is often the case that clients *did* attempt to protect their children some (or even most) of the time, such as by telling them to stay in their room when the abuser became violent or directly intervening when the abuser was aggressive or violent toward them. In some cases, the client may not have been aware their child was being harmed, such as when their partner was sexually abusing the child in secret, and therefore they could not have intervened. At the same time, there are typically incidents in which clients could have intervened but did not and instead stood by as the abuser insulted, threatened, or hit their child. In addition, clients often blame themselves for having put their children at risk simply by being in an abusive relationship even if their partner never directly harmed them.

Overall, it is important to help clients develop a balanced and accurate view of their own efforts to protect their children that acknowledges both what they did and did not do, as well as what they could and could not have done given the reality of the abusive situation they were in. If clients are placing unrealistic expectations on themselves, such as thinking they should have been able to physically overpower their much larger and stronger partner, then you can help them adjust these expectations and grieve the fact that they may have been powerless to protect their children in some situations. If there are incidents in which clients did not attempt to protect their children from harm, you can help them validate how their decisions in those moments were understandable even if they regret them now. If some portion of clients' guilt is justified (e.g., when their lack of intervention in certain incidents violates their values as a parent), helping them to make repairs, radically accept their past behavior, and work to let go of their self-judgments may be useful. In addition, it is important to acknowledge the role of the abuser in these situations and ensure that the client views their partner as having primary responsibility for any harm that was done to children.

Recognizing Warning Signs

A common belief reported by clients who have experienced IPV is that they do not trust themselves to pick partners in the future who will not be abusive, and, as a result, they may avoid getting into new relationships. This is particularly true among clients who have been abused by multiple dating partners or spouses. As a result of these past experiences, clients often say that they always pick "bad" partners and feel unable to identify warning signs that a person is likely to become abusive. While processing past experiences of IPV, you can provide education about warning signs for IPV and help clients to identify red flags that may have been present early in the relationship or before their partner first became acutely violent. This may include behaviors that were directed at the client, such as jealousy, calling them names, wanting them to "check in" multiple times per day, degrading them in front of other people, not respecting their requests, and being critical of their friends or family. Warning signs may also include more general characteristics that are associated with perpetration of IPV, such as abusing alcohol or drugs, having a history of violence, and behaving disrespectfully or aggressively toward others. You can also help clients to think through what they will do if they see these red flags in future relationships. In some cases, clients may actively be in relationships with partners who are exhibiting these types of warning signs, in which case you can help them to clarify their relationship goals, identify their personal limits, and plan how they will respond if these limits are crossed. Overall, the goal is to help clients both increase their awareness of common warning signs for IPV and enhance their sense of control over whether they are likely to end up in another abusive relationship in the future.

Concluding Comments

Clients in need of DBT PE have typically experienced multiple traumas in a variety of life contexts that most often include interpersonal traumas of a sexual, physical, and/or psychological nature. Although each client's experience of trauma is unique, clients who have experienced the same type of trauma often have similar beliefs and emotions about these events. Therefore, being knowledgeable about these common trauma types and typical reactions to them will prepare you to more effectively validate and normalize clients' experiences and help clients to develop more accurate and helpful beliefs about the meaning of these deeply painful experiences.

CHAPTER 17

Treating Diverse Populations

As therapists, it is critical that we deliver treatment in a way that is sensitive to and informed by the unique characteristics and cultural backgrounds of our clients. When delivering DBT PE, we very often work with clients whose traumatic experiences are deeply intertwined with aspects of their identity, such as their age, sex, race, sexual orientation, gender identity, and veteran status, and are indicative of the prejudices, stereotypes, and inequities of the broader culture within which they occurred. In addition, the ways in which clients respond to and make meaning of their traumatic experiences are often influenced by the values, beliefs, and expectations of the specific cultural groups to which they belong. Therefore, understanding the influence of cultural factors on clients' experiences of and responses to trauma—and tailoring treatment accordingly—is a critical element of providing effective DBT PE. At the same time, there is limited research with many client populations to date, both in terms of studies of DBT PE specifically, as well as studies of standard DBT and PE more broadly. We simply do not know enough yet from an empirical standpoint about how to make DBT PE as effective as possible for clients from diverse sociocultural groups.

This chapter is intended to be a starting point that reflects the current knowledge base and ideally spurs conversations and research that will help us to better understand how to deliver DBT PE effectively to all clients who need it. Because earlier chapters have largely focused on adult civilian women (the population with whom DBT PE was originally developed and researched), this chapter focuses on adolescents; males; veterans; and racial, ethnic, sexual, and gender minorities. The information included here integrates psychological theories and research on the experience, impact, and treatment of trauma in these sociocultural groups, as well as the collective clinical wisdom of individuals who specialize in working with these client populations. For each population, I describe common trauma experiences, review relevant treatment research, and highlight issues that may be useful to consider when delivering DBT PE to individuals from these groups. Of course, this is not meant to imply that all clients who share a certain characteristic, such as age or sexual orientation, will have similar experiences or need treatment to be tailored in the same way. Additionally, many clients belong to multiple groups, such as being both transgender and a person of color, and therapists need to take into account these intersecting identities to understand the complexity of clients' experiences.

It is also important to emphasize that DBT PE is not formally adapted for different client populations, but rather the goal is to adhere to the standard structure and procedures of DBT PE while tailoring the delivery of treatment to the characteristics of each client. This reflects DBT PE's case formulation-based approach to treatment that requires therapists to identify the specific factors that are contributing to PTSD for a given client and then deliver *in vivo* exposure, imaginal exposure, and processing in an individualized way to target these unique mechanisms. In this process, it is incumbent upon therapists to assess the potential role of factors related to the client's identity and culture in their experience of and responses to trauma. It is my hope that the information in this chapter helps you to ask informed questions, develop effective treatment plans, and deliver DBT PE in a culturally sensitive manner with clients from diverse populations.

Adolescents

Trauma Exposure and PTSD

Most adolescents have been exposed to potentially traumatic events. The U.S. National Survey of Children's Exposure to Violence (Finkelhor, Turner, Shattuck, & Hamby, 2015) found that among youth ages 14–17, 63% had been physically assaulted, primarily at the hands of peers (42%) and siblings (29%), and these experiences were more common among males than females. In addition, 75% of youth had experienced relational aggression and bullying, and 30% had been physically intimidated. Most youth had witnessed violence (68%), particularly assaults in their communities (58%) or families (32%). Females were at higher risk of experiencing sexual offenses, particularly sexual harassment (20%), sexual assault (14%), and rape or attempted rape (13%)—less than 6% of males had experienced these sexual offenses. Finally, 38% of youth reported child maltreatment (e.g., sexual, physical, or emotional abuse) by an adult caregiver. Although a majority of adolescents have been exposed to potentially traumatic events, most do not develop PTSD. In the U.S. general population, the lifetime and current (past 30 days) rates of PTSD among adolescents ages 13–18 are 5% and 2%, respectively (Kessler et al., 2012; Merikangas et al., 2010). The lifetime rate of PTSD is 8% among girls and 2% among boys and increases with age: ages 13–14 (4%), ages 15–16 (5%), and ages 17–18 (7%; Merikangas et al., 2010).

Research Evidence

Although DBT was originally developed for adults, it has since been adapted for adolescents (DBT-A; Miller, Rathus, & Linehan, 2007; Rathus & Miller, 2015) and is widely used to treat suicidal, self-injuring, and multiproblem teens. Meta-analytic research indicates that DBT-A is effective in reducing suicide attempts, NSSI, suicidal ideation, and borderline personality disorder (BPD) symptoms (Kothgassner et al., 2021). DBT-A uses the same treatment modes, strategies, protocols, and primary targets as DBT for adults while also incorporating several adaptations, such as including parents and caregivers in DBT skills training groups; adding a skills module for teen–family interactions, called Walking the Middle Path; conducting periodic family sessions; including secondary targets specific to adolescents and families; and shortening the length of treatment (typically to 6 months). Similarly, PE has been adapted for adolescents (PE-A; Foa, Chrestman, & Gilboa-Schechtman, 2008) and two randomized controlled trials (RCTs) have shown it to be effective in improving PTSD severity, depression, and functioning among adolescents ages 12–18 who have experienced single-event traumas (Gilboa-Schechtman et al., 2010) and child sexual abuse (Foa et al., 2013). PE-A includes the same core procedures as standard PE for adults but adds a pretreatment preparation module (one to three sessions) focused on motivational enhancement and case management and includes parent meetings prior to and weekly or biweekly during treatment.

To date, there is limited research on DBT PE with adolescents. A pre–post study by Kaplan, Aguirre, and Galen (2015) included 13 adolescent girls with PTSD related to child sexual abuse who were receiving DBT in residential and/or partial hospital settings. Of these adolescent clients, 100% initiated DBT PE during DBT, 69% completed it, and at the time of discharge, those who completed DBT PE were below a clinical cutoff for PTSD on average, whereas those who did not complete DBT PE were not. In my own study of DBT + DBT PE in public mental health settings, five adolescents receiving DBT in a residential treatment facility participated of whom 100% initiated DBT PE, 60% completed it, and 60% achieved diagnostic remission from PTSD by posttreatment (Harned et al., 2021).

Treatment Considerations

Bolstered by these initial positive findings of studies of DBT PE with adolescents, as well as the larger evidence base for DBT-A and PE-A, many therapists have begun to use DBT PE with their adolescent DBT clients with PTSD. As the research on DBT PE with adolescents continues to accumulate, it is recommended that therapists using DBT PE with adolescents follow the same protocol that has been used in studies of adults while also incorporating several strategies from DBT-A and PE-A to tailor the treatment to adolescent clients.

Parental Involvement

The most significant modification when delivering DBT PE to adolescents is that parents and other caregivers are involved in the treatment. However, the degree to which parents are involved varies widely depending on the age of the client, the nature of the parent–child relationship, and the preferences of both the client and parent(s). Prior to starting DBT PE, parents are typically already involved in treatment since this is a standard part of DBT-A. As part of preparing to start DBT PE, parents are oriented to DBT PE in a family session, and if needed, parental consent to have their child receive DBT PE is obtained (see Chapter 7). In the first few sessions of DBT PE before imaginal exposure is started, an additional orientation session can be held that focuses on sharing more detailed information about the rationale and procedures of DBT PE, identifying ways in which parents can provide support, and addressing parent behaviors that may interfere with the treatment (see Chapter 10). During DBT PE, family sessions are typically conducted as needed and the content of these sessions shifts to focusing on sharing information about how the teen is progressing in DBT PE, providing coaching to parents about how to be most helpful to their teen as they engage in the treatment, and addressing any parental concerns or environmental barriers that arise. In sum, although the level and type of parental involvement during DBT PE can vary widely, the goal is to find an effective balance that respects adolescents' desire for privacy while also allowing parents to be involved in ways that will facilitate their teen's progress in treatment.

It is also important to acknowledge that additional complexities regarding parental involvement may arise for adolescents whose parents are the perpetrators of their past trauma and/or continue to engage in abusive or invalidating behaviors toward the client. Not only will this likely raise challenging issues related to mandatory reporting, but PTSD is also likely to be harder to treat when parental mistreatment is ongoing. As with other forms of ongoing trauma, the first priority needs to be ensuring the physical safety of the client. Once safety has been achieved, PTSD can be treated, including when traumatic invalidation by parents is ongoing (see Chapter 16). Whenever possible, it is preferable to work with parents to target and change ongoing invalidation, ideally prior to starting DBT PE. However, if efforts to change these behaviors have been unsuccessful and parents continue to regularly behave in invalidating or other problematic ways toward the adolescent, it may be wise to limit their involvement in DBT PE. In such cases, it may be helpful to strategize with the client about how to minimize the likelihood that their parents will interfere with their ability to make progress in treatment.

Addressing Motivational Issues

Unlike adult clients who usually self-initiate treatment, adolescent clients are typically referred for treatment by a parent or other adult. Some adolescents may be motivated for treatment even if they did not initiate it, whereas others may be firmly opposed to therapy and it may take considerable time and effort to get them willing to engage in DBT. Even the most motivated adolescent clients may balk at the idea of doing a trauma-focused treatment, such as DBT PE, especially given the increased out-of-session time required for exposure homework, and those who remain unsure about whether they want to be in therapy at all may be particularly likely to veto this suggestion. As a result, you may need to spend more time addressing adolescent clients' concerns and working to build their motivation to engage in DBT PE. Given their younger age, it may be helpful to emphasize the benefits of treating PTSD now rather than waiting for it to get worse: Addressing PTSD as an adolescent is like putting money in the bank toward a better future. You may also need to regularly assess and address motivation during DBT PE and prepare in advance with the teen for what they will do if motivation begins to drop. Teens may also benefit from extra support as they first start doing exposure. For example, in PE-A, adolescents complete their first *in vivo* exposure task in session (rather than on their own) so that the therapist is present to provide support and reinforcement. Parents may also be useful allies and can help to cheerlead and encourage their teen's efforts to complete exposure tasks outside of sessions.

Some adolescents with PTSD may refuse to engage in DBT PE (or trauma-focused treatment more broadly). This may be more likely among teen clients for whom PTSD has not yet caused significant problems in their lives and who do not view it as a serious impediment to reaching their goals. In such cases, you can highlight the potential negative consequences of continuing to live with PTSD (e.g., it is likely to eventually impact them and their relationships in ways that are upsetting), while also accepting adolescents' choice not to treat their PTSD if they do not want to. If this occurs, the best outcome may be that you lay the groundwork for future therapy by educating adolescent clients about the availability of evidence-based treatments for PTSD and encouraging them to pursue such treatments in the future if needed.

Modifying Language

In general, therapists should modify their language as needed to fit the needs of the client. With adolescents, this may involve simplifying certain terms to make them easier to understand. For example, in PE-A *in vivo* exposure is called "real-life experiments," imaginal exposure is "recounting the memory," hot spots are "worst moments," and SUDS is a "stress thermometer."

In addition, the examples and metaphors you use should be adapted to be age appropriate and relevant for adolescents. When using the DBT PE handouts with adolescents, you should explain the content using language that is easy for clients to understand and assess their comprehension of the information being presented. As when working with adults, if there is a form (e.g., the Exposure Recording Form) that a client is struggling to understand or complete, you can choose to simplify it if needed. It is also important to note that many adolescent clients are perfectly capable of understanding and using complex terms, as well as completing the standard DBT PE handouts such that few if any modifications may be necessary.

Extending Treatment

If adolescents are being treated within a DBT-A program that lasts 6 months, it may be challenging or impossible to deliver both Stage 1 DBT and Stage 2 DBT PE within this shorter treatment model. Therefore, you will need to plan for the possibility that more time will be needed and consider whether and how it will be possible to extend treatment to allow for DBT PE to be completed. Of note, the DBT PE portion of treatment is likely to be similar to or possibly shorter in length than when used with adults (for whom the average is 13 sessions), as adolescents may have fewer traumas that require targeting, as well as less-entrenched avoidance behaviors and trauma-related beliefs.

Males

Trauma Exposure and PTSD

Males are at higher risk for exposure to potentially traumatic events than females. In the U.S. general population, 61% of males and 51% of females experience at least one traumatic event in their lifetime and males are more likely to be exposed to multiple (three or more) traumas (Kessler et al., 1995). Meta-analytic research indicates that males are more likely to experience accidents, physical assaults, combat or war, disasters, serious illness or injury, and witnessing death or injury to others; females are more likely to experience child sexual abuse and adult sexual assault; and both sexes are equally likely to experience child physical abuse and neglect (Tolin & Foa, 2006). Despite higher rates of trauma exposure, males are significantly less likely to develop PTSD than females. The estimated lifetime prevalence of PTSD is 3–5% for males and 8–10% for females (Kessler et al., 1995; McLean, Asnaani, Litz, & Hofmann, 2011). For males, the types of traumatic events that are most likely to result in PTSD are rape (65%), combat (39%), child neglect (24%), and child physical abuse (22%; Kessler et al., 1995).

Research Evidence

Although DBT was originally developed and researched with females, multiple RCTs of DBT have now been conducted with mixed-sex samples of adolescents and adults (e.g., McCauley et al., 2018; McMain et al., 2009; Rosenfeld et al., 2019). Similarly, PE was originally developed and researched among female sexual assault survivors but has since been studied in mixed-sex samples of adolescents and adults with various trauma types (e.g., Foa et al., 2018; Gilboa-Schechtman et al., 2010; Zoellner, Roy-Byrne, Mavissakalian, & Feeny, 2019). In addition, cognitive-behavioral treatments for PTSD have been shown to be comparably effective for males and females (e.g., Felmingham & Bryant, 2012; Galovski, Blain, Chappuis, & Fletcher,

2013). To date, males have been included in two studies of the integrated DBT + DBT PE treatment, including a study of veterans with BPD traits receiving treatment in a U.S. Department of Veterans Affairs (VA) medical center (51% male; Meyers et al., 2017) and a study of adolescents and adults receiving DBT in public mental health agencies (17% male; Harned, Schmidt et al., 2021). In this latter study, males and females showed comparable rates of improvement in PTSD and other outcomes during treatment (Harned, Schmidt et al., 2021). (The impact of client sex on outcomes was not evaluated in the Meyers et al., 2017, study.)

Treatment Considerations

Males are a diverse group and vary considerably in the degree to which they choose to adhere to traditional gender role norms. In this section, I focus on males who exhibit values and behaviors consistent with traditional masculinity, as this has been shown to be related to the development of more severe PTSD (Neilson, Singh, Harper, & Teng, 2020).

Psychoeducation about Traditional Masculinity and PTSD

In many Western cultures, traditional masculine gender role norms emphasize power, strength, emotional control, and self-reliance, and disparage behaviors that connote weakness, such as expressing vulnerable emotions or seeking help. When adhered to in a rigid manner, these gender role norms may contribute to decreased well-being and PTSD. In particular, emotional stoicism and control, a key aspect of traditional masculinity, is associated with more severe PTSD among trauma-exposed men (Neilson et al., 2020). If male clients exhibit these traits, you should provide psychoeducation aimed at destigmatizing the experience and expression of emotions. In DBT, this is often done by teaching clients about the functions of emotions and framing them as neither good nor bad, masculine nor feminine, but rather a universal and critical part of the human experience. It is also important to educate clients about the link between emotional avoidance and PTSD. Overall, the goal is to help traditionally masculine clients understand that their efforts to control their emotions, while understandable based on their gender socialization, are making their PTSD worse and their emotions less controllable in the long run.

Addressing Ambivalence about Therapy

Endorsement of traditional masculinity ideologies is also likely to decrease treatment seeking due to beliefs that men should be able to solve problems on their own and that asking for help is a sign of weakness. As a result, many male clients may experience shame about seeking mental health treatment and express ambivalence about being in therapy. The desire to quit therapy may be particularly likely to increase during and after sessions in which they express emotions that make them feel weak or out of control, as this may contribute to shame and self-judgment. Males who ascribe to traditional gender norms may be particularly reluctant to do DBT PE given its focus on disclosing trauma and experiencing emotions, such as fear, sadness, guilt, and shame, that are considered antithetical to traditional masculinity. You may need to spend extra time addressing male clients' concerns and building their motivation to engage in DBT PE. In this process, it may be useful to appeal to traditionally masculine values as reasons to do DBT PE—for example, the treatment requires courage and strength, it helps them gain control over their trauma memories and emotions, and it increases their sense of competence by enabling them to engage in normative life activities with less emotional distress.

Increasing Willingness and Ability to Experience Emotions

The sixth criterion for establishing readiness for DBT PE—demonstrating the willingness and ability to experience intense emotions without escaping—may be particularly challenging for many male clients. Given that males are often socialized to "suck it up" and to view the expression of emotions (other than anger) as unmanly, weak, and cowardly, they may be particularly unwilling to experience emotions. It can be helpful to explicitly counteract male clients' expectations of being viewed as weak if they express emotions by clearly giving them permission to experience emotions in session, actively reinforcing their efforts to do so, and framing their willingness to allow emotions as indicative of bravery and strength. Male therapists may also serve as important role models by strategically modeling the expression of vulnerable emotions. In general, it can be helpful to expose clients to positive models of male emotionality, such as videos or movies in which men endorse the need to experience emotions or receive positive feedback after expressing vulnerable emotions. Male clients may also have particularly pronounced skills deficits in emotion regulation and require more teaching and coaching about how to experience emotions effectively. These skills can be practiced in session including using informal exposure to help clients gain confidence in their skills prior to starting DBT PE.

Targeting Problematic Beliefs Related to Traditional Masculinity

During DBT PE, male clients may express a variety of problematic beliefs that stem from traditional male gender role norms. Males often judge themselves for having PTSD and believe that feeling distressed as a result of trauma means they have failed to live up to masculine standards. Males are also more likely to have unrealistic expectations about their ability to protect themselves and others from harm and to remain strong and in control in dangerous situations. This may lead them to feel as if they did not live up to male role expectations during a traumatic event, as well as to view the experience of trauma itself as emasculating. Interpersonal traumas in which males were victimized by another person may be especially likely to threaten their gender identity and make them believe they are no longer "real men." Sexual victimization is often particularly stigmatized, as it is antithetical to the expectation of male sexual dominance and power, and instead is associated with femininity and weakness. When heterosexual males are sexually assaulted by other males, this may also threaten their sexual identity and lead to heightened concerns about being perceived as gay. If the experience of trauma threatens males' gender or sexual identity, they may believe they need to engage in hypermasculine behaviors to reestablish their masculinity and heterosexuality, such as aggression, frequent sex with females, and other risky or daring behaviors.

When clients' traditionally masculine beliefs are contributing to their PTSD or reducing the effectiveness of treatment, these beliefs need to be actively targeted. This is often done during processing by helping clients to develop realistic expectations for their own behavior during traumatic events, generate nonjudgmental ways of understanding their responses that they view as weak or unmanly, normalize the experience of distress and PTSD in reaction to trauma, and find adaptive ways to increase their sense of control and competence that are not risky or destructive. In addition, clients can be asked to consider whether holding these traditionally masculine beliefs may be ineffective in some ways—for example, beliefs about the importance of emotional stoicism may be negatively impacting their relationships with romantic partners and children. *In vivo* exposure tasks can be designed to specifically test and disconfirm their expectancies about what will happen if they violate stereotypes of traditional masculinity by doing things such as asking for help, expressing vulnerable emotions, and acknowledging weaknesses within supportive relationships. These opportunities to try new styles of interacting with people in their lives can provide important information to help clients decide which masculine gender role norms they find helpful and want to maintain, and which they find unhelpful and may no longer want to adhere to in general or in certain contexts.

Veterans

Trauma Exposure and PTSD

Veterans are likely to have experienced both military and nonmilitary traumas. A nationally representative survey of U.S. veterans found that 34% had been exposed to combat and 38% had seen someone die suddenly or be badly hurt during their military service (Wisco et al., 2014). Meta-analytic research estimates that 31% of military personnel experience sexual harassment (9% of men, 52% of women) and 14% experience sexual assault (2% of men, 24% of women) during their military service (Wilson, 2018). In addition, veterans in the general population report high rates of nonmilitary traumas, such as child sexual abuse (8%), child physical abuse (16%), adult sexual assault (4%), and adult physical assault (15%; Wisco et al., 2014). In a sample of women veterans with BPD who were receiving DBT in a VA, 60% reported child sexual abuse, 65% reported IPV, and 85% reported being raped as an adult (Koons et al., 2001). The high rates of child abuse and IPV among veterans may be due in part to the fact that the military can provide a way to escape abusive home environments. Among U.S. veterans, prevalence estimates of lifetime and current PTSD are 8% and 5%, respectively (Wisco et al., 2014). Lifetime prevalence of PTSD is higher among female veterans (19%) than male veterans (7%) and among younger compared to older veterans (Wisco et al., 2014).

Research Evidence

Clinical practice guidelines developed by the VA and Department of Defense (DoD) recommend DBT for veterans at risk for suicide, particularly those with BPD and recent self-directed violence (VA/DoD, 2019), and PE for veterans with PTSD (VA/DoD, 2017). DBT is increasingly being implemented in the VA system (Landes et al., 2017), and to date has been evaluated in two RCTs conducted with veteran samples. These studies found DBT to outperform treatment as usual among women veterans with BPD (Koons et al., 2001) and to be comparable to enhanced usual care among a predominantly male sample of veterans at high risk for suicide (Goodman et al., 2016). PE has been nationally implemented in the VA system and has been found to be effective in reducing PTSD and depression among veterans treated by trained VA therapists (Eftekhari et al., 2013). Meta-analytic research indicates that exposure-based treatments are associated with very large improvements in PTSD among veterans in the United States and other countries (Haagen, Smid, Knipscheer, & Kleber, 2015).

To date, the integrated DBT and DBT PE treatment has been formally evaluated in an open trial with 33 male and female veterans with PTSD and BPD traits receiving care in a 12-week intensive outpatient program at a VA medical center. Results indicated that veterans experienced large improvements in PTSD, dysfunctional coping, and use of DBT skills, as well as moderate decreases in suicidal ideation (Meyers et al., 2017). Additional program evaluations of DBT PE with veterans are underway, including in my own DBT program at the Seattle VA where DBT PE is a standard part of the treatment we provide.

Treatment Considerations

In this section, I focus on military-related traumas and common dynamics that arise in their treatment. The information included in this section is derived from the extensive research base on PTSD and its treatment among veterans, recommendations for delivering PE to veterans (e.g., Litz, Lebowitz, Gray, & Nash, 2016; Lorber & Garcia, 2010), and the clinical experience of myself and others who routinely deliver DBT and DBT PE in the VA system.

Understanding the Warrior Ethos

The term *warrior ethos* refers to certain values that are instilled in military training, such as courage, honor, loyalty, selflessness, integrity, and persistence. These values translate to strict expectations for behavior that are shared by many veterans, such as putting the mission first, protecting one another, holding oneself to a high standard, and refusing to accept defeat. It is important to consider how these values may have impacted veterans' behavior at the time of the military traumas they experienced, as well as their interpretations and beliefs about these events now. For example, the warrior ethos expects that service members will never leave a fallen comrade behind, which may cause veterans to hold themselves responsible for the deaths of other service members who they were unable to rescue. Military training also emphasizes the need for strict emotional control in combat situations where being able to "turn off" emotions is seen as adaptive, which may lead veterans to feel intensely ashamed if they felt or expressed fear in combat situations. Veterans may be particularly likely to exhibit cognitive rigidity when they believe their behavior violated the values of the warrior ethos even when their expectations are unrealistic and/or are the source of significant suffering. In such cases, veterans may be unwilling to change their interpretations because that feels like a threat to their identity as a warrior. When this occurs, you can both validate the importance of the values that were instilled in them as part of their military training and encourage them to be more flexible in their thinking (see Chapter 14).

It is also important to note that the warrior ethos overlaps considerably with traditional masculinity ideologies, and these intersecting value systems lead many male veterans to exhibit particularly intensified levels of stereotypically masculine behaviors that may complicate PTSD treatment. Female veterans may also endorse traditionally masculine gender role norms, and efforts to conform to these norms may have helped women to fit in and gain respect in the male-dominated military culture. Therefore, the strategies described in the previous section for addressing these types of traditionally masculine characteristics during DBT PE are often relevant for veterans of all genders.

Normalizing PTSD and Other Difficulties
Caused by Military Service

Given the emphasis on mental toughness and emotional control in military culture, it is not surprising that veterans often judge themselves for having PTSD and other mental health difficulties. They may believe that they should not have been affected by combat or other highly stressful military experiences and view their PTSD as a sign of personal weakness. They may also compare themselves to other service members who they view as stronger or more resilient, including people who may have experienced the same or similar traumatic events and did not appear to be negatively affected by them. This may result in thinking they are the "only one" who suffers in this way. These kinds of self-critical beliefs may have delayed treatment seeking and contribute to efforts to downplay or suppress emotional distress during treatment.

To address this, you can provide validation and psychoeducation focused on normalizing the experience of fear during or as a result of life-threatening experiences, as well as the development of PTSD and other mental health difficulties after traumatic events. In addition, many resources exist that can help to normalize the experience of military-related PTSD among veterans, such as the U.S. National Center for PTSD's AboutFace online video gallery of veterans sharing their experiences with PTSD and PTSD treatment. Other strategies focused on helping veterans to increase self-compassion for their own suffering can also be helpful, such as teaching self-validation and loving-kindness meditation. It may also be useful to have veterans complete *in vivo* exposure tasks to address unjustified shame about their mental health difficulties, such as sharing information about their PTSD with other veterans, family members, and friends who are likely to respond with care and support.

Distinguishing Military versus Civilian Values

The values of military and civilian culture are often quite different, and it is important to help veterans distinguish between the two when processing their military-related traumas. This is particularly true when veterans may have engaged in behavior at the time of a trauma that was consistent with the values of military culture but is inconsistent with civilian values. For example, killing is considered a necessary and moral part of combat, and service members may have felt happy, proud, and excited when they were successful in killing enemy combatants. They may also have used humor to talk about killing others, as well as derogatory terms to dehumanize the enemy, both of which may have helped to make killing less distressing in the moment. In contrast, killing is equated with murder and is considered immoral in civilian life, and those who kill are typically viewed as evil and depraved. In addition, joking or boasting about killing others is typically viewed negatively in civilian culture.

When helping veterans to determine whether emotions like guilt and shame about their behavior at the time of military traumas is justified, it is important to have them evaluate their behavior in the context of the moral code of the environment they were in at the time. In situations in which veterans engaged in behaviors that were consistent with their own and/or the military's values at the time but are inconsistent with the values they hold in a civilian context (e.g., reveling in and enjoying killing), then guilt is unjustified. Similarly, shame about these past behaviors is unjustified in present-day contexts that understand and accept military culture (e.g., when talking with other veterans) but may be justified in contexts that reject violence (e.g., among antiwar activists), as well as if they reemerge out of context in civilian culture (e.g., joking about killing others with civilian coworkers).

Addressing Moral Injury

In the context of war, military service members are likely to be confronted with a variety of moral or ethical dilemmas. When their military experiences included actions that violated their own personal values or the moral codes to which most people ascribe, they may suffer from particularly intense levels of shame, guilt, self-condemnation, and suicidality as a result. This is referred to as "moral injury," which is defined as "perpetrating, failing to prevent, or bearing witness to war zone acts that produce inner conflict because of moral compromise" (Litz et al., 2016, p. 2). These may include perpetration injuries, such as engaging in acts that violate their sense of honor or duty (e.g., killing civilians, torture, unnecessary violence) or perceived inactions that resulted in harm to others (e.g., failing to provide medical aid to an injured civilian, not reporting a rape committed by a fellow service member). Moral injuries may also include betrayal-based injuries in which trusted leaders or other service members engaged in behaviors that violated the person's moral values (e.g., giving orders that resulted in the unnecessary death of fellow service members, engaging in war atrocities). More generally, moral injury can occur when service members experienced a change in belief about the necessity or morality of war during or after their service, which may lead them to condemn their own participation in war or the military more broadly.

Moral injury traumas often raise complex issues related to guilt and shame and the degree to which these emotions may be justified or unjustified by these past actions or inactions. You will need to help veterans carefully evaluate the facts of the event that caused moral injury, the context in which the event occurred, and the moral codes that were relevant in that context. In many cases there were competing moral codes at play, such as the values of "obeying orders" and "protecting civilians," and it may have been impossible to adhere to both simultaneously. If the client's behavior was consistent with one moral code and not another, then it will be important to help them recognize the impossibility of adhering to both moral codes, understand the factors that led them to prioritize one over another, and radically accept their own behavior without judgment. In these cases when guilt is not justified, it may also help to have veterans discuss the morally ambiguous situation with others who were in the same or similar contexts to obtain corrective feedback that helps them to recognize that their behavior was appropriate for that context.

Infrequently, if a veteran chose to engage in or did not intervene to prevent actions that clearly violated the moral code of the context they were in, then some degree of guilt is justified. Similarly, if their actions or inactions are likely to be judged or denounced by important people in their life, then shame may also be justified in some contexts. Strategies for regulating justified guilt and shame are described in detail in Chapter 15 and include things like making repairs, increasing dialectical thinking about themselves and their behavior, and forgiving themselves for their past behavior.

Addressing Traumatic Loss

Many veterans develop PTSD as result of traumatic losses they experienced during their military service. These typically involve witnessing or learning about the violent and sudden death of other service members to whom they felt connected, and often includes feeling responsible for their death and/or guilty for having survived when the other person did not. It is also not unusual for veterans who suffered traumatic losses to believe that they should have been the one to die instead of the person who was killed. Veterans who experienced traumatic losses often exhibit symptoms of prolonged or complicated grief, such as yearning for the deceased person, frequent preoccupying thoughts and memories of the person who died, difficulty accepting the loss, and intense emotional distress when confronted with reminders of the deceased person. Suicidality is also a common reaction to traumatic loss and may be motivated by a desire to "right the wrong" of their own survival or join the deceased person in the afterlife.

The processing of traumatic losses often includes addressing veterans' sense of responsibility and guilt for the death of others. In some cases, the veteran may have directly caused the person's death (e.g., a friendly fire mistake) or contributed to it in some other way (e.g., by not detecting the improvised explosive device [IED] that killed the person), whereas in other cases their sense of responsibility stems from a general belief that it was their duty to protect other service members no matter what. It can be helpful to normalize the tendency to feel responsible for the death of others during war and highlight that this often helps people feel as if they have some control over their own and others' fate in the future. At the same time, you need to help veterans evaluate the degree to which they and others (including the military organization more broadly) may hold some responsibility for the person's death, and to reduce their guilt to a level that matches the amount of responsibility that can reasonably be attributed to their own actions or inactions. In addition, it is important to grieve the loss of the person and increase radical acceptance of their death. Several adapted versions of PE have been developed for military traumatic loss (Litz et al., 2016), as well as complicated grief more broadly (Shear, 2015), that include other strategies that may be useful to incorporate, such as discussing positive and negative memories of the deceased to develop a realistic rather than idealized view of the person, having a pretend conversation with the person, and finding pleasurable activities to engage in with people who are still alive.

Addressing Military Sexual Trauma

Military sexual trauma (MST) is a term used to refer to experiences of sexual assault or sexual harassment during military service by other military personnel and/or civilians. Experiences of MST have many similar dynamics as those discussed in Chapter 16 related to sexual assault more broadly, while also potentially having some unique characteristics related to the military context in which they occurred. MST is overwhelmingly perpetrated by males against female military personnel and occurs both at work during duty hours, as well as outside of work on the military installation. In the military, MST both reflects and contributes to the broader sexist culture in which female service members are frequently devalued and treated as inferior to their male counterparts. In addition, victims of MST often have to continue to interact with the person(s) who sexually assaulted or harassed them as part of their jobs and have limited options for escape. If the perpetrator is a superior, their authority over the person extends beyond their work duties to include all aspects of their life both on and off duty, giving them an unusual amount of control. Although less common, men also experience MST, which may be particularly stigmatized and is likely to be experienced as a threat to their masculinity (see the section "Males" above).

For both female and male victims, the experience of being sexually assaulted or harassed by a fellow service member is also likely to jeopardize the person's sense of being part of a collective, cohesive unit and to result in feelings of betrayal both by the person(s) directly involved in the MST, as well as the military organization more broadly. Given that military life provides a great sense of community and connection for its members (which is a common reason that many individuals choose to join the military), feeling alienated from this community can be a particularly painful outcome of MST. In treatment, you therefore need to be prepared to address issues that commonly arise when treating sexual traumas more broadly (e.g., self-blame, issues of consent), as well as experiences that may be more common in MST (e.g., the inability to escape, feelings of betrayal, and alienation from one's community).

Racial and Ethnic Minorities

This section focuses on treating PTSD among individuals from racial and ethnic minority groups in the U.S. since this is where DBT PE has been developed and researched to date. According to the most recent U.S. Census (2019), non-Latinx White people comprise the majority of the population (60.1%) and ethnoracial minority groups include people who identify as

Latinx (18.5%), Black and African American (13.4%), Asian (5.9%), American Indian and Alaska Native (1.3%), and Native Hawaiian and Other Pacific Islander (0.2%). For brevity, I refer to non-Latinx White people as "White" and Black and African American people as "Black" for the remainder of this section. The terms *people of color* and *clients of color* are used to refer to all people who do not identify as non-Latinx White.

Trauma Exposure and PTSD

Differences in rates of trauma exposure have been observed across racial and ethnic groups. Some epidemiological studies have found that the rate of trauma exposure is the same among White and Black people (84%; Alegría et al., 2013), whereas other studies found a higher rate of trauma exposure among White (84%) than Black (76%) people (Roberts, Gilman, Breslau, Breslau, & Koenen, 2011). Studies consistently find that Latinx (68–79%) and Asian (66–71%) people report a lower rate of trauma exposure than White and Black people (Alegría et al., 2013; Roberts et al., 2011). Differences also exist in the types of trauma that are experienced across racial and ethnic groups. White people are significantly more likely than other racial groups to experience nonassaultive traumas, such as accidents, illnesses, and unexpected deaths (Alegría et al., 2013; Roberts et al., 2011). In contrast, Black and Latinx people have significantly higher exposure to witnessing domestic violence as children (Roberts et al., 2011) and Black people are more likely to witness violence in general (Alegría et al., 2013). Compared to White people, Black people are also more likely to experience IPV, stalking, and mugging (Roberts et al., 2011), as well as other forms of personal violence, such as physical assault (Alegría et al., 2013). Rates of child sexual and physical abuse, as well as adult sexual assault and rape, do not differ among White, Black, and Latinx people (Alegría et al., 2013; Roberts et al., 2011). Asian people have the highest rates of exposure to political violence and war-related trauma other than combat, and the lowest rates of exposure to all other trauma types (Alegría et al., 2013; Roberts et al., 2011).

In addition to these widely acknowledged types of trauma, people of color also experience high rates of racial trauma that are often not recognized by researchers and therapists. Although some types of racial trauma (e.g., racially motivated physical assaults) meet the fifth edition of the *Diagnostic and Statistical Manual of Mental Disorders* (DSM-5) definition of trauma (i.e., Criterion A of the PTSD diagnosis), many racist incidents do not (e.g., discrimination, verbal harassment) but can nonetheless have traumatic effects (Bryant-Davis & Ocampo, 2005; Carter, 2007). National estimates indicate that about half of people of color report a lifetime experience of major discrimination (e.g., not being hired for a job or given a promotion, being hassled by the police) and 91% of Black people and 81% of people from other racial/ethnic minority groups report experiences of day-to-day discrimination (e.g., being treated with less courtesy and respect, being called names or insulted; Kessler, Mickelson, & Williams, 1999). The term *racial microaggressions* is often used to describe these types of brief, everyday slights and indignities that communicate hostile, derogatory, or negative messages to a person of color because of their race (Sue et al., 2007). In addition, people of color are regularly vicariously exposed to racial trauma, such as exposure to stories and videos of police killings of Black people (e.g., Bor, Venkataramani, Williams, & Tsai, 2018). The cumulative effects of exposure to direct and vicarious racism can negatively impact psychological well-being (e.g., Bor et al., 2018; Harrell, 2000), including causing symptoms of PTSD (e.g., Pieterse et al., 2010; Sibrava et al., 2019). In DBT PE, racial trauma is conceptualized as a form of traumatic invalidation that is based on race. Table 17.1 provides examples of race-based traumatic invalidation and the negative messages these behaviors convey.

TABLE 17.1. Race-Based Traumatic Invalidation

Type of invalidating behavior	Examples	Messages
Criticizing	Being called a racial slur. Racial insults (e.g., "You're just another lazy Black person"). Negative stereotypes (e.g., "Mexicans are rapists and drug dealers"). Racial microaggressions (e.g., "You are a credit to your race").	You are bad/unacceptable. Your people are bad/unacceptable.
Unequal treatment	Discrimination in education, housing, health care, and employment. Being treated with less courtesy or respect than Whites. Receiving poorer service in stores and restaurants. Being stopped by police due to racial profiling.	You are inferior. You are a second-class citizen.
Ignoring	"I don't see color. Your race doesn't matter to me." People acting like you are invisible. Not being called on in classes or meetings. Others not acknowledging the importance of your racial identity.	You do not matter. Your racial identity is not important.
Emotional neglect	Others not seeing you as vulnerable or in need of support. Not being taught the coping skills and tools needed to navigate racism. Being told you're not supposed to feel or express distress in response to racism. Whites being indifferent to the suffering caused by racism.	Your suffering doesn't matter. You are unlovable.
Excluding	"Go back to your own country." Being excluded from important social, educational, or professional activities. People assuming you are not American (e.g., "Where were you born?"). TV shows, movies and books featuring primarily White people.	You do not belong. You are unwanted.
Misinterpreting	Being followed in stores. A White person misreading your sadness as anger. Politicians claiming peaceful protestors against racism are violent agitators. Misconceptions about racial justice movements.	You can't be trusted. You are dangerous.
Controlling	Being told how you should behave to fit in with White culture. To a Black person: "You need to stop talking in slang." To a Latinx person: "You need to stop talking in Spanish." Being told to act subservient to avoid being the target of racism.	Your way of being is wrong. You need to change.
Blaming	Being blamed for being the target of racism (e.g., "You should have just cooperated"). Being accused of causing problems for White people (e.g., "Your people are taking our jobs") Being blamed for inequities caused by systemic racism (e.g., "Anyone who works hard can succeed"). Being criticized for complaining about discrimination (e.g., "Stop playing the race card").	Your problems are your own fault. You cause trouble.
Denying reality	Others denying that they said or did racist things. Being told that you are being treated equally when you are not. Being accused of overreacting to offensive racial comments. People telling you that your perceptions of racism are inaccurate.	You are crazy. You can't trust your perceptions.

The prevalence of PTSD has been found to vary across racial/ethnic groups. Although White people are exposed to trauma at comparable or higher rates than Black people, the lifetime prevalence of PTSD is significantly higher among Black people (8–9%) than White people (6–7%; Alegría et al., 2013; Roberts et al., 2011). Compared to White people, Latinx people exhibit a similar lifetime rate of PTSD (5–7%) despite having lower rates of trauma exposure, whereas Asian people have a significantly lower prevalence of PTSD (2–4%; Alegría et al., 2013; Roberts et al., 2011). PTSD is also likely to have a chronic course among Black and Latinx people, which may be due in part to the added detrimental effects of racial trauma and discrimination (Sibrava et al., 2019).

Research Evidence

Systematic reviews of RCTs of DBT and PE conducted in the U.S. or North America have found that the overall racial/ethnic minority inclusion rates in these studies were 39–41% (Benuto, Bennett, & Casas, 2020; Harned, Coyle, & Garcia, 2022), which is quite similar to the U.S. population (40%; U.S. Census, 2019). In DBT RCTs, 61% of participants were White, 15% were Latinx, 11% were Black, 5% were Asian, 5% were multiracial, <1% were American Indian or Native Alaskan, and 3% were categorized as "other" (Harned et al., 2022). In PE RCTs, 59% of participants were White, 31% were Black, 5% were Latinx, 1% were Asian, and 5% reported race as "other" (Benuto et al., 2020). These data indicate that all racial/ethnic minority groups are well represented in RCTs of DBT, whereas Black individuals, but not other racial/ethnic minority groups, are well represented in RCTs of PE. Although few studies have examined potential racial/ethnic differences in outcomes in DBT or PE, the available research suggests that racial/ethnic minority and White clients show comparable improvements in these treatments (Adrian et al., 2019; McClendon, Dean, & Galovski, 2020)—however, Black and Latinx clients may have lower rates of initiation and retention in PTSD treatments (McClendon et al., 2020).

The inclusion rates of racial/ethnic minorities in published studies of DBT PE are shown in Table 17.2. These data indicate that Black and American Indian individuals are well represented in studies of DBT PE compared to the U.S. population, whereas Latinx and Asian individuals are underrepresented. However, it is also important to note that three out of four of the studies have overrepresented White clients and that much of the racial and ethnic diversity found in these samples is due to one study conducted in the Philadelphia public mental health system (Harned, Schmidt et al., 2021). In this study, racial/ethnic minority clients comprised the majority of the sample (65%) and results indicated that they were equally likely to initiate and show improvement in PTSD and other outcomes during DBT PE as White clients. However, among

TABLE 17.2. Inclusion of Racial and Ethnic-Minority Clients in Studies of DBT PE

	White	Black	Asian	American Indian	Multiracial	Latinx
Harned et al. (2012)	9 (69.2%)	0 (0%)	1 (7.7%)	0 (0%)	3 (23.1%)	2 (15.4%)
Harned et al. (2014)	21 (80.8%)	0 (0%)	1 (3.8%)	0 (0%)	4 (15.4%)	0 (0%)
Meyers et al. (2017)	25 (75.8%)	1 (3.0%)	1 (3.0%)	5 (15.2%)	1 (3.0%)	0 (0%)
Harned, Schmidt, et al. (2021)	12 (35.2%)	14 (41.2%)	0 (0%)	0 (0%)	4 (11.8%)	9 (26.5%)
Totals	67 (59.3%)	15 (13.3%)	3 (2.7%)	5 (4.4%)	12 (10.6%)	11 (9.7%)

clients who received DBT alone (i.e., without DBT PE), White clients experienced significant improvements in PTSD, whereas racial/ethnic minority clients did not. These findings suggest that racial/ethnic minority and White clients are likely to benefit comparably from DBT PE, while also highlighting the importance of providing DBT PE to clients from minority groups.

Treatment Considerations

Considerations for providing DBT PE to racial and ethnic minority clients are derived from existing theory and research on racism-related stress and trauma (e.g., Bryant-Davis & Ocampo, 2005; Carter, 2007; Harrell, 2000), as well as recommendations for tailoring PE to Black clients in particular (Williams et al., 2014). In this section, I focus specifically on issues relevant to providing DBT PE to clients of color—however, it is critical that DBT PE is delivered within a broader context of culturally sensitive care in which issues of race, ethnicity, and culture are routinely considered in assessment and treatment, including their potential impact on the therapy relationship.

Assessing and Targeting Racial Trauma

Given the prevalence of experiences of racism in the lives of people of color, it is critical to assess for the presence of racial trauma when considering the need for and potential targets of DBT PE. For some clients of color, discrete racist events (e.g., police brutality, physical assaults) may be very clearly linked to symptoms of PTSD. In many cases, however, clients of color may not link PTSD symptoms to racism because they are not related to any specific or extreme event, but rather are the cumulative effect of everyday racism and discrimination. In addition, shame about these racist experiences and their impact (e.g., internalized racism) can prevent clients of color from wanting to disclose these effects. The framework of traumatic invalidation may provide a useful approach to both normalize internalized racism that stems from invalidating racist experiences and assess the types of racist behaviors clients may have experienced that contributed to these self-invalidating beliefs. In addition, there are a number of standardized measures of racial stress and trauma that can be used (see Appendix D).

If clients have PTSD symptoms related to racial trauma, these events can be targeted via imaginal exposure in the same way as other types of trauma. This is a relatively straightforward process when the client has experienced a single or discrete racist incident that is clearly linked to PTSD. However, when PTSD symptoms are the cumulative effect of many everyday experiences of racism, you need to help clients select one or more specific racist events to focus on for imaginal exposure. Using the strategies described in Chapter 8 for selecting a specific event to target from chronic traumas, the goal is to identify events that are both highly distressing and linked to core negative beliefs that clients hold about themselves and, potentially, their race.

Targeting Race-Related Behavioral Avoidance

Clients of color who have experienced racial traumas and racism often avoid situations and cues that remind them of these past experiences, such as people of certain racial or ethnic backgrounds or locations similar to where a racist incident occurred. They may also avoid many everyday situations and activities in which they believe they are likely to experience racism, such as shopping, going to the bank, riding public transportation, and participating in community events. When they have to approach these types of avoided situations, they may engage in behaviors that they believe will reduce the likelihood that others will behave in racist ways, such as wearing certain clothes, talking in certain ways, and acting in a manner that is intended to disconfirm racial stereotypes. These efforts to alter one's self-presentation to fit in with the perceived demands of the social context are often referred to as "shifting" and "code switching," and can include a wide variety of behaviors that are themselves potentially self-invalidating (e.g., altering one's appearance or not self-advocating around White people).

When conducting DBT PE with clients of color, it is important to assess for these types of race-based avoidance and self-altering behaviors by asking questions, such as "Are there places or situations you avoid because you think you are likely to be attacked or discriminated against because of your race?" and "Are there things you either do or don't do that help you to feel safer and less likely to experience racism?" It is important to validate how these types of race-based fears are understandable given the client's past experiences and are likely to be adaptive in some contexts given the reality of racism. At the same time, race-based fears can become overgeneralized and lead to excessive avoidance that causes impairment and maintains PTSD. When this is the case, race-based fears should be targeted via *in vivo* exposure in the same way that other types of overgeneralized fears (e.g., of all men) are routinely targeted with the goal of helping clients to better differentiate between excessive versus adaptive avoidance. In addition, efforts to alter one's self-presentation to match the cultural norms of different contexts may perpetuate shame, self-invalidation, and nonacceptance of the self, and *in vivo* exposure can help clients to make wise-minded decisions about whether and when these behaviors may be effective versus ineffective for their own life-worth-living goals.

As with any *in vivo* exposure task, it is important to select situations that involve acceptable and everyday levels of risk. This means that clients of color should not be asked to approach situations in which there is a high likelihood they will experience racism (e.g., attending a rally for a racist politician). Instead, *in vivo* exposure should focus on approaching situations and activities that people of color routinely participate in without serious negative consequences. If you are not of the same race as the client, it may be difficult to estimate the potential risks of some situations for people of the client's race. If this occurs, clients can be asked to consult their own wise mind and/or ask family members and same-race friends whether they ever do the exposure task or think that it is likely to be dangerous. It is also important to acknowledge that racism occurs in a wide variety of situations, many of which cannot be predicted in advance. Therefore, if clients do experience a racist incident while engaged in an *in vivo* exposure task—a clearly negative and undesired outcome—it may nonetheless provide an opportunity to evaluate the costs of these aversive experiences and bolster clients' confidence in their ability to cope with and recover from them if they do occur. Clients can then be encouraged to use this information to make wise-minded decisions about whether and how much they want to organize their lives to try to avoid these types of racist experiences.

When designing race-related *in vivo* exposure tasks, it is also important to ensure that situations and activities that are targeted for exposure are likely to improve the client's quality of life and help them reach their life-worth-living goals. For example, clients may want or need to be able to interact with White coworkers, neighbors, and members of their church, or go to public places where people of their race are likely to be in the minority. However, they may not want or need to go to certain stores that sell products they are not interested in or walk in predominantly White residential areas where they do not know anyone. Similarly, clients may want to be able to present as their true selves in some contexts (e.g., with family members, romantic partners, and friends of all races), but may want or need to alter their self-presentation in other contexts (e.g., at school or work) to increase their likelihood of achieving important goals. Overall, the goal is to use *in vivo* exposure to help clients of color develop realistic expectations about the likelihood of racism and discrimination in different contexts, including when they are or are not altering their self-presentation, so that they can make wise-minded decisions about where they want to go and with whom they want to interact. Ideally, this will also enable them to expand their lives in ways that will provide greater opportunities to experience joy, connection, and meaning.

Assessing the Role of Race

During processing, you should consider the potential role of race in clients' experiences of trauma, as well as the emotions and beliefs they have about these events. This is true both for racial traumas (e.g., racist incidents), as well as nonracial traumas (e.g., child abuse, IPV) that may still have a racial component. When assessing the meaning clients of color have made about the traumas they have experienced, you can ask whether they believe any aspects of the event were related to their race. For example, clients may believe that a person of a different race would have been treated differently in the situation (e.g., they would not have been disbelieved) or that others would have responded differently at the time of the event (e.g., bystanders would have offered to help). Clients may also believe that their experiences after a traumatic event were influenced by their race. For example, they may have experienced negative reactions from people to whom they disclosed their traumas, such as having their perceptions of racism challenged or being told not to report traumas perpetrated by people of their own race to avoid making their race "look bad" to others. When this occurs, there is likely to be a double layer of trauma to address, including the traumatic event itself, as well as the subsequent invalidation of those to whom it was disclosed. In addition, clients of color may have encountered racial disparities in their attempts to access medical or mental health treatment, pursue legal action, or obtain financial benefits related to a traumatic event, which may have compounded their trauma-related suffering.

Addressing Guilt and Self-Blame

You should also assess for guilt and self-blame about the racial traumas and inequities that clients of color have experienced. For example, clients who have experienced racial traumas may believe they should have known a racist incident was going to happen and been able to prevent it (e.g., they should not have gone to the store where they were followed), that it occurred because of something they said or did (e.g., the way they were dressed), and/or that it would not have happened if they had behaved differently (e.g., if they had complied with the request to search their bag). These self-blaming beliefs should be targeted in processing with the goal of helping clients to view experiences of racism and discrimination as being due to the person(s) who committed them and not themselves. Clients may also attribute some responsibility for these events to systemic racism, including the systems and institutions that create and maintain racial inequities. As when targeting unjustified guilt more broadly, the goal is to help clients validate their own actions during and after racist events, reduce self-judgment, and shift responsibility to the person(s) and systems that were actually to blame.

Addressing Shame and Internalized Racism

Many racial and ethnic-minority clients also experience race-related shame and self-disgust as a result of the traumas they have experienced. As people of color are repeatedly victimized by racism, they may internalize it and come to believe negative stereotypes and biases about themselves and other people of their race. This insidious consequence of systemic racism may lead clients of color to feel inferior and inadequate compared to people of other races, to view themselves and others of their race as repulsive and undesirable, and to believe they are bad or worthless because of their race. In some cases, clients of color may have difficulty acknowledging these internalized racist beliefs due to self-judgment (e.g., believing this means they are disloyal to their race). It is important to normalize beliefs indicative of internalized racism when clients raise them, potentially hypothesize that they may be present when they do not, and generally allow clients to discuss these sensitive issues at their own pace. When negative racial beliefs are targeted in processing, you can help clients of color to consider how these beliefs developed and have been maintained by repeated personal experiences of racism, as well as the broader racist culture. In addition, opposite action can be used to reduce unjustified shame and self-disgust by having clients of color share their experiences of racism with supportive people who will challenge their negative beliefs about themselves. Clients can also be exposed to other sources of corrective information about race and racism, such as positive racial role models, antiracist books and movies, and educational information that directly challenges racist beliefs. Overall, the goal is to help clients of color reduce race-related shame and disgust and, ideally, to come to value their race as part of their larger identity.

Coping with Ongoing Racism

The unfortunate and distressing reality is that racism remains ubiquitous in our culture; therefore, clients of color who have PTSD related to racial traumas or other types of trauma that had a racial component are highly likely to experience racism and discrimination again. Although stressors related to racism cannot be eliminated in the short term, you can help clients of color consider strategies for increasing safety (e.g., reducing the likelihood of encountering violence) and decreasing exposure to racism (e.g., minimizing contact with people known to be racist). When faced with experiences of racism, clients can use the DBT pros and cons skill to decide whether to use change- and/or acceptance-based strategies to address these experiences, as well as the DBT skill of evaluating options for whether or how intensely to ask for change depending on the situation. In addition, the DBT cope ahead skill can be used to identify and mentally rehearse strategies for coping with racism and discrimination in specific situations in which it may occur. Depending on the context, this may include a wide variety of skills, such as STOP to prevent ineffective responses, DEAR MAN to ask for desired changes, opposite action for anger to gently avoid the racist person, crisis survival skills to get through the situation without making it worse, and check the facts to reduce self-blame.

Other effective coping strategies may include getting support from people and organizations within one's community, as well as possibly from people from other racial/ethnic groups, including White allies. Clients may also want to consider strategies for seeking justice or repairs, such as reporting the incident to a person in authority, filing formal complaints, or pursuing legal action. For some clients of color, participating in activism and movements that aim to change racist and discriminatory policies, institutions, and systems can also provide an experience of empowerment and help to counteract feelings of hopelessness in the face of ongoing racism. Engaging in activism against racism can also be an important value-driven activity that contributes to building a life worth living in the long term. Finally, therapists should consider personally engaging in activism for racial justice, rather than placing the burden on clients of color to either advocate for themselves or tolerate ongoing racism and inequality.

Sexual and Gender Minorities

This section focuses on treating PTSD among people who identify as a sexual and/or gender minority (SGM), including lesbian, gay, bisexual, and other nonheterosexual (e.g., queer, asexual, pansexual) sexual orientations, as well as transgender or other gender-diverse (e.g., nonbinary, gender fluid, genderqueer) identities. Although sexual orientation and gender identity are distinct constructs, there is considerable overlap in the types of trauma experienced by people who identify as SGM, as well as the issues that should be taken into consideration when delivering DBT PE to these individuals.

Trauma Exposure and PTSD

SGM individuals have higher rates of exposure to trauma than heterosexual and cisgender people. A large nationally representative survey of adults in the United States found that people who identify as a sexual minority had a significantly elevated risk of exposure to nearly every trauma type except war-related traumas (Roberts, Austin, Corliss, Vandermorris, & Koenen, 2010). These disparities were particularly large for child maltreatment and interpersonal violence, which were more than twice as high among lesbian (28 and 60%, respectively) and bisexual women (31 and 54%, respectively) than heterosexual women (13 and 26%, respectively). Gay and bisexual men did not differ from heterosexual men in rates of child maltreatment but did experience significantly higher rates of unwanted sex (12–18% vs. 2%, respectively). In addition, gay men were significantly more likely to be exposed to other forms of interpersonal violence (51%) than heterosexual men (25%). Elevated rates of trauma exposure have also been found among individuals who identify as a gender minority. The 2015 U.S. Transgender Survey found that 47% of transgender people had been sexually assaulted and 54% had experienced IPV (James et al., 2016). SGM individuals who are also people of color experience even higher rates of trauma than their White SGM peers (e.g., Balsam, Lehavot, Beadnell, & Circo, 2010; James et al., 2016). In addition, SGM military service members are a particularly at-risk group, with research indicating an increased risk of MST in this population, including sexual harassment (sexual minority = 81%, transgender = 84%), stalking (sexual minority = 39%, transgender = 30%), and sexual assault (sexual minority = 26%, transgender = 30%) (Schuyler et al., 2020).

In addition to these widely recognized types of trauma, SGM individuals also frequently experience chronic invalidation at both systemic and interpersonal levels. Similar to racist incidents, anti-SGM prejudice can include events that meet Criterion A of the DSM-5 PTSD diagnosis (e.g., hate crimes that involve physical or sexual violence), as well as other types of invalidating and highly stressful events (e.g., discrimination, rejection, being outed). Meta-analytic research indicates that sexual minority individuals report high rates of mistreatment based on sexual orientation, such as verbal harassment (55%), being excluded from social groups (44%), discrimination (41%), verbal/emotional abuse by family members (40%), school bullying and victimization (33%), and workplace discrimination (25%) (Katz-Wise & Hyde, 2012). According to the U.S. Transgender Survey, 77% of transgender individuals experienced some form of gender identity-related mistreatment (e.g., verbal harassment, discrimination) at school, and in the past year, many had experienced mistreatment at work (23%), in places of public accommodation (31%), in airport security (43%), and in public restrooms (24%) (James et al., 2016). Consistent with the minority stress model (Meyer, 2003), these types of discriminatory experiences have been shown to increase risk for mental health problems, such as emotion dysregulation, anxiety, depression, and suicidality (e.g., Hatzenbuehler, 2009; Mustanski, Andrews, Herrick, Stall, & Schnarrs, 2014), as well as PTSD symptoms (e.g., Bandermann & Szymanski, 2014; Reisner et al., 2016; Szymanski & Balsam, 2011). Therefore, within DBT PE, discrimination and rejection on the basis of SGM identities that has resulted in significant PTSD symptoms is conceptualized as a form of traumatic invalidation that may require targeting via imaginal exposure and processing. Table 17.3 provides examples of SGM identity-related traumatic invalidation and the negative messages these experiences convey.

Epidemiological research indicates that among trauma-exposed adults the lifetime rate of PTSD is higher among lesbian (18%) and bisexual (26%) women than heterosexual (13%) women, as well as among gay (13%) and bisexual (9%) men than heterosexual (5%) men (Roberts et al., 2010). These disparities in PTSD are almost completely explained by the higher rate and younger age of onset of trauma exposure among sexual minority individuals (Roberts et al., 2010). To date, no epidemiological studies have examined rates of PTSD among gender minority individuals—however, prevalence estimates of PTSD in samples of transgender people range from 18 to 61% (Rowe, Santos, McFarland, & Wilson, 2015; Shipherd, Maguen, Skidmore, & Abramovitz, 2011; Valera, Sawyer, & Schiraldi, 2001). In addition, higher gender nonconformity increases the risk of child abuse and lifetime PTSD, and PTSD is particularly elevated among individuals who are both highly gender nonconforming and a sexual minority (e.g., 59–75% of gender-nonconforming lesbian and gay people; Roberts, Rosario, Corliss, Koenen, & Austin, 2012).

Research Evidence

A systematic review of DBT RCTs in the U.S. found that sexual minority individuals are well represented in these studies (27% of the samples; Harned et al., 2022). However, gender identity has rarely been assessed in DBT RCTs and none have evaluated whether SGM identities impact treatment outcomes (Harned et al., 2022). Similarly, there is a lack of knowledge about the generalizability of findings of PE RCTs to SGM individuals. Three studies of DBT PE have assessed sexual orientation and transgender identity (see Table 17.4). Overall, 38% of clients in these studies identified as a sexual minority and 1% identified as transgender. In addition, one study found that although sexual minority clients had more severe PTSD and emotion dysregulation than heterosexual clients, they were equally likely to initiate and benefit from DBT PE (Harned, Schmidt et al., 2021).

Treatment Considerations

In this section, clinical considerations for tailoring DBT PE to SGM clients are provided that are derived from existing theory and research about SGM-related stress and trauma (e.g., Hatzenbuehler, 2009; Hendricks & Testa, 2012; Meyer, 2003), as well as recommendations for providing DBT (Pantalone, Sloan, & Carmel, 2019) and evidence-based treatments for PTSD (e.g., Livingston, Berke, Scholl, Ruben, & Shipherd, 2020; Pantalone, Valentine, & Shipherd, 2017; Shipherd, Berke, & Livingston, 2019) to SGM clients. While the focus is on the delivery of DBT PE specifically, it is critical that DBT PE is provided within a broader treatment environment that is inclusive and affirmative for SGM clients and in which issues related to sexuality and gender are considered throughout assessment and treatment.

TABLE 17.3. Sexual and Gender Identity-Related Traumatic Invalidation

Type of invalidating behavior	Examples	Messages
Criticizing	Being told your feelings of same-sex attraction are immoral or wrong. Being bullied, insulted, or verbally harassed due to your sexual or gender identity. Negative stereotypes (e.g., "Bisexuals just want to have sex with everyone"). Microaggressions (e.g., "I like you even though you are gay").	You are bad/unacceptable. People like you are bad/unacceptable.
Unequal treatment	Institutional discrimination in housing, education, and employment. Receiving poorer-quality health care due to providers lacking knowledge about appropriate care for transgender people. Being denied benefits or services due to your sexual or gender identity. Being fired or denied a promotion due to your sexual or gender identity.	You are inferior. You are a second-class citizen.
Ignoring	Having your sexual or gender identity dismissed as trivial or irrelevant. People assuming you are heterosexual. People ignoring requests to use your name or pronouns. Others not acknowledging the importance of your sexual or gender identity.	You do not matter. Your sexual or gender identity is not important.
Emotional neglect	Being denied insurance coverage for gender-affirmative surgical procedures. Not receiving care or support because of your sexual or gender identity. Not being taught the coping skills and tools needed to navigate discrimination. Being told you talk about sexual and gender identity-related bias too much.	Your suffering doesn't matter. You are unlovable.
Excluding	Being kicked out of your home or religious community due to your identity. Gender-binary public restrooms. TV shows, movies, and books featuring primarily cisgender heterosexual people. Having your same-sex romantic partner excluded from family events.	You do not belong. You are unwanted.
Misinterpreting	Others not wanting you near their children due to fears that you will molest them. Same-sex heterosexual friends misreading friendliness as sexual advances. Being accused of being a sexual predator for using a bathroom that matches your gender identity. Police assuming that transgender women of color are sex workers.	You can't be trusted. You are dangerous.
Controlling	Being told how you should behave to fit in with heteronormative culture. To a transgender woman: "You need to stop wearing women's clothing." To a lesbian: "You need to wear more feminine clothing." People threatening to "out" you if you do not change.	Your way of being is wrong. You need to change.

(continued)

TABLE 17.3. *(continued)*

Type of invalidating behavior	Examples	Messages
Blaming	Being blamed for the traumas one has experienced (e.g., "You were raped because you are so promiscuous"). Being blamed for being the target of transphobia (e.g., "You deserve it for attempting to be a woman"). Being blamed for others' negative reactions (e.g., "You make your coworkers uncomfortable"). Being blamed for societal problems (e.g., "Gay men are responsible for the HIV epidemic").	Your problems are your own fault. You cause trouble.
Denying reality	Being told that homophobic incidents you experienced never happened. People denying that they treat you differently because of your sexual or gender identity. Being told you are crazy for thinking someone is biased against you. Others saying you are overreacting to offensive jokes about LGBT people.	You are crazy. You can't trust your perceptions.

Assessing for SGM Identity-Related Traumas

It is important to consider the potential role of different types of negative events related to clients' sexual and gender identities in causing PTSD symptoms, including both Criterion A traumas and traumatic invalidation. This can be relatively straightforward when clients have experienced discrete homophobic or transphobic incidents (e.g., physical attacks, rapes) or other extreme invalidating events (e.g., being forced to receive conversion therapy) that are clearly linked to PTSD. In some cases, traumatic invalidation may be directly linked to Criterion A traumas, such as being denied a rape kit due to being transgender or being blamed for being sexually abused due to being gay. However, when PTSD is related to chronic and/or cumulative experiences of SGM identity-related invalidation, clients may not recognize these types of experiences as potentially linked to PTSD. You can assess this by orienting clients to the construct of traumatic invalidation and evaluating its applicability to their experiences of SGM identity-related invalidation. There are also a variety of standardized self-report measures that can be used to assess experiences of SGM identity-related discrimination and rejection (see Appendix D).

TABLE 17.4. Inclusion of Sexual and Gender Minority Clients in Studies of DBT PE

	Sexual orientation					Gender identity
	Heterosexual	Lesbian	Gay	Bisexual	Other	Transgender
Harned et al. (2012)	6 (46.1%)	2 (15.4%)	0 (0%)	1 (7.7%)	4 (30.8%)	0 (0%)
Harned et al. (2014)	20 (76.9%)	0 (0%)	0 (0%)	4 (15.4%)	2 (7.7%)	0 (0%)
Harned, Schmidt, et al. (2021)	19 (55.9%)	7 (20.6%)	2 (5.9%)	5 (14.7%)	1 (2.9%)	1 (2.9%)
Totals	45 (61.6%)	9 (12.3%)	2 (2.7%)	10 (13.7%)	7 (9.6%)	1 (1.4%)

To target SGM identity-related traumatic invalidation via imaginal exposure and processing, you need to work with clients to identify one or more discrete events on which to focus. These may include invalidation by specific people (e.g., parents), groups (e.g., peers in middle school), and/or institutions (e.g., a church). Ideally, these events should be ones that are highly distressing, linked to PTSD symptoms, and related to the core negative beliefs the client has internalized about their sexual and/or gender identity. Strategies for identifying single events from chronic experiences of invalidation are described in detail in Chapter 8.

Addressing SGM Identity-Related Behavioral Avoidance

Clients who have experienced traumas and discriminatory experiences related to their sexual or gender identity are likely to engage in behavioral avoidance in an effort to reduce their risk of revictimization, such as avoiding situations in which they believe they are likely to be harassed or discriminated against (e.g., public restrooms, gyms, medical appointments). In addition, SGM individuals may modify their behavior to reduce the risk they will be mistreated (e.g., avoiding holding hands with a same-sex partner in public, not wearing clothing that matches their gender identity). You can assess these types of behavioral avoidance by asking questions, such as "Are there situations or activities you avoid because you are afraid of being harmed or mistreated due to your sexual or gender identity?" and "Are there things you either do or don't do to reduce the likelihood people will discover your sexual or gender identity?"

These forms of behavioral avoidance are consistent with two processes identified in minority stress theory as contributing to adverse mental health outcomes: efforts to conceal one's identity and expectations of rejection by members of the dominant culture (Meyer, 2003). In the context of PTSD, these psychological processes may maintain trauma-related distress if they contribute to excessive behavioral avoidance (e.g., of all heterosexual people or of any situation in which they may be required to show their driver's license). At the same time, avoiding some situations or keeping one's identity hidden in some contexts is adaptive when there is a real risk of harm or rejection, and it is essential that you validate this reality. In DBT PE, *in vivo* exposure can be used to help SGM clients differentiate between situations in which avoidance fueled by identity concealment and rejection expectancies is adaptive and those in which it is not and may be contributing to ongoing distress and impairment.

To design effective *in vivo* exposure tasks, it is first necessary to carefully evaluate the client's feared outcomes of approaching the avoided situation. When avoidance is due to fear (e.g., of violence or other serious harm), situations should be selected for exposure that will enable clients to learn that the avoided situations are generally unlikely to result in physical harm. An important variable to consider is the degree to which clients may disclose or express their sexual or gender identity during the task, as this is likely to both increase fear, as well as the risk of potential harm. The goal is to identify situations and activities that SGM people regularly engage in without any serious negative consequences, including at least some situations in which their identities are known or assumed. If you do not identify as the same sexual or gender identity as your client, it may be challenging to help clients estimate the actual likelihood of being harmed in some situations, particularly those in which clients may disclose or express their identity. When there is doubt, clients may be asked to consult their wise mind and/or ask acquaintances who share their sexual or gender identity about their perceptions of potential danger.

It is also important to discuss the possibility that less overtly harmful forms of mistreatment may occur during *in vivo* exposure tasks, such as invalidation or verbal harassment. You can help clients use the DBT cope ahead skill to plan for how they will respond if this occurs.

In this way, if clients experience some type of invalidation during an *in vivo* exposure task (e.g., they are insulted or treated with disrespect), it may provide a useful—albeit undesired—opportunity to evaluate the costs of being the target of such behavior and help clients build confidence in their ability to cope with such experiences when they do occur. Given the highly unfortunate reality that these types of prejudice events can neither be entirely predicted nor avoided, this may help clients to make a wise mind decision about whether the costs of continuing to avoid certain situations in which these types of invalidation may sometimes occur might outweigh the potential benefits.

When avoidance is due to shame about one's identity, the goal of *in vivo* exposure is to create experiences that disconfirm expectancies of being rejected by others. Therefore, *in vivo* exposure for shame-related avoidance typically involves tasks related to sharing rather than concealing information about one's sexual orientation, gender identity, or sex assigned at birth. This can include direct disclosures (e.g., telling others about one's sexual orientation, requesting that others use one's chosen name and pronouns) or indirect disclosures (e.g., wearing a rainbow pin, dressing according to one's gender identity). As with any shame-related exposure, it is critical to try to identify people with whom shame does not fit the facts (i.e., who are likely to respond to such disclosures with acceptance rather than rejection). Given the high degree of stigmatization of SGM individuals, the threat of rejection or even victimization is often realistic, and the risk of expectancies being confirmed rather than disproven may be high in many contexts. Therefore, decisions about identity disclosure must be guided by the client's values and wise mind (e.g., after careful consideration of the pros and cons of disclosing to a specific person). Additionally, it is important to acknowledge that the person may respond negatively to their disclosure and to use the cope ahead skill to prepare in advance for this possibility.

In general, the process of identity disclosure is highly individual, context dependent, and must be under the control of the client. If clients decide to keep their identity or sex assigned at birth hidden with certain people or in certain contexts, you can validate this choice as understandable, and when the risk of rejection is estimated to be high, as a wise self-protective strategy. For SGM clients who have few people in their lives who are accepting of their identity, it is also important to help them find communities and develop relationships with people who know and accept their identity. Thus, you should be familiar with local resources that may help clients to build connections with similar and accepting others (e.g., transgender support groups and sexual minority community organizations).

Addressing Guilt and Self-Blame

During processing, you should assess whether clients feel guilty about or blame themselves for the SGM identity-related traumatic and invalidating events they have experienced. For example, clients may believe they should have known the event was going to happen and been able to prevent it (e.g., they should have assumed the person was prejudiced), that they did something to provoke the mistreatment (e.g., initiate a conversation with a same-sex stranger), that it would not have happened if they had behaved differently (e.g., if they had not shared their opinion about marriage equality), or that they should have done something different during or after the incident (e.g., confront the person). As when targeting self-blaming beliefs more broadly, the goal is to help clients identify the understandable reasons they acted in the ways they did at the time of the event and shift attributions of responsibility from themselves to the person(s) who mistreated them. In some cases, clients may have chosen to enter potentially risky situations (e.g., going home with a stranger) or done things that may have increased their risk of being victimized (e.g., concealing their sex assigned at birth prior to sexual intimacy with a new partner). These decisions must also be understood in context and differentiated from being responsible for others' actions. At times, it may be accurate that an episode of anti-SGM violence or prejudice was prompted by something the client did (e.g., flirting with someone of the same sex), and when this is the case, it is important to help clients recognize that this does not justify the mistreatment or make the event their fault. Instead, responsibility lies with the offender, as well as potentially the broader culture that stigmatizes and perpetuates discrimination against SGM people.

Addressing Shame and Internalized Stigma

Many SGM clients experience shame about their sexual or gender identity in general and as a result of the traumas they have experienced. Often this shame is driven by internalized stigma, which involves absorbing negative messages from the environment and consequently self-invalidating one's sexual or gender identity. Internalized stigma is identified in minority stress theory as a common reaction to trauma that is likely to contribute to distress (Meyer, 2003). One way this may happen is if SGM clients interpret their traumatic and discriminatory experiences as meaning that they are bad, unacceptable, inferior, or undesirable because they are not heterosexual or cisgender, or perhaps even that they deserved to be victimized as punishment for their sexual or gender identity. As with other types of self-invalidating beliefs, it is often useful to help clients understand how these negative beliefs about their sexual or gender identity developed and have been maintained as a result of chronic invalidation and rejection. For example, were there specific people or events that led them to begin to think about themselves as bad or inferior because of their sexual or gender identity? These discussions may help SGM clients to see that their negative self-evaluations are not facts but are instead interpretations learned from the prejudiced social, familial, and cultural environments in which they have lived. During processing, more self-validating ways of making meaning of past traumas should be generated with the goal of reducing shame and internalized stigma and increasing self-acceptance.

Addressing Concerns about Links between Sexuality and Past Sexual Trauma

Many sexual minority clients who have experienced sexual abuse or assault question whether their sexual orientation was caused by or related to their sexual trauma. For example, lesbians who were sexually assaulted by men may wonder whether they became attracted to women because their trauma made them fear and avoid men. On the other hand, sexual minority clients who were sexually abused by a person of the same sex may similarly wonder whether they became interested in same-sex partners because of these experiences. These questions reflect an assumption that being a sexual minority is caused rather than naturally occurring, whereas being heterosexual is often assumed to be natural and biologically determined. One way to address this issue, therefore, is to highlight this assumption (and potential double standard) and encourage clients to thoughtfully evaluate their causality hypothesis. It may also be helpful to inform clients that research on this topic is inconclusive—for example, some studies find that child sexual abuse is correlated with identifying as a sexual minority later in life and some do not.

    In general, clients should be encouraged to find their own wise mind perspective on this issue. To that end, it may be helpful to think through the timing of when their sexual trauma(s) occurred in relation to when they experienced their first same-sex attraction or began to think they may not be heterosexual. If awareness of their sexuality emerged after their sexual trauma, how exactly do they think these experiences may have been related? Is it possible they may have come to identify as a sexual minority even if they had not experienced sexual trauma? Is it possible their sexuality is innate and may have predated sexual trauma even if they were not yet aware of it? While some clients may find it helpful to think through these types of questions, it is also important to emphasize that there does not need to be a reason (trauma or otherwise) that people are not heterosexual. Indeed, the idea that being a sexual minority requires an explanation (whereas being heterosexual does not) is itself reflective of heterosexist bias. Moreover, there is a risk that the process of searching for an explanation for one's sexuality can become a source of distress and rumination in and of itself, and instead it may be more effective to accept one's sexual identity without needing to know whether or how it was caused.

It is also important to assess the meaning that clients are making of potential links between their past sexual trauma and current sexuality. For example, what would it mean to them if their trauma had caused them to be gay? Often this question reveals some type of self-invalidation or internalized homophobia, such as that being gay is as an unnatural, damaged, or dysfunctional identity (e.g., a negative consequence of past trauma similar to PTSD), rather than a positive identity that can be naturally occurring. When this is the case, it is important to help clients reduce self-judgment and increase self-acceptance of their sexuality regardless of whether it was influenced by past trauma. In some cases, clients may believe that if their sexuality was shaped by past trauma, that it may not be real. For example, clients may wonder whether their preference for same-sex partners is actually PTSD-related avoidance of heterosexual relationships rather than their "true" sexual identity. In these cases, *in vivo* exposure may help clients to better distinguish between trauma cues and their sexuality. For example, clients who identify as lesbian could complete *in vivo* exposures related to reducing fear and avoidance of men, including potential sex-related cues (e.g., photos of nude men). If habituation to men occurs and they remain attracted to women, this may help to reduce concerns that their sexuality is due to avoidance of men. More generally, clients should be encouraged to identify what feels "right" for them in terms of their sexual orientation and *in vivo* exposure may be one strategy that helps to achieve this broader goal.

Coping with Ongoing Bias and Discrimination

Given the painful reality that bias and discrimination against sexual and gender minorities remains common, it is highly likely that SGM clients will experience additional discrimination and invalidation in their lives. This discrimination may occur by members of the dominant culture (e.g., people who are cisgender and heterosexual), members of one's own community (e.g., bias against bisexual people by lesbian or gay individuals), or members of other minority communities (e.g., bias against transgender people by cisgender sexual minority individuals). Although some strategies may help to reduce the likelihood of experiencing these types of events (e.g., minimizing contact with family members known to be homophobic), it is likely impossible to eliminate these types of experiences entirely, which makes it important to ensure that clients have the skills needed to cope with these experiences effectively when they do occur. To that end, you should assess the strategies clients typically use when they encounter anti-SGM prejudice, help them evaluate the effectiveness of these strategies, and when needed, suggest additional skills that may be useful. Since there is no single response that is appropriate in all contexts, it is also important to ensure that clients have multiple options for responding, including both change- and acceptance-focused strategies, and that they know how to determine which strategies are likely to be most effective in a given situation. The DBT cope ahead skill can also be used to prepare for discrimination and invalidation in specific future situations in which it may occur (e.g., when interacting with a health care provider or going through airport security).

In addition, SGM clients should be encouraged to seek support from other SGM people, as well as non-SGM allies who can provide validation and emotional support in the aftermath of discriminatory experiences. This can also help to facilitate reappraisal of these experiences as not being their fault or unique to them, but rather as an all-too-common experience of SGM people that is fueled by a culture that stigmatizes and discriminates against sexual and gender minorities. To that end, some clients may find it empowering and meaningful to participate in activism or social movements that advocate for the rights of SGM people, as well as events that celebrate these groups, such as annual Pride marches. Similarly, you should consider participating in activism against SGM discrimination and prejudice at both institutional and interpersonal levels, including within the organization in which you work.

Concluding Comments

DBT PE can be used with individuals from any sociocultural group and should be delivered in a manner that is sensitive to and informed by each client's unique characteristics. Thus, it is critical that you consider the impact of factors such as age, sex, veteran status, race, ethnicity, sexual orientation, and gender identity on clients' experiences of and responses to trauma and tailor treatment accordingly. This ensures not only that DBT PE is delivered in a culturally competent manner to individual clients but may also contribute to reducing broader disparities among marginalized populations that are likely to include a disproportionate number of people with PTSD.

PART V

NEXT STEPS

CHAPTER 18

Stage 3 and Beyond

Upon completing DBT PE, you and your client will need to regroup and ask yourselves "What's next?" If Stage 1 is about getting out of the hell of behavioral dyscontrol and Stage 2 is about resolving the misery caused by past trauma, then Stage 3 is about how to have a better future. Broadly speaking, I conceptualize this final stage of treatment as helping clients to change the consequences of an emotionally avoidant and self-invalidating way of living. The combination of being terrified of their emotions and hypercritical of themselves has often greatly limited clients' lives and kept them from attempting to reach important goals, or in many cases, even setting goals in the first place. Stage 3 is the time for clients to free themselves from these past trauma-related shackles and begin taking concrete steps to improve the reality of their present lives so they can have a better future. Bolstered by the learning that occurred during DBT PE—that they are worthwhile people who can do hard things even when they cause intense emotions—clients are now in a position of being able to set and achieve life goals that may have previously seemed impossible. Therefore, even more than in the prior stages of treatment, Stage 3 is about actively building a life that feels worth living.

It is worth noting that for many years I avoided calling this last stage of treatment "Stage 3," and I still feel somewhat hesitant to do so. This is because Stage 3 of DBT has not yet been formally defined or developed, and I do not want to appear as if I have done so when I have not. My intent has always been to develop Stage 2 of DBT, particularly in terms of the primary goal of reducing posttraumatic stress, and to leave the task of developing Stage 3 to someone else. At the same time, I believe that what generally occurs in this last stage of treatment after DBT PE is complete is consistent with the brief definition of Stage 3 provided in the DBT manual. In particular, Stage 3 is described as focusing on "developing the ability to trust the self; to validate one's own opinions, emotions, and actions; and, in general, to respect oneself independently of the therapist. Work on the patient's individual goals also occurs largely during this stage" (Linehan, 1993, p. 172). In the integrated DBT + DBT PE treatment, this final stage focuses on helping clients to achieve their remaining goals now that they are no longer limited by PTSD, which often includes continuing to strengthen and generalize their newly formed beliefs about themselves as valid people who deserve respect. Given this, I think it is reasonable to refer to this as Stage 3 of DBT while also acknowledging that this is murky territory. It is also important to note that clients may be able to achieve the goals of Stage 3 in treatments other than DBT that are less intensive (e.g., cognitive-behavioral therapy or interpersonally focused treatments) and/or they may no longer need any treatment at all.

Structuring Treatment in Stage 3

Once DBT PE is complete, clients may continue to receive DBT focused on addressing any residual life problems. At this point, individual therapy sessions return to the less intensive format of standard DBT (usually 1 hour per week) rather than the longer and/or more frequent sessions that are typically used when DBT and DBT PE are delivered concurrently. Clients may or may not receive DBT group skills training in this stage depending on their needs. As with the earlier stages of treatment, the duration of Stage 3 is flexible and will vary depending on the number and severity of clients' remaining problems, as well as more pragmatic issues, like the amount of time left in the treatment contract. In my original studies in which treatment was limited to 1 year, this third stage of treatment lasted 19 weeks on average. (As a reminder, Stage 1 took an average of 20 weeks and Stage 2 [i.e., DBT PE] lasted an average of 13 weeks.) However, these are averages and the actual duration of each stage of treatment is based on the client's progress, not on predetermined or fixed treatment lengths.

In Stage 3, individual therapy sessions are structured according to the standard DBT target hierarchy. Given that life-threatening behaviors are no longer present and therapy-interfering behaviors are usually mild or absent, the primary focus of Stage 3 is on addressing problems that are interfering with clients having the quality of life they wish to have. The specific quality-of-life problems that are addressed and the order in which they are targeted is determined by the client's goals and preferences. Our role as therapists is to offer consultation to clients as they work to identify and clarify their goals, and then to use DBT strategies to help them achieve the goals they select. This allows for a flexible and individualized approach to treatment while at the same time ensuring that it remains adherent to the evidence-based principles and procedures of DBT.

Common Client Goals in Stage 3

Given that this last stage of treatment focuses on applying DBT to goals that are selected by the client, the first task is typically to help clients identify their remaining treatment goals. Some clients will already be quite clear about their goals, whereas others will find this to be a challenging task that requires them to think outside the small box of their prior lives. For example, clients may need to ask themselves questions like "What do I want my life to be like now that I don't have PTSD?" and "Who do I want to be now that I no longer feel defined by my past?" The DBT skill of accumulating positive emotions in the long term by identifying one's values and using these to select specific goals and action steps can be a useful framework for helping clients identify their goals.

As an example, I once treated a woman who had been abused starting in early childhood and had lived a life dominated by dysfunction and instability prior to DBT. When we reached Stage 3, she had only a vague sense of her goals as she had never allowed herself to really consider that her future could be different from her past. After talking about potential goals in session, I assigned her homework to clarify her values and identify goals that would make these values a consistent part of her life. She arrived at our next session and excitedly told me that she had decided she wanted to turn her passion for art and creativity into a career, which was particularly poignant given that her parents had constantly criticized and devalued her interest in art. She had identified several goals related to this value, which included building relationships with people who shared her creative interests, finishing her degree in design, and eventually starting her own design business—none of which had ever seemed like realistic or valid choices to her in the past. I eagerly agreed to this plan and we set off to help her begin to achieve these goals. Although each client will have their own unique life-worth-living goals, these goals often fall within the following general categories.

Strengthening a Positive Self-Concept

As has been discussed in detail in earlier chapters, intense self-hatred and self-criticism are the norm among clients who receive this treatment and are typically directly linked to the trauma and invalidation they have experienced in their lives. As a result of the trauma processing that occurs during DBT PE, clients begin to view themselves with more compassion and to be able to validate how their emotions and behaviors both in the past and present are understandable. On the dialectic between the extremes of self-hatred and self-love, DBT PE often helps clients get past the midpoint and onto the side of a positive self-concept. However, these changes may still be somewhat tenuous with clients periodically reverting to old habits of self-invalidation or being prone to agreeing with invalidating comments made about them by others. Thus, helping clients to further strengthen and generalize their new positive beliefs about themselves is often a target of the last stage of treatment and can be achieved with a wide variety of strategies, such as replacing self-invalidating thoughts with more validating ones; identifying and frequently reminding oneself of one's positive qualities; acting as if one is deserving of love and respect; practicing loving-kindness meditation toward oneself; using opposite action to reduce negative self-directed emotions, like shame and disgust; and asking to be treated with respect by others.

Ending Destructive Relationships and Developing Validating Ones

A common consequence of developing a more positive self-concept is that clients become aware, often painfully so, of the ways in which people in their current life may be invalidating and mistreating them. Whereas in the past being mistreated by others often did not raise alarms because it was congruent with clients' negative beliefs about themselves as being bad and worthless, being treated poorly becomes harder and harder to ignore or justify once clients start to view themselves as deserving of respect and kindness. Thus, during and after DBT PE, many clients come to the painful realization that they are being mistreated by important people in their lives (e.g., partners, close friends, family members). In Stage 3, clients often set goals related to being unwilling to tolerate mistreatment by others, asking people in their lives to treat them with greater respect and care, and disengaging from or ending relationships with people who continue to mistreat them. This happens often enough that in my current team we have jokingly adopted the new skill (coined by the advice columnist and activist Dan Savage) of "DTMFA," which stands for Dump the Mother-F**ker Already. All joking aside, detaching from or ending destructive marriages, friendships, and relationships, including with past abusers with whom clients may still have contact, is often an agonizing process, but ultimately a much needed and positive change in many of our clients' lives.

In addition, nearly all clients identify goals related to building new relationships and connections with others that are mutually rewarding and in which they feel accepted, cared for, and respected. As a result of PTSD-related avoidance, as well as negative beliefs about themselves and others, many clients have cut themselves off from other people and have been leading very isolated lives with few if any friends or close connections. In addition, many clients have sworn off dating or romantic relationships altogether and have instead resigned themselves to being alone their entire lives. As PTSD improves and beliefs and emotions that fuel isolation change, clients often become increasingly interested in pursuing new relationships. Thus, in this last stage of treatment we often help clients figure out how to meet new people; choose friends who are compatible in their lifestyle, needs, and values; nurture these new connections; and take steps to find an effective and rewarding romantic relationship if desired.

Engaging in Productive and Meaningful Activities

PTSD is often associated with significant functional impairment and disability. After PTSD has been resolved, many clients therefore set goals related to improving their ability to participate productively in school, work, household, and/or recreational activities. For many clients, achieving these types of functional goals may take years—for example, obtaining a college degree, achieving full financial independence, or getting a black belt in martial arts. However, considerable progress can often be made toward achieving these goals during the last stage of treatment, such as choosing a career path that will eventually lead to living wage employment, applying for jobs, taking a college course, or becoming an active member of an organized recreational activity (e.g., volunteer organization, sports team, special interest club).

Treating Residual Disorders

Although it is not uncommon for PTSD treatment to resolve other disorders that were related to or being maintained by PTSD (e.g., depression, substance use disorders, eating disorders, other anxiety disorders), there may still be disorders in need of treatment after DBT PE is complete. If this is the case, you can provide another targeted treatment for the residual disorder, including potentially integrating another evidence-based protocol into DBT if needed.

Finding Meaning and a Sense of Purpose

Finally, many clients express a desire to find meaning in the traumas they have experienced and/or a sense of purpose that can motivate them as they move forward in their life. For many clients, this takes the form of helping others or giving back in some way that can reduce the suffering of others. Many clients I have worked with have decided to pursue careers in mental health, volunteer in organizations that provide support to people with similar life experiences (e.g., veterans, rape survivors), participate in protests or advocacy groups that fight against social injustices, or raise money for people in need. In addition, some clients find meaning in their own suffering by identifying how it has helped them to grow in positive ways in their life. For example, some clients believe that their traumas have enabled them to be loving parents, to persist through overwhelming obstacles, or to have deep empathy for the suffering of others. Although not all clients may wish to find this type of meaning or purpose from their traumatic experiences, for those who do this can be an important task of the last stage of treatment that can help them find greater peace and a sense of meaning after trauma.

Concluding Comments

DBT with the DBT PE protocol is intended to be a comprehensive treatment for people with PTSD who have a severe overall level of disorder characterized by pervasive dysregulation of behavior, emotion, cognition, self-concept, and relationships. Clients often begin treatment with a seemingly insurmountable number of complex problems, many of which are being fueled by their unresolved traumas. This treatment is designed not only to treat their PTSD but also the wide-ranging impacts of a lifetime of trauma and invalidation, including the severe and often life-threatening problems that initially make them inappropriate for trauma-focused treatment. The overarching goal is for clients to finish treatment with a life they now experience as worth living, rather than one that makes them want to be dead. In the last stage of treatment, we can help clients make significant progress toward achieving their remaining life-worth-living goals, while also helping them to build the skills, confidence, and support they need to continue pursuing these goals on their own. Building a new life from one that was profoundly shaped by trauma is a lifelong journey, and by the end of treatment, clients will hopefully be well down the path to finding a more fulfilling and meaningful future.

What Is Posttraumatic Stress Disorder?

Posttraumatic stress disorder (PTSD) may develop after a person has experienced, witnessed, or learned about one or more traumatic events. PTSD symptoms may start immediately after a traumatic event or they may not appear until years later. They can also vary in intensity over time. For example, you may have more PTSD symptoms around anniversary dates of past traumatic events or when you are under high stress.

There are 20 PTSD symptoms that fall into four categories. You do not have to have all of these symptoms to have PTSD. These symptoms cause significant distress and can make it difficult to function in your daily life.

INTRUSIVE MEMORIES

Frequent thoughts, memories, or images of traumatic events.

☐ Repeated unwanted distressing memories of past traumatic events.

☐ Suddenly acting or feeling like a traumatic event is happening again (flashbacks).

☐ Upsetting dreams or nightmares about past traumatic events.

☐ Feeling very emotionally upset when something reminds you of a traumatic event.

☐ Intense physical reactions when something reminds you of a traumatic event.

AVOIDANCE

Frequent efforts to avoid things associated with traumatic events.

☐ Avoiding thoughts or feelings about past traumatic events.

☐ Avoiding people, places, activities, or things that remind you of past traumatic events.

CHANGES IN THINKING AND EMOTIONS

Negative changes in thinking and mood that began or worsened after the traumatic event.

☐ Difficulty remembering important parts of what happened during the traumatic event.

☐ Strong negative beliefs about yourself, others, or the world (e.g., "I am bad," "People can't be trusted," "The world is dangerous").

☐ Blaming yourself for the trauma or blaming someone else who was not directly responsible.

☐ Intense and long-lasting emotions, such as fear, anger, guilt, shame, and sadness.

☐ No longer being interested in activities you used to enjoy.

☐ Feeling distant or cut off from other people.

☐ Difficulty experiencing positive emotions, such as happiness, love, and excitement.

(continued)

Changes in Arousal and Reactivity
Constantly feeling under threat and on edge.

☐ Frequent irritability, anger outbursts, or aggressive behavior toward others.

☐ Self-destructive or reckless behavior (e.g., self-harm, substance use, risky driving).

☐ Being very alert or on guard for potential danger.

☐ Being jumpy or easily startled.

☐ Difficulty concentrating on tasks, such as school, work, reading, or watching TV.

☐ Trouble falling or staying asleep.

Some people with PTSD also experience frequent dissociation. If this is true for you, you may have the dissociative subtype of PTSD.

DISSOCIATION
Frequently feeling disconnected from yourself and things around you.

☐ Feeling detached or separated from yourself or like you are watching yourself from outside of your body.

☐ Feeling like people and things around you are foggy, unreal, or far away.

What Is Traumatic Invalidation?

Traumatic invalidation occurs when a person's environment repeatedly or intensely communicates that their characteristics, behaviors, or emotional reactions are unacceptable. Traumatic invalidation is typically done by important people, groups, or institutions that the person is close to or dependent on and/or may occur at the cultural level for people from marginalized groups. Invalidating behaviors can take many forms and cause people to develop a variety of negative beliefs about themselves. Often the person's responses to the invalidation are also invalidated, which leads to even more suffering.

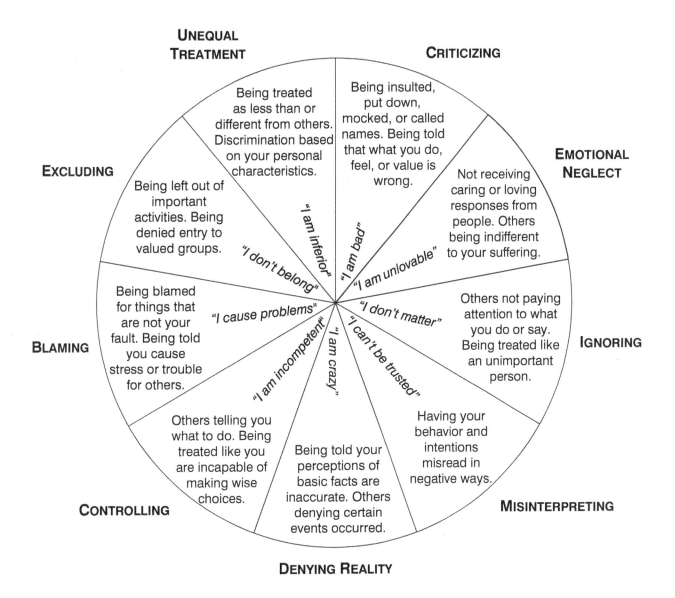

The Impact of Traumatic Invalidation

Experiences of traumatic invalidation cause PTSD symptoms and negatively impact people's beliefs about themselves and their relationships with others.

PTSD SYMPTOMS

Traumatic invalidation results in PTSD symptoms, including intrusions, avoidance, negative changes in cognitions and mood, and increased arousal and reactivity.

- Common examples of PTSD symptoms related to traumatic invalidation include:

  ☐ Avoiding thoughts or reminders of invalidation   ☐ Intrusive memories of invalidation

  ☐ Frequent negative emotions (shame, guilt)   ☐ Distressing dreams about invalidation

  ☐ Being very sensitive to potential invalidation   ☐ Negative beliefs about yourself

  ☐ Intense reactions to reminders of invalidation   ☐ Feeling detached from others

  ☐ Reckless or self-destructive behavior   ☐ Other: _____

SELF-INVALIDATION

Traumatic invalidation teaches people to invalidate themselves in ways that are similar to how they were invalidated by others. These self-critical thoughts occur frequently and often lead to intense feelings of shame and self-hatred.

- Common examples of self-invalidation include:

  ☐ Judging or criticizing yourself   ☐ Thinking your reactions are not valid

  ☐ Treating yourself as if you do not matter   ☐ Blaming yourself for problems

  ☐ Calling yourself names   ☐ Assuming you will do things wrong

  ☐ Ignoring your own needs   ☐ Minimizing things you do well

  ☐ Thinking you should be different than you are   ☐ Other: _____

NOT TRUSTING YOURSELF

Another painful outcome of traumatic invalidation is that it teaches people to doubt themselves and believe they cannot be trusted to make wise choices. Often people will feel as if they do not possess any inner wisdom and must rely on others to tell them what to do.

- Common examples of not trusting yourself include:

  ☐ Thinking you do not have a wise mind   ☐ Avoiding taking on responsibilities

  ☐ Basing your behavior on what others do   ☐ Doubting your perceptions of reality

  ☐ Feeling unable to do things on your own   ☐ Making your reactions match others'

  ☐ Asking others to make decisions for you   ☐ Other: _____

(continued)

UNREALISTIC STANDARDS

Traumatic invalidation often teaches people to hold themselves to strict and perfectionistic standards that are not realistic and lead them to constantly feel as if they are failing or not good enough.

- Common examples of having unrealistic standards include:

☐ Having strict rules for your own behavior   ☐ Thinking you must do things perfectly

☐ Holding yourself to others' high standards   ☐ Minimizing the difficulty of tasks

☐ Trying to appear flawless   ☐ Harshly criticizing yourself for errors

☐ Frequently feeling like a failure   ☐ Setting unrealistic goals for yourself

☐ Avoiding activities that you are not good at   ☐ Other: _____

PERVASIVE INSECURITY

Traumatic invalidation often results in a pervasive sense of insecurity in relationships. People often expect that others will reject them and have difficulty trusting and feeling safe around people.

- Common examples of pervasive insecurity include:

☐ Expecting people to reject or hurt you   ☐ Trying hard to please people

☐ Changing to fit what you think others will like   ☐ Difficulty trusting other people

☐ Feeling like you can't rely on other people   ☐ Frequent fears of abandonment

☐ Asking for reassurance that you are liked   ☐ Feeling on guard when around people

☐ Assuming your presence is unwanted   ☐ Other: _____

FEELING INVALID

The experience of being broadly and frequently rejected often threatens people's psychological integrity and makes them feel as if they are not a valid, reasonable, or legitimate person.

- Common examples of feeling invalid include:

☐ Believing you are inherently bad   ☐ Feeling different from everyone else

☐ Thinking you should not take up space   ☐ Questioning your own humanity

☐ Feeling like you do not fit in anywhere   ☐ Believing you should not exist

☐ Thinking something is innately wrong with you   ☐ Feeling invisible

☐ Feeling like you do not matter   ☐ Other: _____

What Is DBT PE?

The Dialectical Behavior Therapy Prolonged Exposure (DBT PE) protocol is a treatment for PTSD that is designed to be added to DBT. It is based on prolonged exposure therapy, a first-line evidence-based treatment for PTSD, and has been adapted to fit the needs and characteristics of typical DBT clients.

How Does It Work?

People with PTSD often avoid emotions, thoughts, and situations that remind them of the traumas they have experienced. Although avoidance reduces distress in the short run, it keeps you from recovering from PTSD in the long run. DBT PE works by helping you to gradually approach trauma-related memories and situations so that PTSD will improve and you will gain more control over your life.

What Is Involved?

DBT PE uses three core procedures to treat PTSD:

1. *In vivo* **exposure** involves confronting situations you avoid in real life. You will be asked to gradually approach people, places, and things you have been avoiding because they remind you of your trauma, feel dangerous, or bring up distressing emotions. This will help you learn that these situations are not harmful and you can cope with them, which will make them less distressing.
2. **Imaginal exposure** involves repeatedly describing traumatic events out loud during your therapy sessions. By talking and thinking in detail about what happened to you, your trauma memories will become less overwhelming and will be less likely to come up unexpectedly at other times.
3. **Processing** involves talking with your therapist about the emotions and thoughts that arise as a result of imaginal exposure. The goal is to help you gain a new perspective about the traumas you have experienced that will cause you less distress and enable you to change unhelpful trauma-related patterns in your life.

How Long Does It Last?

The length of DBT PE varies across people but typically lasts between 12 and 16 sessions. The number of sessions you need will be determined based on your progress during treatment.

How Is DBT PE Combined with DBT?

The combined DBT and DBT PE treatment occurs in three stages. First, DBT is used to help you gain control over impulsive and self-damaging behaviors and learn coping skills to better tolerate and regulate your emotions. Once these goals are achieved, you will advance to the second stage of treatment in which DBT PE is used to treat your PTSD. DBT PE sessions are typically delivered in addition to your regular DBT individual and group sessions, which means that you may have more frequent and/or longer sessions during this stage of treatment. After DBT PE is complete, you will return to receiving DBT alone to address whatever goals are important to you at that time. For many clients, this third stage of treatment focuses on increasing self-respect and building a life that is no longer limited by PTSD.

(continued)

Who Is Appropriate?

DBT PE is intended for people who have multiple problems in addition to PTSD that make it difficult or unsafe to immediately engage in trauma-focused treatment. Most people who receive DBT PE struggle with a variety of complex problems, such as suicidal, self-harming, and other damaging behaviors; multiple psychological disorders; emotion dysregulation; and difficulties functioning in daily life. To be appropriate to start DBT PE, you first have to stop engaging in suicidal and self-harming behaviors, participate effectively in therapy, and learn skills to experience and tolerate intense emotions. DBT is used to help people achieve these readiness goals so that they can receive DBT PE.

What If I Have Experienced Multiple Traumas?

Most people who receive DBT PE have experienced multiple traumas that often started in childhood. DBT PE can be used to treat any type of trauma, but some of the most common types are child sexual and physical abuse, rape, intimate partner violence, and traumatic invalidation. You will decide which traumas you want to focus on in treatment based on which ones are currently causing you the most distress. Typically, two to three traumas are addressed during DBT PE to achieve significant improvement in PTSD, but this varies by person.

What If I Can't Remember the Trauma Clearly?

It is very common for people to have difficulty remembering all the details of their traumatic experiences. For many people who receive DBT PE, their trauma memories are quite fragmented, have significant gaps, and are foggy in places. DBT PE can be used as long as you have at least some memory of the trauma(s) that you have experienced. You do not need to remember all of the details for the treatment to work.

Is It Effective?

About 70% of people who complete DBT PE experience significant improvements in their PTSD. DBT PE has also been shown to result in improvements in other problems that are related to PTSD, such as depression, dissociation, anxiety, shame, guilt, emotion regulation, and difficulty functioning in relationships and other activities of daily living.

What Are the Risks?

DBT PE has been shown to be safe to deliver. In fact, research suggests that people who receive DBT PE during DBT are less likely to attempt suicide and self-harm than people who receive DBT alone. Some people may experience temporary increases in distress at the beginning of DBT PE, such as increases in urges to engage in problem behaviors, dissociation, or emotion dysregulation. If this occurs, it typically lasts for no more than a few weeks before PTSD begins to improve and distress decreases.

What Will I Be Expected to Do?

During DBT PE, you will be asked to complete imaginal exposure and processing during your therapy sessions. You will also be given homework to complete *in vivo* exposure exercises and listen to recordings of your imaginal exposure on your own between sessions.

Getting Ready to Start DBT PE

To be eligible to begin DBT PE, you will need to meet the following six readiness criteria that are intended to ensure that you will be able to complete PTSD treatment effectively and safely.

Target start date for DBT PE: _____

READINESS CRITERIA	WHAT YOU NEED TO DO TO GET READY
1. Not at imminent risk of suicide.	
2. No recent suicide attempts or nonsuicidal self-injury.	Date of last episode: _____
3. Able to control suicidal and self-injurious behaviors in the presence of things that make you want to engage in those behaviors.	
4. No serious therapy-interfering behaviors.	
5. PTSD is your highest-priority quality-of-life target.	
6. Able and willing to experience intense emotions without escaping.	

How PTSD Is Maintained

People with PTSD often have problematic beliefs about themselves, others, and emotions that developed because of the trauma they experienced. These beliefs cause them to interpret trauma cues negatively (e.g., "I'm not safe"), which sets off strong emotions (e.g., fear). These emotions are often intensely distressing and lead to additional negative interpretations (e.g., "I can't tolerate this"). To get relief from this distress and increase a sense of safety, the person then engages in some type of avoidance. This avoidance provides temporary relief but keeps PTSD going in the long run by preventing new learning about the accuracy of interpretations and problematic beliefs.

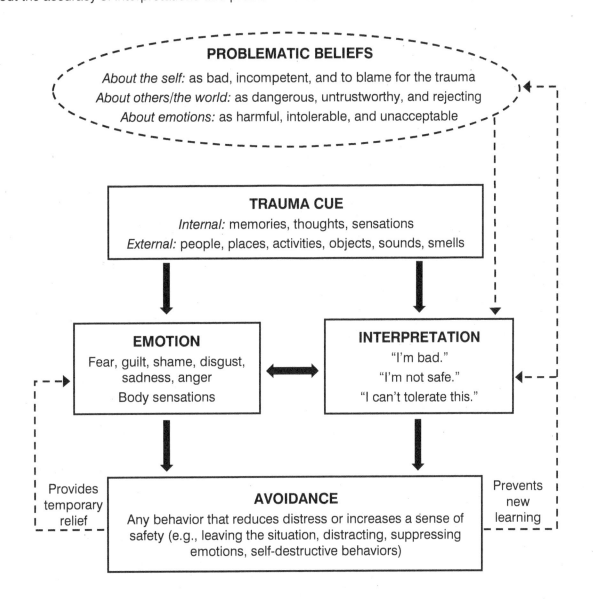

How DBT PE Works to Reduce PTSD

Because avoidance interferes with recovering from PTSD, the way to reduce PTSD is to stop avoiding. In DBT PE, this is done by using *in vivo* exposure, imaginal exposure, and processing to approach rather than avoid situations, memories, and emotions that are associated with your trauma. This will make it possible to correct the problematic interpretations and beliefs that are setting off your strong emotional responses. Over time, this corrective learning will reduce the intensity of your emotions and your PTSD will improve.

Imaginal Exposure
Approaching avoided trauma memories by describing them out loud and in detail

In Vivo Exposure
Approaching safe but avoided situations, people, and things in real life

Processing
Talking about and evaluating trauma-related emotions and beliefs

Corrective Learning
Change problematic beliefs.
Develop a more helpful perspective about the meaning of the trauma.
Reduce the intensity of trauma-related emotions in the long term.

Improved PTSD

Post-Exposure Skills Plan

Doing exposure, either in session or as homework, is likely to elicit intense emotions and may lead to urges to engage in problem behaviors. List below any skills you can use after doing exposure to manage intense emotions you may have, as well as ensure that you do not engage in problem behaviors.

Skills to Use

1.	
2.	
3.	
4.	
5.	
6.	
7.	
8.	
9.	
10.	

Problem Behaviors to Be Avoided

1.	
2.	
3.	
4.	
5.	

Dialectical Reactions to Trauma

Emotional Flooding
"I am overwhelmed by my emotions."
(intrusive trauma memories, thoughts, and images; intense emotional and physical reactions to trauma reminders)

Reckless Dyscontrol
"I am dangerous and out of control."
(suicide attempts and self-injury; substance use; binge eating; excessive risk taking; impulsive decision making)

Desperate Connection
"I can't tolerate being alone."
(fear of abandonment; being overly trusting; becoming quickly attached; frequent sexual behavior with people not known well)

Undercontrolled
– –
Overcontrolled

Detached Independence
"I am better off alone."
(pushing people away; not sharing personal information; avoiding emotional and physical intimacy; refusing help)

Emotional Numbness
"I don't have any emotions."
(shutting off emotions; feeling numb or empty inside; depression and emotional flatness; dissociation)

Rigid Control
"The world is dangerous and out of control."
(on guard; taking excessive precautions; perfectionism; extreme orderliness; inhibiting spontaneity; hyperarousal)

Understanding Your Reactions to Trauma

Trauma has a significant and lasting impact on people's emotions, behaviors, and relationships. People who have experienced trauma have a wide range of reactions that may change from one extreme to another over time. In addition, many trauma survivors have multiple, seemingly opposite reactions at the same time.

Emotional Reactions

Many people have difficult emotional reactions after experiencing trauma. They may have frequent intense emotions, including fear, anger, guilt, shame, disgust, and sadness. These emotions may occur in response to things that remind them of their trauma, or they may be present most of the time. It is also common for people who have experienced trauma to feel numb or emotionally shut down. Often people try not to have emotions by avoiding things that are likely to be upsetting and they may feel unable to have emotions even when they want to. Many people who have experienced trauma go back and forth between being numb and being flooded with intense emotion.

Check off the emotional reactions you have experienced:

Emotional Flooding	Emotional Numbness
☐ Overwhelming fear and anxiety	☐ Feeling numb, empty, or dead inside
☐ Extreme anger	☐ Difficulty feeling emotions intensely or at all
☐ Intense guilt and shame	☐ Shutting off emotions once they start
☐ Frequent disgust at self or others	☐ Depression and emotional flatness
☐ Long-lasting sadness and despair	☐ Unable to feel positive emotions (love, joy)
☐ Distressing thoughts and memories of trauma	☐ Feeling disconnected from yourself or as if things around you are unreal (dissociation)
☐ Feeling as if you are reexperiencing the trauma (flashbacks)	☐ Avoiding things likely to cause you to have emotions
☐ Intense emotional and/or physical distress when reminded of the trauma	☐ Avoiding thinking or talking about your trauma
☐ "I am overwhelmed by my emotions."	☐ "I don't have any emotions."
☐ Other:	☐ Other:

Behavioral Reactions

Many people who have experienced trauma engage in reckless behaviors that are potentially damaging to themselves or others, such as suicide attempts, self-injury, substance use, binge eating, unsafe sex, physical aggression, and reckless driving. People may take excessive risks and act impulsively without thinking things through. On the other hand, many trauma survivors take excessive precautions and have difficulty acting spontaneously. They may keep tight control over their behavior in an effort to protect themselves from potential danger. They often have a strong need for things to be predictable and orderly and may engage in a lot of planning and preparation before taking action. Many people who have experienced trauma are reckless and impulsive some of the time and hypervigilant and overly controlled at other times.

(continued)

Check off the behavioral reactions you have experienced:

Reckless Dyscontrol	Rigid Control
☐ Suicide attempts and self-injury	☐ Extreme cleanliness or orderliness
☐ Other self-damaging behaviors (e.g., substance use, binge eating, gambling)	☐ Following strict or perfectionistic rules for your own behavior
☐ Taking excessive risks (e.g., reckless driving, unsafe sex, shoplifting)	☐ Taking excessive precautions (e.g., actions intended to prevent or minimize danger)
☐ Acting on impulse without thinking things through	☐ Excessive planning or preparation before taking action
☐ Doing things with little or no planning	☐ Not allowing yourself to be spontaneous
☐ Ignoring or minimizing potential risks	☐ Constantly being on guard for potential risks
☐ Making important decisions quickly	☐ Difficulty making even small decisions
☐ Restlessness, hyperactivity, and difficulty completing tasks	☐ Hyperarousal (e.g., irritability, poor sleep, easily startled, difficulty concentrating)
☐ "I am dangerous and out of control."	☐ "The world is dangerous and out of control."
☐ Other:	☐ Other:

Interpersonal Reactions

People who have experienced trauma often have a strong need to be in relationships, even if those relationships are problematic, and they feel very afraid of being alone. They may become easily attached, share personal information quickly, and have frequent sexual encounters with people they do not know well. On the other hand, many trauma survivors are uncomfortable with close relationships, avoid sexual and emotional intimacy, and try not to become attached to people. They may try to appear strong and deny needing others' help or support. People often alternate between seeking close relationships and detaching from and not trusting people.

Check off the interpersonal reactions you have experienced:

Desperate Connection	Detached Independence
☐ Being overly trusting	☐ Not trusting people
☐ Sharing personal information quickly	☐ Not sharing personal information
☐ Frequent sexual behavior with people you do not know well	☐ Avoiding sexual and physical intimacy
☐ Easily becoming attached to people	☐ Trying not to become attached to people
☐ Regularly putting other people's needs ahead of your own	☐ Refusing to accept help or support from others when it is offered
☐ Not standing up for yourself when people treat you poorly	☐ Pushing people away when they express love or care toward you
☐ Behaving in a clingy or needy way with people	☐ Behaving as if you are self-sufficient and do not need people
☐ Feeling very afraid when you think a relationship is going to end	☐ Feeling very afraid when you feel connected or close to someone
☐ Quickly starting a new relationship when another relationship ends	☐ Doing things to try to get people to leave you alone
☐ "I can't tolerate being alone."	☐ "I am better off alone."
☐ Other:	☐ Other:

Common Avoided Situations

People with PTSD typically avoid a wide variety of situations that cause emotional distress, such as certain activities, places, people, objects, sounds, and smells. *In vivo* exposure is designed to help you gradually approach rather than avoid these situations so that you can learn that they are safe and you can cope with the emotions they bring up. The more you approach these situations, the less distress they will cause, and the more you will feel in control of your life and able to do things that are important to you.

Situations That Are Reminders of a Trauma

People with PTSD often avoid things that remind them of their trauma. Check off trauma reminders that you avoid.

- ☐ People who resemble a perpetrator (e.g., in terms of age, gender, race, or hair color)
- ☐ Locations similar to where a trauma occurred (e.g., hospitals, schools, public garages)
- ☐ Sounds present at the time of a trauma (e.g., music, sirens, shouting, gunfire)
- ☐ Clothes similar to what was worn during a trauma (e.g., shorts, a certain color)
- ☐ Objects that are associated with a trauma (e.g., knives, foods, rope)
- ☐ Smells present during a trauma (e.g., alcohol, cologne, smoke)
- ☐ Activities similar to a trauma (e.g., sexual intimacy, driving, sleeping)
- ☐ Articles, books, TV shows, or movies that describe a similar trauma
- ☐ Photos of people involved in the trauma or of yourself at the age at which it occurred
- ☐ Other: _____

Situations Viewed as Dangerous

People with PTSD avoid many situations they believe are likely to be dangerous. Check off situations you avoid that feel dangerous.

- ☐ Crowds
- ☐ New or unfamiliar places
- ☐ Sitting far away from an exit
- ☐ Walking outside alone
- ☐ Talking to people you do not know well
- ☐ Going to bed without checking the locks
- ☐ Riding public transportation
- ☐ Being home alone
- ☐ Open or enclosed spaces
- ☐ Other: _____

Situations Avoided Due to Depression

People with PTSD often find it hard to do certain activities due to depression. Check off activities you avoid due to depression.

- ☐ Hobbies
- ☐ Socializing with friends or family
- ☐ Exercise
- ☐ Pleasurable activities
- ☐ Household tasks
- ☐ Leaving the house
- ☐ School or work tasks
- ☐ Taking trips or vacations
- ☐ Self-care
- ☐ Other: _____

(continued)

Situations That Cause Unjustified Shame

People with PTSD often avoid situations that make them feel ashamed of the type of person they are, their abilities, or their way of interacting with others. Check off situations you avoid because they cause you to feel shame.

Being Genuine
- ☐ Showing your emotions
- ☐ Expressing your opinion
- ☐ Disclosing your trauma history
- ☐ Sharing personal information
- ☐ Disagreeing with others
- ☐ Talking about your interests
- ☐ Other: _____
  _____

Being Deserving
- ☐ Asking for what you want
- ☐ Saying no to unwanted requests
- ☐ Doing something kind for yourself
- ☐ Taking up physical space
- ☐ Putting your needs ahead of others
- ☐ Taking a break or relaxing
- ☐ Other: _____
  _____

Being Imperfect
- ☐ Making a mistake
- ☐ Being late
- ☐ Asking for help
- ☐ Not doing your best
- ☐ Making a mess
- ☐ Leaving things undone
- ☐ Other: _____
  _____

Being Competent
- ☐ Accepting praise
- ☐ Giving advice
- ☐ Talking about your strengths
- ☐ Sharing your successes
- ☐ Taking on a leadership role
- ☐ Behaving skillfully in a difficult situation
- ☐ Other: _____
  _____

Being Vulnerable
- ☐ Showing emotions that feel weak
- ☐ Talking about things you're afraid of
- ☐ Accepting help and support
- ☐ Being open when you are struggling
- ☐ Expressing care for other people
- ☐ Acting as if you need people
- ☐ Other: _____
  _____

Being Seen
- ☐ Having your photo taken
- ☐ Wearing revealing clothing
- ☐ Making eye contact with others
- ☐ Looking at yourself in the mirror
- ☐ Eating or speaking in front of people
- ☐ Doing things that call attention to you
- ☐ Other: _____
  _____

In Vivo Exposure Hierarchy

Name: _____ Date: _____

The *in vivo* exposure hierarchy is a list of situations (e.g., people, places, objects, activities) you are currently avoiding and would like to be able to have in your life. These can include:

- Situations that remind you of past traumatic events
- Situations that feel dangerous or unsafe but that are not objectively harmful
- Activities that you used to enjoy but have stopped doing due to depression
- Situations that cause you to feel unjustified shame

Avoided Situations	SUDS (Session 2)	SUDS (Final Session)
1.		
2.		
3.		
4.		
5.		
6.		
7.		
8.		
9.		
10.		
11.		
12.		
13.		
14.		
15.		

Exposure Recording Form

Name: _____ Date: _____

Time started: _____ Time stopped: _____

Situation practiced: _____

Exposure type (circle one): Imaginal / *In vivo*   Location (circle one): In session / Homework

Probability and Cost Estimates

What is the worst that could happen in this situation? *(Be as specific as possible.)*	How likely is it that this will happen? (0–100)		How bad would it be if this happened? (0–100)		Did this happen?
	Before	**After**	**Before**	**After**	**Y or N**
1.					
2.					
3.					

SUDS, Urges, and Dissociation

	SUDS (0–100)	Urge to kill myself (0–5)	Urge to self-harm (0–5)	Urge to quit therapy (0–5)	Urge to use substances (0–5)	Dissociation (0–100)
Before						
Peak						
After						

Specific Emotions and Radical Acceptance

	Fear (0–100)	Guilt (0–100)	Shame (0–100)	Disgust (0–100)	Anger (0–100)	Sadness (0–100)	Joy (0–100)	Radical acceptance (0–100)
Before								
After								

What did you learn during this exposure task?

_____

_____

_____

DBT PE Handout 8A

Exposure Recording Form

Name: _____

The form contains columns for:

- What's the worst that could happen?
- How likely is it? (0–100): Pre / Post
- How bad would it be? (0–100): Pre / Post
- Did it happen? Y/N
- SUDS, URGES, DISSOCIATION: Pre / Peak / Post
  - SUDS (0–100)
  - Suicide (0–5)
  - Self-harm (0–5)
  - Quit therapy (0–5)
  - Substances (0–5)
  - Dissociation (0–100)
- EMOTIONS & ACCEPTANCE: Pre / Post
  - Fear (0–100)
  - Guilt (0–100)
  - Shame (0–100)
  - Disgust (0–100)
  - Anger (0–100)
  - Sadness (0–100)
  - Joy (0–100)
  - Radical acceptance (0–100)

Repeated blocks (each with):

DATE: ___ START: ___ STOP: ___ SITUATION: ___ *IN VIVO/IMAGINAL*

	Pre	Peak	Post
1.			
2.			
3.			

What did you learn? _____

(This block is repeated four times on the form.)

How to Do Exposure Homework

The following guidelines are intended to help you complete *in vivo* and imaginal exposure homework effectively. *Remember:* The more exposure homework you do and the more effectively you do it, the faster and better the treatment will work!

BEFORE STARTING THE EXPOSURE TASK

Get Prepared

- **Plan a specific time and place** to complete the exposure task. Try to choose a time when you are unlikely to be interrupted.
- **Locate materials** you will need to complete the exposure task.
  - For *in vivo* exposure, you may need to find or get certain materials that are trauma reminders (e.g., specific objects, sounds, smells).
  - For imaginal exposure, you will need the device on which you recorded your session and headphones.
  - Get a blank Exposure Recording Form
- Have your **Post-Exposure Skills Plan** handy as well as anything you might need to use the skills on your plan (e.g., an ice pack).

Complete the Exposure Recording Form

- **Feared outcomes:** List up to three things you are most afraid could happen during the exposure. Try to identify the worst things you think might happen. Be as specific as possible about what you think could happen and focus on outcomes that could be observed by others whenever possible. For example:
  - Instead of "I will go crazy," you might write, "I will scream and fall on the floor."
  - Instead of "People will think I'm stupid," you might write, "People will say critical things to me."
  - Instead of "I will feel too sad," you might write, "I will cry nonstop for hours."
- For each of the feared outcomes you listed, complete a **before/pre** rating of your:
  - **Probability estimate** (0–100): What is the likelihood that this could happen during or as a result of the exposure task?
  - **Cost estimate** (0–100): How bad would it be if this happened?
- Complete the rest of the **before** ratings to indicate how you are feeling as you get ready to complete the exposure task:
  - **SUDS (Subjective Units of Distress Scale)** (0–100): overall level of distress
  - **Urges** (0–5): urges to kill yourself, self-harm, quit therapy, and use substances
  - **Dissociation** (0–100): current level of dissociation
  - **Specific emotions** (0–100): current levels of fear, guilt, shame, disgust, anger, and sadness *related to the traumatic event*, as well as joy *related to completing this particular exposure task*
  - **Radical acceptance** (0–100): how much you radically accept that the trauma you are working on occurred

(continued)

DURING THE EXPOSURE TASK

- **Participate one-mindfully.** When doing exposure, just do exposure. For example, do not do exposure while driving, watching TV, or listening to music. As much as possible, focus your complete attention on the exposure task.
- **Allow emotions** to be experienced fully during the exposure task. Try not to block, suppress, or push away your emotions. Allow your emotions to come and go naturally without acting on them.
- **Avoid avoidance.** Be on the lookout for avoidance. Avoidance can be subtle (e.g., thinking about something else during the exposure, carrying something that makes you feel safer) or obvious (e.g., stopping the exposure early, not looking at the cue). When you notice yourself avoiding, encourage yourself to do the exposure task all the way instead.
- **Continue until you achieve your goals.** To be most effective, these goals should be achievable (difficult but not unmanageable) and based on specific behavior(s) you will perform during the exposure (e.g., listening to an imaginal exposure recording for 30 minutes or initiating conversation with three strangers at a party). Consult with your therapist about what these goals should be.

AFTER COMPLETING THE EXPOSURE TASK

- Congratulate yourself for doing something difficult!
- Use your **Post-Exposure Skills Plan**, if needed.

Complete the Exposure Recording Form

- For each of the feared outcomes, fill in the **after/post** ratings for:
  - **Probability estimates (0–100):** What is the likelihood that this will happen when you do this exposure task again in the future?
  - **Cost estimates (0–100):** How bad would it be if it did happen when you do this exposure task again in the future?
  - **Actual occurrence (Yes/No):** Did this actually happen?
- Fill in the **peak** (highest) and **after/post** ratings for:
  - SUDS (0–100)
  - Urges (0–5)
  - Dissociation (0–100)
- Fill in the **after/post** ratings for:
  - Specific emotions (0–100)
  - Radical acceptance (0–100)
- Write **what you learned** during the exposure task. For example, you may have learned that the things you predicted did not actually happen. Or you may have learned that the things that happened were not as bad as you thought they would be and you were able to cope with them.

Asking for Support during DBT PE

You may find it helpful to ask people in your life to provide support as you complete DBT PE. If you choose to do this, you will need to think through what types of support you would find helpful, as well as who in your life is likely to be willing and able to provide this support. The list below includes a variety of ways a person might provide support, but it is not expected that one person could fulfill all these roles. Check off the types of support that you would like to ask for.

THINGS THAT MAY BE HELPFUL

Being a Cheerleader

☐ Encouraging you to complete exposure tasks rather than avoid
☐ Communicating belief in your ability to succeed
☐ Validating how hard it is to do exposure tasks
☐ Praising your efforts to approach feared situations
☐ Celebrating your successes

Being a Confidant

☐ Listening to you talk about your struggles
☐ Encouraging you to share and express your emotions
☐ Validating the experiences and emotions that you share
☐ Being open to hearing about your trauma if you want to talk about it
☐ Keeping the information that you share private

Being a Coach

☐ Helping you prepare to complete exposure tasks
☐ Assisting you during exposure tasks when asked
☐ Helping you to use your Post-Exposure Skills Plan when needed

Being an Assistant

☐ Taking over chores or other tasks to free up your time to do exposure
☐ Providing transportation to/from sessions or places you will be doing exposure
☐ Helping you to find or purchase things you need to do exposure
☐ Keeping people or pets away from you while you are doing exposure

Other things that may be helpful:

_____

_____

_____

(continued)

You may also have concerns that certain people in your life may do things that would be unhelpful during DBT PE. If this is true, you may want to ask those people *not* to do things that would make it harder for you to do DBT PE and/or that might make the treatment less effective. Check off the things that you would like to ask certain people *not* to do.

THINGS THAT MAY BE UNHELPFUL

☐ Judging or making fun of you for your fears
☐ Criticizing you for having urges to avoid doing exposure
☐ Minimizing the difficulty of approaching feared situations
☐ Invalidating your emotions that come up as a result of exposure
☐ Encouraging you to avoid or not to do exposure
☐ Trying to force you to do exposure
☐ Insisting that you tell them about your trauma
☐ Demanding to know what you are working on in treatment
☐ Expressing high anxiety or worry about you or your treatment
☐ Interrupting or distracting you while you are doing exposure
☐ Being excessively reassuring or soothing while you are doing exposure
☐ Listening to your imaginal exposure recordings or looking at your homework forms
☐ Pressuring you to take legal action against perpetrators

Other things that may be unhelpful:

_____

_____

MAKING YOUR REQUEST

Once you are clear who you want to ask for support and what you want to ask for, then you can use the DEAR MAN and GIVE skills to make your request. You may want to prepare a script in advance using the steps below and practice it before talking to the person.

1. **D**escribe the situation.
2. **E**xpress feelings/opinions.
3. **A**ssert your request.
4. **R**einforcing comments.
5. **M**indful and **A**ppearing confident comments (if needed).
6. **N**egotiating comments (if needed).
7. **V**alidating comments.
8. **E**asy manner comments.

You may also want to write down the things you want to avoid saying or doing.

Goals of Relapse Prevention

CONTINUE DOING EXPOSURE

- Identify *in vivo* and imaginal exposure tasks to continue practicing.
- Plan in advance for how you will do exposure.
- Guide yourself through completing exposure tasks effectively.

ADOPT AN EXPOSURE LIFESTYLE

- Notice when urges to avoid arise and choose to approach instead.
- Practice random acts of exposure and be willing to try new things.
- Allow yourself to experience emotions fully.

IDENTIFY AND REDUCE RISK FACTORS

- Decrease emotional vulnerability and build resilience to stress.
- Minimize the use of avoidant coping strategies.
- Anticipate and prepare for high-risk situations.

MANAGE RELAPSES EFFECTIVELY

- Identify and validate the reasons why PTSD has increased.
- Brainstorm solutions that are likely to help reduce PTSD.
- Stay motivated to keep trying solutions until PTSD decreases again.

Become Your Own Exposure Therapist

After completing DBT PE, it is recommended that you continue practicing *in vivo* and imaginal exposure on your own. This can help you to make even more gains while also reducing the likelihood that PTSD will increase in the future. When doing exposure, follow the guidelines on *DBT PE Handout 13* to make it as effective as possible.

In Vivo Exposure

Which *in vivo* exposure tasks would you like to continue practicing on your own? Consider choosing situations and activities that still cause moderate to high levels of distress and/or that you are still avoiding and would like to be able to do more often.

In Vivo Tasks	Current SUDS
1.	
2.	
3.	
4.	
5.	
6.	
7.	
8.	
9.	
10.	

Imaginal Exposure

Which trauma memories would it be helpful to continue processing on your own? This could involve periodically listening to imaginal exposure recordings you made during DBT PE, making new recordings on your own, and/or describing a trauma out loud without recording it.

Target Trauma(s)	Current SUDS
1.	
2.	
3.	

Guidelines for Doing Exposure Effectively

PREPARE TO DO EXPOSURE

- **Select exposure tasks that will test your beliefs.** Identify what you are most afraid will happen if you approach the things you are avoiding. Pick an exposure task that will allow you to find out whether the negative outcomes you expect actually occur.

- **Make sure the exposure task is safe.** Use wise mind to be sure that you choose exposure tasks that have little to no risk of actual harm. Consult a person you trust if needed.

- **Plan a time and place to complete the exposure.** Try to choose a time when you are unlikely to be interrupted. If you are doing exposure at a specific location, figure out how you will get there and back.

- **Locate materials you will need.** For imaginal exposure, you will need your recording device and headphones. For *in vivo* exposure, you may need to find materials in advance (e.g., specific trauma reminders).

- **Set specific goals for the exposure.** To be most effective, the goals should be:
  - **Achievable:** exposure tasks should be difficult, but not unmanageable.
  - **Objective:** goals should be based on specific behavior(s) you will engage in during the exposure (e.g., listen to an imaginal exposure recording for 30 minutes, initiate a conversation with a stranger).

- **Make a Post-Exposure Skills Plan.** Identify skills you will use, if needed, to cope effectively with urges or emotions that may be present after the exposure is done.

DO EXPOSURE EFFECTIVELY

- **Practice one-mindfulness.** When doing exposure, do exposure. Focus your complete attention on the exposure task and avoid distractions.

- **Avoid avoidance.** Watch out for avoidance during exposure. Avoidance can be anything you do, intentionally or unintentionally, that prevents or reduces emotions during exposure (e.g., closing your eyes, taking medications, thinking about other things). If you notice avoidance, coach yourself to do exposure all the way instead.

- **Experience your emotions.** Don't try to block or suppress your emotions. Don't try to hold on to your emotions. Allow your emotions to run their natural course.

- **Don't stop until you have reached your goals.** Continue the exposure until you achieve the specific goals you set in advance.

- **Track your progress.** Use the Exposure Recording Form (DBT PE Handout 8 or 8A) to rate your feared outcomes, SUDS, urges, and emotions before and after completing an exposure task. Look for patterns of change over time, such as decreases in SUDS and unjustified emotions.

- **Repeat the exposure task until it no longer causes much distress.** As a general guideline, keep practicing an exposure task until your peak SUDS are about a 30 or less.

Adopt an Exposure Lifestyle

Adopting an exposure lifestyle involves noticing when you have urges to avoid safe but uncomfortable situations and choosing to approach instead. Living an exposure lifestyle will make it less likely that PTSD will return and can help to increase joy and meaning in your life.

A way to remember these skills is to remember the word **FREE**.

Fight fear

(Do) **R**andom acts of exposure

Expand your world

Embrace emotions

Fight fear	When fear shows up, CHECK THE FACTS to determine whether it is justified. When fear does not fit the facts, use OPPOSITE ACTION and approach things that make you afraid ALL THE WAY without avoiding. Don't let fear limit your freedom!
(Do) **R**andom acts of exposure	NOTICE URGES TO AVOID and spontaneously choose to approach instead. LOOK FOR OPPORTUNITIES to randomly practice exposure and seize the moment when it arises. Use WISE MIND to decide when it is effective to approach rather than avoid.
Expand your world	Be WILLING to do new things that make you uncomfortable. Try new activities, explore new places, and meet new people. SAY YES to things that are likely to INCREASE JOY and create new possibilities in your life. Let go of self-consciousness and PARTICIPATE fully in these new experiences.
Embrace emotions	Allow yourself to EXPERIENCE EMOTIONS rather than trying to block or get rid of them. Let your emotions come and go naturally like a wave. Use MINDFULNESS of current emotion to notice where you feel your emotions in your body. RADICALLY ACCEPT your emotions to achieve FREEDOM from suffering.

Practicing the FREE Skill

Track your efforts to adopt an exposure lifestyle by using the FREE skill. Describe two situations that you wanted to avoid and how you used the FREE skill to approach instead.

SITUATION 1: Rate urges to avoid (0–100)   Before: _____   After: _____

Situation I wanted to avoid (who, what, when, where):

Check the FREE skills you used:
- ☐ Fight fear
- ☐ (Do) Random acts of exposure
- ☐ Expand your world
- ☐ Embrace emotions

Describe what you did:

Describe the outcome of using the FREE skill: What did you learn?

SITUATION 2: Rate urges to avoid (0–100)   Before: _____   After: _____

Situation I wanted to avoid (who, what, when, where):

Check the FREE skills you used:
- ☐ Fight fear
- ☐ (Do) Random acts of exposure
- ☐ Expand your world
- ☐ Embrace emotions

Describe what you did:

Describe the outcome of using the FREE skill: What did you learn?

Risk Factors for a Relapse of PTSD

It is important to be aware of the factors that may increase your risk of a relapse of PTSD. The goal is to notice when increases in these risk factors occur and act quickly to address them before PTSD has a chance to return.

EMOTIONAL VULNERABILITY

Increases in PTSD often occur at times when people are particularly vulnerable to negative emotions and more sensitive to stressful events.

- Check off the vulnerability factors that are likely to be risk factors for you:

  ☐ Not getting enough sleep   ☐ Eating too much or too little
  ☐ High stress and life demands   ☐ Not doing things that build mastery
  ☐ Not treating physical illnesses   ☐ Few pleasurable or valued activities
  ☐ Using alcohol or drugs   ☐ Not taking prescribed medications
  ☐ Not exercising   ☐ Other: _____

Notice when emotional vulnerability is increasing and use the ABC PLEASE skills to decrease your vulnerability and build resilience to stress.

AVOIDANT COPING

PTSD is fueled by avoidance of painful emotions, thoughts, and situations, and relying on avoidance to cope increases the risk of a relapse of PTSD.

- Check off the avoidant coping strategies that are likely to be risk factors for you:

  ☐ Suppressing emotions   ☐ Avoiding situations that cause distress
  ☐ Isolating from friends and family   ☐ Trying not to think about painful events
  ☐ Dissociating   ☐ Not actively solving problems
  ☐ Refusing to accept reality   ☐ Other: _____

Notice when your use of avoidant coping strategies is increasing and use exposure and the FREE skill to reduce avoidance and approach instead.

HIGH-RISK SITUATIONS

High-risk situations are events that cause high stress and may prompt an increase in PTSD.

- Check off the high-risk situations that are likely to be risk factors for you:

  ☐ Anniversary dates of traumatic events
  ☐ Contact with perpetrators of past trauma (e.g., at family gatherings)
  ☐ Situations that remind you of past trauma (e.g., visiting the location of a trauma)
  ☐ Negative life stressors (e.g., relationship breakups, financial problems)
  ☐ Positive life stressors (e.g., starting a new school or job, moving)
  ☐ Other: _____

Anticipate high-risk situations and use the COPE AHEAD skill to rehearse coping effectively with these situations before they occur.

Reducing the Risk of a Relapse of PTSD

Write down what you did each day to decrease emotional vulnerability and avoid avoidance.   Week starting: _____

Day	DECREASE EMOTIONAL VULNERABILITY			AVOID AVOIDANCE
	Accumulate positives	Build mastery	PLEASE skills	Exposure and FREE skills

PREPARE FOR HIGH-RISK SITUATIONS: Write down an upcoming high-risk situation and how you used **Cope Ahead** to prepare for it.

Future high-risk situation	How I imagined coping effectively (describe)

Guidelines for Managing Increases in PTSD

Many people who have recovered from PTSD experience increases in symptoms at times. Follow these steps to prevent an increase in PTSD from becoming a full-blown relapse.

Step 1. Identify and validate the factors that contributed to PTSD increasing.

ASK: What are the understandable reasons that PTSD has increased?

Examples of common contributing factors are listed on DBT PE Handout 16.

- DON'T JUDGE yourself or the reasons why your PTSD has increased.
- VALIDATE how it makes sense that PTSD has increased even though you wish it had not.
- COMMIT to changing and/or coping effectively with the factors that have contributed to this increase in PTSD.

Step 2. Brainstorm solutions.

ASK: What skills and strategies might help to address the reasons my PTSD has increased?

Examples of skills that may be helpful:

- Radically accept that PTSD has increased
- Do *in vivo* exposure to safe but avoided situations
- Do imaginal exposure to distressing trauma memories
- Adopt an exposure lifestyle with the FREE skill
- Practice mindfulness of current emotions
- Check the facts about unhelpful trauma-related beliefs
- Use opposite action to reduce unwanted emotions
- Reduce vulnerability with ABC PLEASE skills
- Problem-solve situations that are causing stress
- Use DEAR MAN to ask for help or say no

Step 3. Choose solutions to work on now.

Be specific about what you will do. Break solutions into small steps, if needed.

Examples: Listen to an imaginal exposure recording four times. Do daily *in vivo* exposure to a trauma reminder. Spend time with a friend. Avoid alcohol. Exercise three times/week.

Step 4. Keep yourself motivated.

- Use SELF-ENCOURAGEMENT to motivate yourself to keep trying solutions until PTSD decreases.
- REMIND yourself that you have successfully reduced your PTSD before and you can do it again now.
- REWARD yourself for small steps toward your goals.
- SEEK TREATMENT or return for a few booster sessions with an ex-therapist, if needed.

Managing an Increase in PTSD

If you notice an increase in PTSD symptoms, complete these steps to figure out how to get these symptoms to decrease again. See *DBT PE Handout 18* for ideas.

1. **IDENTIFY CONTRIBUTING FACTORS:** What are the understandable reasons that PTSD has increased or returned (e.g., vulnerability factors, avoidant coping, high-risk situations)?

   _____

   _____

   _____

   _____

   _____

2. **BRAINSTORM SOLUTIONS:** What skills or strategies may help to address the factors that contributed to the increase in PTSD? List as many potential solutions as you can.

   _____

   _____

   _____

   _____

   _____

   _____

   _____

3. **CHOOSE SOLUTIONS:** Which solutions seem best? Try them and track the outcome.

Solution	✓ Done	Outcome
1.		
2.		
3.		
4.		
5.		
6.		
7.		

4. **KEEP YOURSELF MOTIVATED:** What strategies can you use to stay motivated to keep working hard until your PTSD decreases?

   _____

   _____

   _____

Troubleshooting Problems during DBT PE

Follow these six troubleshooting steps if progress is slow or limited during DBT PE.

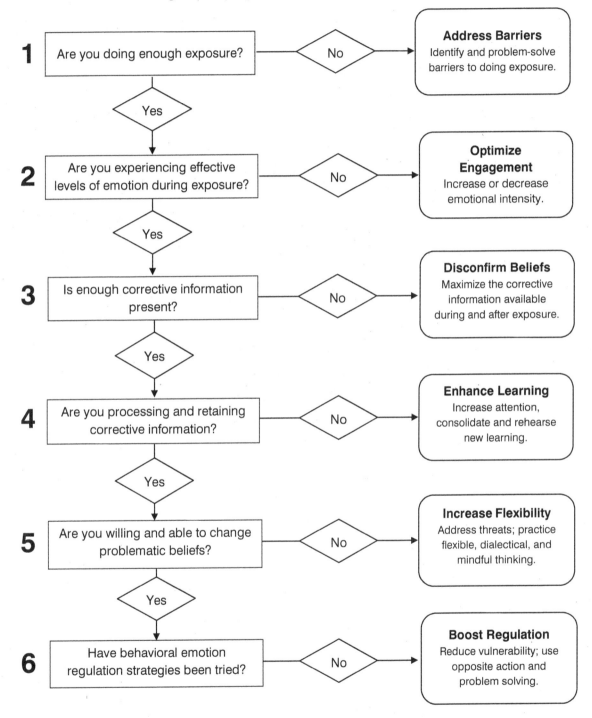

1 Are you doing enough exposure? — **No** → **Address Barriers** Identify and problem-solve barriers to doing exposure.

Yes ↓

2 Are you experiencing effective levels of emotion during exposure? — **No** → **Optimize Engagement** Increase or decrease emotional intensity.

Yes ↓

3 Is enough corrective information present? — **No** → **Disconfirm Beliefs** Maximize the corrective information available during and after exposure.

Yes ↓

4 Are you processing and retaining corrective information? — **No** → **Enhance Learning** Increase attention, consolidate and rehearse new learning.

Yes ↓

5 Are you willing and able to change problematic beliefs? — **No** → **Increase Flexibility** Address threats; practice flexible, dialectical, and mindful thinking.

Yes ↓

6 Have behavioral emotion regulation strategies been tried? — **No** → **Boost Regulation** Reduce vulnerability; use opposite action and problem solving.

Preparing to Resume DBT PE

At times, DBT PE may need to be paused because a problem has occurred that makes it unsafe or ineffective to continue. If DBT PE is paused, the goal is for this to be as brief as possible and for you to continue with DBT PE as soon as the problem has been resolved. Before DBT PE can be resumed, you will need to meet the following criteria that are intended to reduce the likelihood that the problem will happen again.

Behavior That Caused DBT PE to Be Paused:_____

_____

CRITERIA FOR RESUMING	WHAT YOU NEED TO DO TO RESUME DBT PE
1. If the behavior was a suicide attempt or nonsuicidal self-injury, it must no longer be occurring.	Date of last episode: _____
2. For other types of behavior, you must be able to control it enough that it will not interfere with DBT PE.	
3. You need to solve the problems that contributed to the behavior.	
4. You must be committed to preventing the behavior from happening again.	
5. When others were harmed by the behavior, you will need to make repairs.	

APPENDIX B

THERAPIST FORMS

DBT PE Case Formulation Worksheet

Client: _____ Date completed: _____

PTSD
Describe the type, severity, and duration of the client's PTSD symptoms.

TRAUMA HISTORY		
Briefly describe the client's history of trauma. For each trauma type, specify the client's age(s) at the time the trauma occurred and the perpetrator (if applicable). If known, rank-order the traumas by the severity of PTSD symptoms they currently cause.		
Trauma type	**Age(s)**	**Perpetrator (if any)**
1.		
2.		
3.		
4.		
5.		
6.		
7.		

(continued)

Trauma type	Age(s)	Perpetrator (if any)
8.		
9.		
10.		

TRAUMA CUES

Describe the primary internal and external trauma cues the client avoids.

MECHANISMS

A. **Problematic beliefs and emotions:** List the primary problematic beliefs and associated emotions that are hypothesized to be maintaining the client's PTSD.

Problematic beliefs: about the self, others, the world, and emotions	Emotions
1.	
2.	
3.	
4.	
5.	
6.	
7.	

(continued)

B. **Avoidance:** Describe the primary avoidance strategies the client uses to increase a sense of safety and/or reduce aversive emotions when confronted with trauma cues.

ORIGINS OF MECHANISMS

Briefly describe how the client learned or acquired the hypothesized mechanisms. Consider the role of the invalidating environment and biologically based emotional vulnerability.

Trauma Interview

Client: _____ Date: _____

INTERVIEWER: I'm going to ask you some questions about the traumas you have experienced, but you will not need to go into a lot of detail in describing your traumas today. Our main goal is to work together to figure out which traumas we will focus on during treatment and to pick the traumatic event that we will target first with imaginal exposure. I will then ask you some more specific questions about this first target trauma and your current responses to it.

SECTION 1. ASSESSMENT OF TRAUMA HISTORY

INTERVIEWER: First, I want to know about the traumas you have experienced in your life. These can include events that happened one time that were highly distressing, as well as repeated events that together caused you to feel very upset. All that I need is a brief description of the type of trauma, your age at the time, and who the perpetrator was if relevant. You do not need to tell me exactly what happened or go into a lot of detail in describing these traumas. I will start by listing the traumas I already know about. [*Briefly summarize the trauma information you know.*] Is that right? Are there any other traumas to add?

Additional probe questions as needed:
- Have you ever experienced or witnessed other events involving sexual abuse or assault, serious injury, or actual or threatened death?
- Have you ever experienced severe or repetitive invalidation, such as being criticized, ignored, emotionally neglected, or blamed by a person or group that was important to you?
- Have you had highly distressing experiences of being discriminated against or mistreated due to aspects of your identity, such as your race, sexual orientation, gender, or religion?

1. Lifetime trauma history

Brief description of trauma	Age(s)	Perpetrator (if any)

(continued)

SECTION 2. IDENTIFICATION OF TARGET TRAUMAS

INTERVIEWER: Of all these traumatic experiences that have happened to you [*summarize traumatic events endorsed by client*], which [*up to three*] currently bother you the most? Which one(s) cause you the most distress? [*Use additional probe questions as needed if the client has difficulty identifying the most distressing events; e.g., Which one(s) come up most often in your thoughts, nightmares, and flashbacks? Which one(s) upset you the most when you are reminded of them? Which one(s) make you feel the worst about yourself? Which one(s) cause the most problems or interfere in your life the most?*]

2. List up to three target traumas the client identifies, from most to least distressing:

     a. _____

     b. _____

     c. _____

Note to clinician: Target traumas must be specific, discrete events and cannot be general types of chronic trauma. For traumas that occurred repeatedly, consider the following factors when selecting specific events to target:

- Level of distress: prefer to target the most distressing event over less distressing events.
- Representativeness: prefer to target events that are representative of the typical way in which the type of trauma usually occurred (e.g., the perpetrator's behavior and the client's response).
- Link to beliefs: prefer to target events that are closely linked to the client's primary problematic beliefs about the self and others (e.g., that are viewed as the strongest proof the beliefs are true).
- Memory quality: prefer to target events that are remembered clearly (e.g., that progress as a story with a beginning, middle, and end) over those that are unclear or fragmented.

INTERVIEWER: Considering these [*up to three*] traumas you have identified, in what order do you want to target them with imaginal exposure? Which one do you want to start with? [*Discuss the potential pros and cons of starting with the most distressing versus a less distressing trauma; e.g., starting with the most distressing trauma often leads to the most rapid relief, may be more likely to generalize to other less distressing traumas, and may decrease the overall length of treatment; starting with a less distressing trauma may enable the client to build mastery with imaginal exposure before targeting the more distressing traumas.*]

3. Ordering of target traumas for imaginal exposure:

     First target trauma: _____

     Second target trauma: _____

     Third target trauma: _____

Note to clinician: Although it is generally recommended to start with the most distressing trauma first, clients may elect to start with a lesser distressing trauma if they prefer.

(*continued*)

SECTION 3. TRAUMA NARRATIVE AND PRIOR DISCLOSURE EXPERIENCES

INTERVIEWER: Now that we have picked the first trauma that we will target, the next thing we need to do is decide where the story of this traumatic event will start and end for the imaginal exposure. [*Ideally, the starting point will be right before anything scary or upsetting started to happen, and the end point will be after the event is over and the client was out of immediate danger. If clients do not remember the event clearly, these points will be the first and last things they can remember.*]

4. Overall, how long do you estimate the entire event lasted from start to finish? _____

5. Identifying start and end points for the imaginal exposure narrative

   a. Thinking of that entire experience, what were you doing right before you first felt afraid or as if something bad was about to happen? _____
   _____
   _____

   b. At what point did the danger end or at what point did you feel some relief, even if it was only temporary? _____
   _____
   _____

INTERVIEWER: Now I'm going to ask you some questions about your prior experiences, if any, of sharing information about this trauma with other people. The reason I'm asking these questions is because it is helpful for me to know if you have ever talked about this trauma before and, if so, how other people have responded.

6. Who, if anyone, knows about this trauma? How did they find out? _____
   _____
   _____
   _____
   _____
   _____
   _____

7. If other people know about the trauma, how have they responded? _____
   _____
   _____
   _____
   _____
   _____
   _____

(continued)

SECTION 4. BELIEFS, EMOTIONS, AND RADICAL ACCEPTANCE

INTERVIEWER: In this final section, I'm going to ask you questions to understand how you think and feel about this event now. This information will help us to figure out what may be keeping your PTSD going and what we will need to change for your PTSD to improve. I'm going to start by asking you some questions about who, if anyone, you blame for the occurrence of this trauma. I want you to know that there are no right or wrong answers, and it is not necessary that you blame anyone.

8. Who or what do you blame for what happened to you?	How much blame do you assign (*must total 100%*)?	How is the person or entity to blame?
a. Myself		
b. Perpetrator		
c. Family member		
d. Friend or acquaintance		
e. The environment		
f. An organization		
g. The culture		
h. Other: _____		

INTERVIEWER: Now I am going to ask you some questions about the emotions you currently have when you think about this trauma. You may have multiple emotions when you think about what happened to you. Again, there are no right or wrong answers, and there is no correct way to feel.

9. What emotions do you currently have about this event?	Intensity of emotion (0–100)	What is it about this event that makes you feel [*insert emotion*]?
a. Fear		
b. Sadness		
c. Anger		
d. Guilt		
e. Shame		
f. Disgust		

10. How much do you radically accept that this event happened to you (0–100)? _____
    (*Note that radical acceptance does not mean that you approve of or like what happened to you. Instead, it simply means that you accept that it occurred.*)

Therapist Imaginal Exposure Recording Form

Client: _____ Therapist: _____

Date: _____ Exposure #: _____ Session #: _____

Description of exposure: _____

Time	SUDS	Notes

Imaginal Exposure Progress Monitoring Form

Client: _____   Therapist: _____

Session #	Memory #	Description of the Imaginal Exposure	Primary Targets in Processing	Peak SUDS	Post Fear	Post Guilt	Post Shame	Post Disgust	Post Anger	Post Sad	Post RA	PTSD Score

Note. RA, radical acceptance.

APPENDIX C

SESSION CHECKLISTS

DBT PE Session 1 Checklist

Therapist: _____ Client: _____ Date: _____

Session Components	Yes	No
1. Review the DBT diary card and set an agenda for the session.	☐	☐

2. Explain that PTSD is maintained by avoidance of trauma cues, including:
  a. Distressing thoughts, memories, and emotions about the trauma
  b. People, situations, and things that prompt distressing thoughts and emotions associated with the trauma
	
	☐
	☐
		
		☐
		☐

3. Explain that PTSD is maintained by problematic beliefs about:
  a. Others and the world (e.g., as untrustworthy, rejecting, and dangerous)
  b. Oneself (e.g., as bad, incompetent, and to blame)
  c. Emotions (e.g., as harmful, intolerable, and unacceptable)
	
	☐
	☐
	☐
		
		☐
		☐
		☐

4. Describe how problematic beliefs and avoidance transact to maintain PTSD (DBT PE Handout 1):
  a. Negative beliefs cause people to interpret trauma cues in unhelpful and inaccurate ways that set off intense emotions.
  b. Avoidance provides temporary relief but keeps PTSD going in the long run by preventing new learning.
	
	☐
	
	☐
		
		☐
		
		☐

5. Orient to the core treatment procedures (DBT PE Handout 2):
  a. *In vivo* exposure is used to approach safe but avoided situations to learn they are not dangerous and can be coped with.
  b. Imaginal exposure involves describing traumatic events out loud so they become less distressing.
  c. Processing is used to gain a new perspective on the meaning of past trauma.
	
	☐
	
	☐
	
	☐
		
		☐
		
		☐
		
		☐

6. Complete the Trauma Interview (Therapist Form 2) and select the first target trauma.	☐	☐

7. Ask for and strengthen commitments to:
  a. Not attempt suicide or self-injure
  b. Actively participate in DBT PE, including completing homework
  c. Not engage in other escape-related problem behaviors immediately before, during, or after sessions or exposure homework
	
	☐
	☐
	☐
		
		☐
		☐
		☐

8. Create a Post-Exposure Skills Plan (DBT PE Handout 3) that includes a balance of acceptance and change skills.	☐	☐

9. Assign homework:
  a. Review the rationale for treatment (DBT PE Handouts 1 and 2).
  b. Practice skills from the Post-Exposure Skills Plan daily and add more skills, if needed (DBT PE Handout 3).
  c. Listen to the session recording once.
  d. Make a plan for after the first imaginal exposure session.
	
	☐
	☐
	
	☐
	☐
		
		☐
		☐
		
		☐
		☐

DBT PE Session 2 Checklist

Therapist: _____ Client: _____ Date: _____

Session Components	Yes	No
1. Review the DBT diary card and set an agenda for the session.	☐	☐
2. Review homework, give feedback, and address homework noncompletion (if needed).	☐	☐
3. Describe the dialectical reactions to trauma and elicit and normalize examples from the client (DBT PE Handouts 4 and 5).	☐	☐
4. Explain that behavioral avoidance works temporarily to reduce distress, but maintains PTSD in the long run by preventing new learning.	☐	☐
5. Orient to the rationale for *in vivo* exposure and how it works to reduce PTSD by: a. Breaking the habit of reducing distress by avoidance or escape b. Disconfirming beliefs about the expected outcome of exposure to avoided situations c. Increasing the ability to tolerate intense emotions d. Reducing the intensity of distress over time (habituation) e. Building mastery and confidence f. Improving quality of life and increasing joy	☐ ☐ ☐ ☐ ☐ ☐	☐ ☐ ☐ ☐ ☐ ☐
6. Create the *in vivo* exposure hierarchy (DBT PE Handout 7) and identify at least five specific avoided situations with at least two in the midrange (SUDS = 40–60). If needed, review DBT PE Handout 6 for ideas.	☐	☐
7. Select at least two *in vivo* exposure tasks for homework and give specific instructions on how to complete them.	☐	☐
8. Orient to the Exposure Recording Form (DBT PE Handout 8 or 8A).	☐	☐
9. Assign homework: a. Review Dialectical Reactions to Trauma (DBT PE Handout 4) and Understanding Your Reactions to Trauma (DBT PE Handout 5). b. Review Common Avoided Situations (DBT PE Handout 6) and add to the *In Vivo* Exposure Hierarchy, if needed (DBT PE Handout 7). c. Read the instructions for doing exposure homework (DBT PE Handout 9). d. Complete the assigned *in vivo* exposure tasks (at least one per day) and fill out an Exposure Recording Form (DBT PE Handout 8 or 8A) each time. e. Practice skills from the Post-Exposure Skills Plan (DBT PE Handout 3) as needed. f. Listen to the session recording once.	☐ ☐ ☐ ☐ ☐ ☐	☐ ☐ ☐ ☐ ☐ ☐

DBT PE Session 3 Checklist

Therapist: _____ Client: _____ Date: _____

Session Components	Yes	No
1. Review the DBT diary card and set an agenda for the session.	☐	☐
2. Review homework, give feedback, and address homework noncompletion (if needed).	☐	☐
3. Explain that cognitive avoidance works temporarily to reduce distress, but maintains PTSD in the long run by preventing new learning about the trauma.	☐	☐
4. Use a metaphor to explain why it is important to process trauma.	☐	☐
5. Explain that imaginal exposure and processing work to reduce PTSD by: a. Learning that thinking and talking about the trauma is safe b. Organizing the trauma memory into a coherent narrative c. Increasing the ability to tolerate intense emotions d. Reducing the intensity of distress over time (habituation) e. Building mastery and enhancing control f. Gaining a new and more helpful perspective on the trauma and its meaning	☐ ☐ ☐ ☐ ☐ ☐	☐ ☐ ☐ ☐ ☐ ☐
6. Give instructions on how to do imaginal exposure (eyes closed/present tense, describe in detail without avoiding, stick to the facts, repeat the story).	☐	☐
7. Describe the therapist's role during imaginal exposure (listening without responding, assessing SUDS, encouraging, coaching as needed).	☐	☐
8. Ask client to complete the "before" ratings on the Exposure Recording Form (DBT PE Handout 8 or 8A).	☐	☐
9. Conduct imaginal exposure for 20–45 minutes.	☐	☐
10. During imaginal exposure: a. Monitor SUDS about every 5 minutes. b. Provide reinforcement. c. Provide coaching (if needed).	☐ ☐ ☐	☐ ☐ ☐
11. Ask client to complete the "peak" and "after" ratings on the Exposure Recording Form.	☐	☐
12. Conduct processing for 15–30 minutes.	☐	☐
13. During processing: a. Target specific emotions and problematic beliefs that are maintaining PTSD. b. Help the client to acquire, strengthen, and generalize new learning. c. Use a variety of DBT acceptance, change, and dialectical strategies to promote change.	☐ ☐ ☐	☐ ☐ ☐
14. Assign homework: a. Complete *in vivo* exposure tasks (ideally daily) and fill out an Exposure Recording Form (DBT PE Handout 8 or 8A) each time. b. Listen to the imaginal exposure recording (ideally daily) and fill out an Exposure Recording Form (DBT PE Handout 8 or 8A) each time. c. Use the Post-Exposure Skills Plan (DBT PE Handout 3) (as needed). d. Listen to the entire session recording one time.	☐ ☐ ☐ ☐	☐ ☐ ☐ ☐

DBT PE Sessions 4+ Checklist

Therapist: _____ Client: _____ Date: _____

Session Components	Yes	No
1. Review the DBT diary card and set an agenda for the session.	☐	☐
2. Review homework, give feedback, and address homework noncompletion (if needed).	☐	☐
3. If advancing to hot spots, orient to the rationale for focusing imaginal exposure on hot spots and help client select a hot spot to target. ☐ N/A	☐	☐
4. If advancing to a new trauma memory, help client select the next trauma. ☐ N/A	☐	☐
5. Orient to the imaginal exposure planned for that session and give instructions about how to optimize its effectiveness.	☐	☐
6. Ask client to complete the "before" ratings on the Exposure Recording Form (DBT PE Handout 8 or 8A).	☐	☐
7. Conduct imaginal exposure for 20–45 minutes.	☐	☐
8. During imaginal exposure: a. Monitor SUDS about every 5 minutes. b. Provide reinforcement. c. Provided coaching (if needed).	☐ ☐ ☐	☐ ☐ ☐
9. Ask client to complete the "peak" and "after" ratings on the Exposure Recording Form.	☐	☐
10. Conduct processing for 20–45 minutes.	☐	☐
11. During processing: a. Target specific emotions and problematic beliefs that are maintaining PTSD. b. Help the client to acquire, strengthen, and generalize new learning. c. Use a variety of DBT acceptance, change, and dialectical strategies to promote change.	☐ ☐ ☐	☐ ☐ ☐
12. Assign homework: a. Complete *in vivo* exposure tasks (ideally daily) and fill out an Exposure Recording Form (DBT PE Handout 8 or 8A) each time. b. Listen to the imaginal exposure recording (ideally daily) and fill out an Exposure Recording Form (DBT PE Handout 8 or 8A) each time. c. Use the Post-Exposure Skills Plan (DPT PE Handout 3) (as needed). d. Listen to the entire session recording one time.	☐ ☐ ☐ ☐	☐ ☐ ☐ ☐

DBT PE Final Session Checklist

Therapist: _____ Client: _____ Date: _____

Session Components	Yes	No
1. Review the DBT diary card and set an agenda for the session.	☐	☐
2. Review homework, give feedback, and address homework noncompletion (if needed).	☐	☐
3. Orient to the imaginal exposure planned for that session.	☐	☐
4. Ask client to complete the "before" ratings on the Exposure Recording Form (DBT PE Handout 8 or 8A).	☐	☐
5. Conduct imaginal exposure by having the client recount the full trauma memory one time.	☐	☐
6. Ask client to complete the "peak" and "after" ratings on the Exposure Recording Form.	☐	☐
7. Review progress with imaginal exposure and processing, including key changes in emotions and beliefs that have occurred.	☐	☐
8. Ask client to rate current SUDS for each item on the *in vivo* exposure hierarchy (DBT PE Handout 7).	☐	☐
9. Review progress with *in vivo* exposure, including key changes in emotions and beliefs that have occurred.	☐	☐
10. Review the goals of relapse prevention and management (DBT PE Handout 11).	☐	☐
11. Explain the importance of continuing to do exposure: a. Ask client to identify *in vivo* and imaginal exposure tasks to keep working on (DBT PE Handout 12). b. Discuss guidelines for doing exposure effectively (DBT PE Handout 13).	☐ ☐	☐ ☐
12. Teach the FREE skill (DBT PE Handouts 14 and 15).	☐	☐
13. Identify risk factors for a relapse of PTSD (DBT PE Handouts 16 and 17).	☐	☐
14. Discuss how to manage an increase in PTSD (DBT PE Handouts 18 and 19).	☐	☐
15. Assign homework to practice the FREE skill (DBT PE Handout 15).	☐	☐

APPENDIX D

POTENTIAL SCREENING AND OUTCOME MONITORING MEASURES

Measure	Type	No. of items	Content	Reference
PTSD				
PTSD Checklist for DSM-5 (PCL-5)	SR	20	Assesses the 20 DSM-5 PTSD symptoms.	Weathers, F. W., Litz, B. T., Keane, T. M., Palmieri, P. A., Marx, B. P., & Schnurr, P. P. (2013). *The PTSD Checklist for DSM-5 (PCL-5)*. National Center for PTSD. https://www.ptsd.va.gov/professional/assessment/documents/PCL5_Standard_form.PDF
PTSD Symptom Scale—Interview for DSM-5 (PSS-I-5)	I	24	Screens for Criterion A trauma and assesses the frequency and intensity of the 20 DSM-5 PTSD symptoms.	Foa, E. B., McLean, C. P., Zang, Y., Zong, J., Rauch, S., Porter, K., . . . Kauffman, B. (2016). Psychometric properties of the Posttraumatic Stress Disorder Symptoms Scale Interview for DSM-5 (PSSI-5). *Psychological Assessment, 28*, 1159–1165.
Clinician- Administered PTSD Scale for DSM-5 (CAPS-5)	I	30	Assesses the 20 DSM-5 PTSD symptoms, as well as their onset, duration, and impact on functioning.	Weathers, F. W., Blake, D. D., Schnurr, P. P., Kaloupek, D. G., Marx, B. P., & Keane, T. M. (2013). *The Clinician-Administered PTSD Scale for DSM-5 (CAPS-5)*. National Center for PTSD. https://www.ptsd.va.gov/professional/assessment/adult-int/caps.asp
Exposure to Potentially Traumatic Events				
Life Events Checklist for DSM-5 (LEC-5)	SR	16	Screens lifetime exposure to various Criterion A traumas.	Weathers, F. W., Blake, D. D., Schnurr, P. P., Kaloupek, D. G., Marx, B. P., & Keane, T. M. (2013). *The Life Events Checklist for DSM-5 (LEC-5)*. National Center for PTSD. https://www.ptsd.va.gov/professional/assessment/documents/LEC5_Standard_Self-report.PDF
Invalidating Childhood Environment Scale (ICES)	SR	18	Assesses parental invalidation during childhood.	Mountford, V., Corstorphine, E., Tomlinson, S., & Waller, G. (2007). Development of a measure to assess invalidating childhood environments in the eating disorders. *Eating Behaviors, 8*, 48–58.
Everyday Discrimination Scale (EDS)	SR	9	Screens types and frequency of everyday discrimination based on race/ethnicity, sexual orientation, etc.	Williams, D. R., Yu, Y., Jackson, J. S., & Anderson, N. B. (1997). Racial differences in physical and mental health: Socio-economic status, stress and discrimination. *Journal of Health Psychology, 2*, 335–351.

(continued)

Note. SR, self-report; I, interview.

Measure	Type	No. of items	Content	Reference
Mechanisms of Change in PTSD				
Posttraumatic Cognitions Inventory (PTCI)	SR	36	Assesses negative beliefs about the self, the world, and self-blame.	Foa, E. B., Ehlers, A., Clark, D. M., Tolin, D. F., & Orsillo, S. M. (1999). The Posttraumatic Cognitions Inventory (PTCI): Development and validation. *Psychological Assessment, 11,* 303–314.
Trauma-Related Guilt Inventory (TRGI)	SR	32	Assesses global guilt and guilt cognitions related to hindsight bias, wrongdoing, and lack of justification.	Kubany, E. S., Haynes, S. N., Abueg, F. R., Manke, F. P., Brennan, J. M., & Stahura, C. (1996). Development and validation of the Trauma-Related Guilt Inventory (TRGI). *Psychological Assessment, 8,* 428–444.
Trauma-Related Shame Inventory (TRSI)	SR	24	Assesses internal and external shame related to trauma.	Oktedalen, T., Hagtvet, K. A., Hoffart, A., Langkaas, T. F., & Smucker, M. (2014). The Trauma-Related Shame Inventory: Measuring trauma-related shame among patients with PTSD. *Journal of Psychopathology and Behavioral Assessment, 36,* 600–615.
Trauma-Related Problems				
Dissociative Experiences Scale–II (DES-II)	SR	28	Screens for dissociative disorders.	Carlson, E. B., & Putnam, F. W. (1993). An update on the Dissociative Experience Scale. *Dissociation, 6,* 16–27.
Trauma Symptoms of Discrimination Scale (TSDS)	SR	21	Assesses trauma symptoms resulting from experiences of discrimination.	Williams, M. T., Printz, D. M. B., & DeLapp, R. C. T. (2018). Assessing racial trauma with the Trauma Symptoms of Discrimination Scale. *Psychology of Violence, 8,* 735–747.
Borderline Symptom List–23 (BSL-23)	SR	23	Assesses symptoms typical of borderline personality disorder.	Bohus, M., Kleindienst, N., Limberger, M. F., Stieglitz, R., Domsalla, M., Chapman, A. L., . . . Wolf, M. (2009). The short version of the Borderline Symptom List (BSL-23): Development and initial data on psychometric properties. *Psychopathology, 42,* 32–39.
Difficulties in Emotion Regulation Scale (DERS)	SR	36	Measures multiple aspects of emotion dysregulation.	Gratz, K. L., & Roemer, L. (2004). Multidimensional assessment of emotion regulation and dysregulation: Development, factor structure, and initial validation of the Difficulties in Emotion Regulation Scale. *Journal of Psychopathology and Behavioral Assessment, 26,* 41–54.
Inventory of Complicated Grief (ICG)	SR	19	Assesses indicators of complicated grief, such as anger, disbelief, and intrusive thoughts.	Prigerson, H. G., Maciejewski, P. K., Reynolds, C. F., Bierhals, A. J., Newsom, J. T., Fasiczka, A., . . . Miller, M. (1995). Inventory of Complicated Grief: A scale to measure maladaptive symptoms of loss. *Psychiatry Research, 59,* 65–79.

References

Adrian, M., McCauley, E., Berk, M. S., Asarnow, J. R., Korslund, K., Avina, C., . . . Linehan, M. M. (2019). Predictors and moderators of recurring self-harm in adolescents participating in a comparative treatment trial of psychological interventions. *Journal of Child Psychology and Psychiatry, 60,* 1123–1132.

Alegría, M., Fortuna, L. R., Lin, J. Y., Norris, L. F., Gao, S., Takeuchi, D. T., . . . Valentine, A. (2013). Prevalence, risk, and correlates of posttraumatic stress disorder across ethnic and racial minority groups in the U.S. *Medical Care, 51,* 1114–1123.

American Psychiatric Association. (2013). *Diagnostic and statistical manual of mental disorders* (5th ed.). Arlington, VA: Author.

Balsam, K. F., Lehavot, K., Beadnell, B., & Circo, E. (2010). Childhood abuse and mental health indicators among ethnically diverse lesbian, gay, and bisexual adults. *Journal of Consulting and Clinical Psychology, 78,* 459–468.

Bandermann, K. M., & Szymanski, D. M. (2014). Exploring coping mediators between heterosexist oppression and posttraumatic stress symptoms among lesbian, gay, and bisexual persons. *Psychology of Sexual Orientation and Gender Diversity, 1,* 213–224.

Benuto, L. T., Bennett, N. M., & Casas, J. B. (2020). Minority participation in randomized controlled trials for prolonged exposure therapy: A systematic review of the literature. *Journal of Traumatic Stress, 33,* 420–431.

Bohus, M., Dyer, A. S., Priebe, K., Krüger, A., Kleindienst, N., Schmahl, C., . . . Steil, R. (2013). Dialectical behaviour therapy for post-traumatic stress disorder after childhood sexual abuse in patients with and without borderline personality disorder: A randomised controlled trial. *Psychotherapy and Psychosomatics, 82,* 221–233.

Bohus, M., Kleindienst, N., Hahn, C., Müller-Engelmann, M., Ludäscher, P., . . . Priebe, K. (2020). Dialectical behavior therapy for posttraumatic stress disorder (DBT-PTSD) compared with cognitive processing therapy (CPT) in complex presentations of PTSD in women survivors of childhood abuse: A randomized clinical trial. *JAMA Psychiatry, 77,* 1235–1245.

Bor, J., Venkataramani, A. S., Williams, D. R., & Tsai, A. (2018). Police killings and their spillover effects on the mental health of Black Americans: A population-based, quasi-experimental study. *The Lancet, 392,* 302–310.

Bradley, R., Greene, J., Russ, E., Dutra, L., & Westen, D. (2005). A multidimensional meta-analysis of psychotherapy for PTSD. *American Journal of Psychiatry, 162,* 214–227.

Brand, B. L., Classen, C. C., Lanius, R., Loewenstein, R. J., McNary, S. W., Pain, C., & Putnam, F. W. (2009). A naturalistic study of dissociative identity disorder and dissociative disorder not otherwise specified patients treated by community clinicians. *Psychological Trauma: Theory, Research, Practice, and Policy, 1,* 153–171.

Brand, B. L., Classen, C. C., McNary, S. W., & Zaveri, P. (2009). A review of dissociative disorders treatment studies. *Journal of Nervous and Mental Disease, 197,* 646–654.

Brand, R. M., Hardy, A., Bendall, S., & Thomas, N. (2020). A tale of two outcomes: Remission and exacerbation in the use of trauma-focused imaginal exposure for trauma-related voice-hearing: Key learnings to guide future practice. *Clinical Psychologist, 24,* 176–185.

Brand, R. M., McEnery, C., Rossell, S., Bendall, S., & Thomas, N. (2018). Do trauma-focused psychological interventions have an effect on psychotic symptoms?: A systematic review and meta-analysis. *Schizophrenia Research, 195,* 13–22.

Briere, J., Kaltman, S., & Green, B. L. (2008). Accumulated childhood trauma and symptom complexity. *Journal of Traumatic Stress, 21,* 223–226.

Brown, J. F. (2015). *The emotion regulation skills system for cognitively challenged clients: A DBT-informed approach.* New York: Guilford Press.

Brown, J. F., Brown, M. Z., & Dibiasio, P. (2013). Treating individuals with intellectual disabilities and challenging behaviors with adapted dialectical behavior therapy. *Journal of Mental Health Research in Intellectual Disabilities, 6,* 280–303.

Bryant-Davis, T., & Ocampo, C. (2005). Racist incident-based trauma. *Counseling Psychologist, 33,* 479–500.

Carter, R. T. (2007). Racism and psychological and emotional injury: Recognizing and assessing race-based traumatic stress. *The Counseling Psychologist, 35,* 13–105.

Cloitre, M., Henn-Haase, C., Herman, J. L., Jackson, C., Kaslow, N., Klein, C., . . . Petkova, E. (2014). A multi-site single-blind clinical study to compare the effects of STAIR narrative therapy to treatment as usual among women with PTSD in public sector mental health settings: Study protocol for a randomized controlled trial. *Trials, 15,* 197.

Cloitre, M., Koenen, K. C., Cohen, L. R., & Han, H. (2002). Skills training in affective and interpersonal regulation followed by exposure: A phase-based treatment for PTSD related to childhood abuse. *Journal of Consulting and Clinical Psychology, 70,* 1067–1074.

Cloitre, M., Stolbach, B. C., Herman, J. L., van der Kolk, B., Pynoos, R., Wang, J., & Petkova, E. (2009). A developmental approach to complex PTSD: Childhood and adult cumulative trauma as predictors of symptom complexity. *Journal of Traumatic Stress, 22,* 399–408.

Cooper, A. A., Kline, A. C., Graham, B., Bedard-Gilligan, M., Mello, P. G., Feeny, N. C., & Zoellner, L. A. (2017). Homework "dose," type, and helpfulness as predictors of clinical outcomes in prolonged exposure for PTSD. *Behavior Therapy, 48,* 182–194.

Craske, M. G., Kircanski, K., Zelikowsky, M., Mystkowski, J., Chowdhury, N., & Baker, A. (2008). Optimizing inhibitory learning during exposure therapy. *Behaviour Research and Therapy, 46,* 5–27.

Craske, M. G., Treanor, M., Conway, C., Zbozinek, T., & Vervliet, B. (2014). Maximizing exposure therapy: An inhibitory learning approach. *Behaviour Research and Therapy, 58,* 10–23.

DeCou, C. R., Comtois, K. A., & Landes, S. J. (2018). Dialectical behavior is effective for the treatment of suicidal behavior: A meta-analysis. *Behavior Therapy, 50,* 60–72.

Department of Veterans Affairs/Department of Defense. (2017). *Clinical practice guideline for the management of posttraumatic stress disorder and acute stress disorder.* www.healthquality.va.gov/guidelines/MH/ptsd

Department of Veterans Affairs/Department of Defense. (2019). *Clinical practice guideline for the assessment and management of patients at risk for suicide.* www.healthquality.va.gov/guidelines/mh/srb/index.asp

Dunkley, C. (2020). *Regulating emotion the DBT way: A therapist's guide to opposite action.* London: Routledge.

Eftekhari, A., Ruzek, J. I., Crowley, J. J., Rosen, C. S., Greenbaum, M. A., & Karlin, B. E. (2013).

Effectiveness of national implementation of prolonged exposure therapy in Veterans Affairs care. *JAMA Psychiatry, 70,* 949–955.

Ehlers, A., Grey, N., Wild, J., Stott, R., Liness, S., Deale, A., . . . Clark, D. M. (2013). Implementation of cognitive therapy for PTSD in routine clinical care: Effectiveness and moderators of outcome in a consecutive sample. *Behaviour Research and Therapy, 51,* 742–752.

Feeny, N. C., Zoellner, L. A., & Foa, E. B. (2002). Treatment outcome for chronic PTSD among female assault victims with borderline personality characteristics: A preliminary examination. *Journal of Personality Disorders, 16,* 30–40.

Feeny, N. C., Zoellner, L. A., Mavissakalian, M. R., & Roy-Byrne, P. P. (2009). What would you choose?: Sertraline or prolonged exposure in community and PTSD treatment seeking women. *Depression and Anxiety, 26,* 724–731.

Felmingham, K. L., & Bryant, R. A. (2012). Gender differences in the maintenance of response to cognitive behavior therapy for posttraumatic stress disorder. *Journal of Consulting and Clinical Psychology, 80,* 196–200.

Finkelhor, D., Turner, H. A., Shattuck, A., & Hamby, S. L. (2015). Prevalence of childhood exposure to violence, crime, and abuse: Results from the National Survey of Children's Exposure to Violence. *JAMA Pediatrics, 169,* 746–754.

Fitzpatrick, S., Ip, J., Krantz, L., Zeifman, R., & Kuo, J. R. (2019). Use your words: The role of emotion labeling in regulating emotion in borderline personality disorder. *Behaviour Research and Therapy, 120,* 103447.

Foa, E. B., Chrestman, K. R., & Gilboa-Schechtman, E. (2008). *Prolonged exposure therapy for adolescents with PTSD: Emotional processing of traumatic experiences.* Oxford, UK: Oxford University Press.

Foa, E. B., Dancu, C. V., Hembree, E. A., Jaycox, L. H., Meadows, E. A., & Street, G. P. (1999). A comparison of exposure therapy, stress inoculation training, and their combination for reducing posttraumatic stress disorder in female assault victims. *Journal of Consulting and Clinical Psychology, 67,* 194–200.

Foa, E. B., Ehlers, A., Clark, D. M., Tolin, D. F., & Orsillo, S. M. (1999). The Posttraumatic Cognitions Inventory (PTCI): Development and validation. *Psychological Assessment, 11,* 303–314.

Foa, E. B., Hembree, E. A., Feeny, N. C., Cahill, S. P., Rauch, S. A. M., Riggs, D. S., & Yadin, E. (2005). Randomized trial of prolonged exposure for posttraumatic stress disorder with and without cognitive restructuring: Outcomes at academic and community clinics. *Journal of Consulting and Clinical Psychology, 73,* 953–964.

Foa, E. B., Hembree, E. A., Rothbaum, B. O., & Rauch, S. A. M. (2019). *Prolonged exposure therapy for PTSD: Emotional processing of traumatic experiences* (2nd ed.). Oxford, UK: Oxford University Press.

Foa, E. B., & Kozak, M. J. (1986). Emotional processing of fear: Exposure to corrective information. *Psychological Bulletin, 99,* 20–35.

Foa, E. B., McLean, C. P., Capaldi, S., & Rosenfield, D. (2013). Prolonged exposure vs supportive counseling for sexual abuse-related PTSD in adolescent girls: A randomized clinical trial. *Journal of the American Medical Association, 310,* 2650–2657.

Foa, E. B., McLean, C. P., Zang, Y., Rosenfield, D., Yadin, E., Yarvis, J., . . . Peterson, A. L. (2018). Effect of prolonged exposure therapy delivered over 2 weeks vs 8 weeks vs present-centered therapy on PTSD symptom severity in military personnel: A randomized clinical trial. *JAMA Psychiatry, 319,* 354–364.

Foa, E. B., Riggs, D. S., Massie, E. D., & Yarczower, M. (1995). The impact of fear activation and anger on the efficacy of exposure treatment for posttraumatic stress disorder. *Behavior Therapy, 26,* 487–499.

Foa, E. B., Rothbaum, B. O., Riggs, D. S., & Murdock, T. B. (1991). Treatment of posttraumatic stress disorder in rape victims: A comparison between cognitive-behavioral procedures and counseling. *Journal of Consulting and Clinical Psychology, 59,* 715–723.

Foa, E. B., Zoellner, L. A., Feeny, N. C., Hembree, E. A., & Alvarez-Conrad, J. (2002). Does imaginal exposure exacerbate PTSD symptoms? *Journal of Consulting and Clinical Psychology, 70,* 1022–1028.

Foote, B., & Van Orden, K. (2016). Adapting dialectical behavior therapy for the treatment of dissociative identity disorder. *American Journal of Psychotherapy, 70,* 343–364.

Galovski, T. E., Blain, L. M., Chappuis, C., & Fletcher, T. (2013). Sex differences in recovery from PTSD in male and female interpersonal assault survivors. *Behaviour Research and Therapy, 51,* 247–255.

Gilboa-Schechtman, E., Foa, E. B., Shafran, N., Aderka, I. M., Powers, M. B., Rachamim, L., . . . Apter, A. (2010). Prolonged exposure versus dynamic therapy for adolescent PTSD: A pilot randomized controlled trial. *Journal of the American Academy of Child and Adolescent Psychiatry, 49,* 1034–1042.

Goodman, M., Banthin, D., Blair, N. J., Mascitelli, K. A., Wilsnack, J., Chen, J., . . . New, A. S. (2016). A randomized trial of dialectical behavior therapy in high-risk suicidal veterans. *Journal of Clinical Psychiatry, 77,* e1591–e1600.

Haagen, J. F. G., Smid, G. E., Knipscheer, J. W., & Kleber, R. J. (2015). The efficacy of recommended treatments for veterans with PTSD: A metaregression analysis. *Clinical Psychology Review, 40,* 184–194.

Hagenaars, M. A., van Minnen, A., & Hoogduin, K. A. L. (2010). The impact of dissociation and depression on the efficacy of prolonged exposure treatment for PTSD. *Behaviour Research and Therapy, 48,* 19–27.

Harned, M. S., Chapman, A. L., Dexter-Mazza, E. T., Murray, A., Comtois, K. A., & Linehan, M. M. (2008). Treating co-occurring axis I disorders in recurrently suicidal women with borderline personality disorder: A 2-year randomized trial of dialectical behavior therapy versus community treatment by experts. *Journal of Consulting and Clinical Psychology, 76,* 1068–1075.

Harned, M. S., Coyle, T. N., & Garcia, N. M. (2022). The inclusion of ethnoracial, sexual, and gender minority groups in randomized controlled trials of dialectical behavior therapy: A systematic review of the literature. *Clinical Psychology: Science and Practice.*

Harned, M. S., Fitzpatrick, S., & Schmidt, S. C. (2020). Identifying change targets for PTSD among suicidal and self-injuring women with borderline personality disorder. *Journal of Traumatic Stress, 33,* 610–616.

Harned, M. S., Gallop, R. J., & Valenstein-Mah, H. R. (2018). What changes when?: The course of improvement during a stage-based treatment for suicidal and self-injuring women with borderline personality disorder and PTSD. *Psychotherapy Research, 28,* 761–775.

Harned, M. S., Jackson, S. C., Comtois, K. A., & Linehan, M. M. (2010). Dialectical behavior therapy as a precursor to PTSD treatment for suicidal and/or self-injuring women with borderline personality disorder. *Journal of Traumatic Stress, 23,* 421–429.

Harned, M. S., Korslund, K. E., Foa, E. B., & Linehan, M. M. (2012). Treating PTSD in suicidal and self-injuring women with borderline personality disorder: Development and preliminary evaluation of a dialectical behavior therapy prolonged exposure protocol. *Behaviour Research and Therapy, 50,* 381–386.

Harned, M. S., Korslund, K. E., & Linehan, M. M. (2014). A pilot randomized controlled trial of dialectical behavior therapy with and without the dialectical behavior therapy prolonged exposure protocol for suicidal and self-injuring women with borderline personality disorder and PTSD. *Behaviour Research and Therapy, 55,* 7–17.

Harned, M. S., & Linehan, M. M. (2008). Integrating dialectical behavior therapy and prolonged exposure to treat co-occurring borderline personality disorder and PTSD: Two case studies. *Cognitive and Behavioral Practice, 15,* 263–276.

Harned, M. S., Ritschel, L. A., & Schmidt, S. C. (2021). Effects of workshop training in the dialectical behavior therapy prolonged exposure protocol on clinician beliefs, adoption, and perceived clinical outcomes. *Journal of Traumatic Stress, 34,* 427–439.

Harned, M. S., Rizvi, S. L., & Linehan, M. M. (2010). Impact of co-occurring posttraumatic stress disorder on suicidal women with borderline personality disorder. *American Journal of Psychiatry, 167,* 1210–1217.

Harned, M. S., Ruork, A. K., Liu, J., & Tkachuck, M. A. (2015). Emotional activation and habituation during imaginal exposure for PTSD among women with borderline personality disorder. *Journal of Traumatic Stress, 28,* 253–257.

Harned, M. S., & Schmidt, S. C. (2019). Perspectives on a stage-based treatment for PTSD among dialectical behavior therapy consumers in public mental health settings. *Community Mental Health Journal, 55,* 409–419.

Harned, M. S., Schmidt, S. C., Korslund, K. E., & Gallop, R. J. (2021). Does adding the dialectical behavior therapy prolonged exposure (DBT PE) protocol for PTSD to DBT improve outcomes in public mental health settings?: A pilot nonrandomized effectiveness trial with benchmarking. *Behavior Therapy, 52,* 639–655.

Harned, M. S., Tkachuck, M. A., & Youngberg, K. A. (2013). Treatment preference among suicidal and self-injuring women with borderline personality disorder and PTSD. *Journal of Clinical Psychology, 69,* 749–761.

Harned, M. S., Wilks, C. R., Schmidt, S. C., & Coyle, T. N. (2018). Improving functional outcomes in borderline personality disorder by changing PTSD severity and post-traumatic cognitions. *Behaviour Research and Therapy, 103,* 53–61.

Harrell, S. P. (2000). A multidimensional conceptualization of racism-related stress: Implications for the well-being of people of color. *American Journal of Orthopsychiatry, 70,* 42–57.

Hatzenbuehler, M. L. (2009). How does sexual minority stigma "get under the skin"?: A psychological mediation framework. *Psychological Bulletin, 135,* 707–730.

Hembree, E. A., Foa, E. B., Dorfan, N. M., Street, G. P., Kowalski, J., & Tu, X. (2003). Do patients drop out prematurely from exposure therapy for PTSD? *Journal of Traumatic Stress, 16,* 555–562.

Hendricks, M. L., & Testa, R. J. (2012). A conceptual framework for clinical work with transgender and gender nonconforming clients: An adaptation of the minority stress model. *Professional Psychology: Research and Practice, 43,* 460–467.

International Society for the Study of Trauma and Dissociation. (2011). Guidelines for treating dissociative identity disorder in adults, third revision. *Journal of Trauma and Dissociation, 12,* 115–187.

James, S. E., Herman, J. L., Rankin, S., Keisling, M., Mottet, L., & Anafi, M. (2016). *The report of the 2015 U.S. Transgender Survey.* National Center for Transgender Equality. www.transequality.org/sites/default/files/docs/usts/USTS%20Full%20Report%20-%20FINAL%201.6.17.pdf

Joseph, J. S., & Gray, M. J. (2011). The utility of measuring explanatory flexibility in PTSD research. *Cognitive Therapy Research, 35,* 372–380.

Joseph, J. S., & Gray, M. J. (2014). A pilot intervention targeting attribution style and rigidity following traumatic event exposure. *Psychological Trauma: Theory, Research, Practice, and Policy, 6,* 708–715.

Kaplan, C., Aguirre, B., & Galen, G. (2015, October). *Targeting PTSD in an adolescent BPD population: Pilot data using a DBT+PE protocol.* Paper presented at the McLean Hospital DBT Training Seminar, Belmont, MA.

Katz-Wise, S. L., & Hyde, J. S. (2012). Victimization experiences of lesbian, gay, and bisexual individuals: A meta-analysis. *Journal of Sex Research, 49,* 142–167.

Kehle-Forbes, S. M., Polusny, M. A., Erbes, C. R., & Gerould, H. (2014). Acceptability of prolonged exposure therapy among U.S. Iraq war veterans with PTSD symptomology. *Journal of Traumatic Stress, 27,* 483–487.

Kessler, R. C., Avenevoli, S., Costello, J., Georgiades, K., Green, J. G., Gruber, M. J., . . . Merikangas, K. R. (2012). Prevalence, persistence, and sociodemographic correlates of DSM-IV disorders in the National Comorbidity Survey Replication Adolescent Supplement. *Archives of General Psychiatry, 69,* 372–380.

Kessler, R. C., Mickelson, K. D., & Williams, D. R. (1999). The prevalence, distribution, and mental health correlates of perceived discrimination in the United States. *Journal of Health and Social Behavior, 40,* 208–230.

Kessler, R. C., Sonnega, A., Bromet, E., Hughes, M., & Nelson, C. B. (1995). Posttraumatic stress disorder in the National Comorbidity Survey. *Archives of General Psychiatry, 52,* 1048–1060.

Kircanski, K., Lieberman, M. D., & Craske, M. G. (2012). Feelings into words: Contributions of language to exposure therapy. *Psychological Science, 23,* 1086–1091.

Kleindienst, N., Priebe, K., Görg, N., Dyer, A., Steil, R., Lyssenko, L., . . . Bohus, M. (2016). State dissociation moderates response to dialectical behavior therapy for posttraumatic stress disorder in women with and without borderline personality disorder. *European Journal of Psychotraumatology, 7.*

Koons, C. R., Robins, C. J., Tweed, J. L., Lynch, T. R., Gonzalez, A. M., Morse, J. Q., . . . Bastian, L. A. (2001). Efficacy of dialectical behavior therapy in women veterans with borderline personality disorder. *Behavior Therapy, 32,* 371–390.

Kothgassner, O. D., Goreis, A., Robinson, K., Huscsava, M. M., Schmahl, C., & Plener, P. L. (2021). Efficacy of dialectical behavior therapy for adolescent self-harm and suicidal ideation: A systematic review and meta-analysis. *Psychological Medicine, 51,* 1057–1067.

Krüger, A., Kleindienst, N., Priebe, K., Dyer, A. S., Steil, R., Schmahl, C., & Bohus, M. (2014). Nonsuicidal self-injury during an exposure-based treatment in patients with posttraumatic stress disorder and borderline features. *Behaviour Research and Therapy, 61,* 136–141.

Landes, S. J., Rodriguez, A. L., Smith, B. N., Matthieu, M. M., Trent, L. R., Kemp, J., & Thompson, C. (2017). Barriers, facilitators, and benefits of implementation of dialectical behavior therapy in routine care: Results from a national program evaluation survey in the Veterans Health Administration. *Translational Behavioral Medicine, 7,* 832–844.

LeBouthillier, D. M., McMillan, K. A., Thibodeau, M. A., & Asmundson, G. J. G. (2015). Types and number of traumas associated with suicidal ideation and suicide attempts in PTSD: Findings from a U.S. nationally representative sample. *Journal of Traumatic Stress, 28,* 183–190.

Linehan, M. M. (1993). *Cognitive-behavioral treatment of borderline personality disorder.* New York: Guilford Press.

Linehan, M. M. (1999). Development, evaluation, and dissemination of effective psychosocial treatments: Levels of disorder, stages of care, and stages of treatment research. In M. G. Glantz & C. R. Hartel (Eds.), *Drug abuse: Origins and interventions* (pp. 367–394). Washington, DC: American Psychological Association.

Linehan, M. M. (2015). *DBT skills training manual* (2nd ed.). New York: Guilford Press.

Litz, B. T., Lebowitz, L., Gray, M. J., & Nash, W. P. (2016). *Adaptive disclosure: A new treatment for military trauma, loss, and moral injury.* New York: Guilford Press.

Livingston, N. A., Berke, D., Scholl, J., Ruben, M., & Shipherd, J. C. (2020). Addressing diversity in PTSD treatment: Clinical considerations and guidance for the treatment of PTSD in LGBTQ populations. *Current Treatment Options in Psychiatry, 16,* 1–17.

Lorber, W., & Garcia, H. A. (2010). Not supposed to feel this: Traditional masculinity in psychotherapy with male veterans returning from Afghanistan and Iraq. *Psychotherapy Theory, Research, Practice, and Training, 47,* 296–305.

Marlatt, G. A., & Gordon, J. R. (Eds.). (1985). *Relapse prevention: Maintenance strategies in the treatment of addictive behaviors.* New York: Guilford Press.

Martell, C. R., Dimidjian, S., & Herman-Dunn, R. (2013). *Behavioral activation for depression: A clinician's guide.* New York: Guilford Press.

McCauley, E., Berk, M. S., Asarnow, J. R., Adrian, M., Cohen, J., Korslund, K., . . . Linehan, M. M. (2018). Efficacy of dialectical behavior therapy for adolescents at high risk for suicide: A randomized clinical trial. *JAMA Psychiatry, 75,* 777–785.

McClendon, J., Dean, K. E., & Galovski, T. (2020). Addressing diversity in PTSD treatment: Disparities in treatment engagement and outcome among patients of color. *Current Treatment Options in Psychiatry, 7,* 275–290.

McLaughlin, A. A., Keller, S. M., Feeny, N. C., Youngstrom, E. A., & Zoellner, L. A. (2014). Patterns of therapeutic alliance: Rupture–repair episodes in prolonged exposure for posttraumatic stress disorder. *Journal of Consulting and Clinical Psychology, 82,* 112–121.

McLean, C. P., Asnaani, A., Litz, B. T., & Hofmann, S. G. (2011). Gender differences in anxiety disorders:

Prevalence, course of illness, comorbidity and burden of illness. *Journal of Psychiatric Research, 45,* 1027–1035.

McMain, S. F., Links, P. S., Gnam, W. H., Guimond, T., Cardish, R. J., Korman, L., & Streiner, D. L. (2009). A randomized trial of dialectical behavior therapy versus general psychiatric management for borderline personality disorder. *American Journal of Psychiatry, 166,* 1365–1374.

Mechanic, M. B., Weaver, T. L., & Resick, P. A. (2008). Mental health consequences of intimate partner abuse: A multidimensional assessment of four different forms of abuse. *Violence Against Women, 14,* 634–654.

Merikangas, K., He, J., Burstein, M., Swanson, S. A., Avenevoli, S., Cui, L., . . . Swendsen, J. (2010). Lifetime prevalence of mental disorders in US adolescents: Results from the National Comorbidity Study—Adolescent Supplement (NCS-A). *Journal of the American Academy of Child and Adolescent Psychiatry, 49,* 980–989.

Meyer, I. H. (2003). Prejudice, social stress, and mental health in lesbian, gay, and bisexual populations: Conceptual issues and research evidence. *Psychological Bulletin, 129,* 674–697.

Meyers, L., Voller, E. K., McCallum, E. B., Thuras, P., Shallcross, S., Velasquez, T., & Meis, L. (2017). Treating veterans with PTSD and borderline personality symptoms in a 12-week intensive outpatient setting: Findings from a pilot program. *Journal of Traumatic Stress, 30,* 178–181.

Miga, E. M., Neacsiu, A. D., Lungu, A., Heard, H. L., & Dimeff, L. A. (2019). Dialectical behaviour therapy from 1991–2015: What do we know about clinical efficacy and research quality? In M. Swales (Ed.), *The Oxford handbook of dialectical behaviour therapy* (pp. 467–496). Oxford, UK: Oxford University Press.

Miller, A. L., Rathus, J. H., & Linehan, M. M. (2007). *Dialectical behavior therapy with suicidal adolescents.* New York: Guilford Press.

Mills, K. L., Barrett, E. L., Merz, S., Rosenfeld, J., Ewer, P. L., Sannibale, C., . . . Teesson, M. (2016). Integrated exposure-based therapy for co-occurring post traumatic stress disorder (PTSD) and substance dependence: Predictors of change in PTSD symptom severity. *Journal of Clinical Medicine, 5,* 101.

Morland, L. A., Wells, S. Y., Glassman, L. H., Greene, C. J., Hoffman, J. E., & Rosen, C. S. (2020). Advances in PTSD treatment delivery: Review of findings and clinical considerations for the use of telehealth interventions for PTSD. *Current Treatment Options in Psychiatry, 30,* 1–21.

Morrison, A. P., Renton, J. C., Dunn, H., Williams, S., & Bentall, R. P. (2004). *Cognitive therapy for psychosis: A formulation-based approach.* Sussex, UK: Brunner-Routledge.

Mustanski, B., Andrews, R., Herrick, A., Stall, R., & Schnarrs, P. W. (2014). A syndemic of psychosocial health disparities and associations with risk for attempting suicide among young sexual minority men. *American Journal of Public Health, 104,* 287–294.

Nacasch, N., Huppert, J. D., Su, Y. J., Kivity, Y., Dinshtein, Y., Yeh, R., & Foa, E. B. (2015). Are 60-minute prolonged exposure sessions with 20-minute imaginal exposure to traumatic memories sufficient to successfully treat PTSD?: A randomized noninferiority clinical trial. *Behavior Therapy, 46,* 328–341.

Nagoski, E. (2021). *Come as you are: The surprising new science that will transform your sex life* (2nd ed.). New York: Simon & Schuster.

Neilson, E. C., Singh, R. S., Harper, K. L., & Teng, E. J. (2020). Traditional masculinity ideology, posttraumatic stress disorder (PTSD) symptom severity, and treatment in service members and veterans: A systematic review. *Psychology of Men and Masculinities, 21,* 578–592.

Pantalone, D. W., Sloan, C. A., & Carmel, A. (2019). Dialectical behavior therapy for borderline personality disorder and suicidality among sexual and gender minority individuals. In J. E. Pachankis & S. A. Safren (Eds.), *Handbook of evidence-based mental health practice with sexual and gender minorities* (pp. 408–429). New York: Oxford University Press.

Pantalone, D. W., Valentine, S. E., & Shipherd, J. C. (2017). Working with survivors of trauma in the sexual minority and transgender and gender nonconforming populations. In K. A. DeBord, A. R.

Fischer, K. J. Bieschke, & R. M. Perez (Eds.), *Handbook of sexual orientation and gender diversity in counseling and psychotherapy* (pp. 183–211). Washington, DC: American Psychological Association.

Persons, J. B. (2008). *The case formulation approach to cognitive-behavior therapy.* New York: Guilford Press.

Pieterse, A. L., Carter, R. T., Evans, S. A., & Walter, R. A. (2010). An exploratory examination of the associations among racial and ethnic discrimination, racial climate, and trauma-related symptoms in a college student population. *Journal of Counseling Psychology, 57,* 255–263.

Powers, M. B., Halpern, J. M., Ferenschak, M. P., Gillihan, S. J., & Foa, E. B. (2010). A meta-analytic review of prolonged exposure for posttraumatic stress disorder. *Clinical Psychology Review, 30,* 635–641.

Ragsdale, K. A., Gramlich, M. A., Beidel, D. C., Neer, S. M., Kitsmiller, E. G., & Morrison, K. I. (2018). Does traumatic brain injury attenuate the exposure therapy process? *Behavior Therapy, 49,* 617–630.

Ragsdale, K. A., & Voss Horrell, S. C. (2016). Effectiveness of prolonged exposure and cognitive processing therapy for U.S. veterans with a history of traumatic brain injury. *Journal of Traumatic Stress, 29,* 474–477.

Rathus, J. H., & Miller, A. L. (2015). *DBT skills manual for adolescents.* New York: Guilford Press.

Ready, D. J., Lamp, K., Rauch, S. A. M., Astin, M. C., & Norrholm, S. D. (2020). Extending prolonged exposure for veterans with posttraumatic stress disorder: When is enough really enough? *Psychological Services, 17,* 199–206.

Reisner, S. L., Hughto, J. M. W., Gamarel, K. E., Keuroghlian, A. S., Mizock, L., & Pachankis, J. (2016). Discriminatory experiences associated with posttraumatic stress disorder symptoms among transgender adults. *Journal of Counseling Psychology, 63,* 509–519.

Resick, P. A., Monson, C. M., & Chard, K. M. (2017). *Cognitive processing therapy for PTSD: A comprehensive manual.* New York: Guilford Press.

Rizvi, S. L., Vogt, D. S., & Resick, P. A. (2009). Cognitive and affective predictors of treatment outcome in cognitive processing therapy and prolonged exposure for posttraumatic stress disorder. *Behaviour Research and Therapy, 47,* 737–743.

Roberts, A. L., Austin, S. B., Corliss, H. L., Vandermorris, A. K., & Koenen, K. C. (2010). Pervasive trauma exposure among US sexual orientation minority adults and risk of posttraumatic stress disorder. *American Journal of Public Health, 100,* 2433–2441.

Roberts, A. L., Gilman, S. E., Breslau, J., Breslau, N., & Koenen, K. C. (2011). Race/ethnic differences in exposure to traumatic events, development of post-traumatic stress disorder, and treatment-seeking for post-traumatic stress disorder in the United States. *Psychological Medicine, 41,* 71–83.

Roberts, A. L., Rosario, M., Corliss, H. L., Koenen, K. C., & Austin, S. B. (2012). Elevated risk of posttraumatic stress in sexual minority youths: Mediation by childhood abuse and gender nonconformity. *American Journal of Public Health, 102,* 1587–1593.

Ronconi, J. M., Shiner, B., & Watts, B. V. (2014). Inclusion and exclusion criteria in randomized controlled trials of psychotherapy for PTSD. *Journal of Psychiatric Practice, 20,* 25–37.

Rosenfeld, B., Galietta, M., Foellmi, M., Coupland, S., Turner, Z., Stern, S., . . . Ivanoff, A. (2020). Dialectical behavior therapy (DBT) for the treatment of stalking offenders: A randomized controlled study. *Law and Human Behavior, 43,* 319–328.

Rowe, C., Santos, G. M., McFarland, W., & Wilson, E. C. (2015). Prevalence and correlates of substance use among trans female youth ages 16–24 years in the San Francisco Bay area. *Drug and Alcohol Dependence, 147,* 160–166.

Schultebraucks, K., Qian, M., Abu-Amara, D., Dean, K., Laska, E., Siegel, C., . . . Marmar, C. R. (2021). Pre-deployment risk factors for PTSD in active-duty personnel deployed to Afghanistan: A machine-learning approach for analyzing multivariate predictors. *Molecular Psychiatry, 26,* 5011–5022.

Schuyler, A. C., Klemmer, C., Mamey, M. R., Schrager, S. M., Goldbach, J. T., Holloway, I. W., & Castro,

C. A. (2020). Experiences of sexual harassment, stalking, and sexual assault during military service among LGBT and non-LGBT service members. *Journal of Interpersonal Violence, 33,* 257–266.

Shapiro, F. (2001). *Eye movement desensitization and reprocessing: Basic principles, protocols, and procedures* (2nd ed.). New York: Guilford Press.

Shear, M. K. (2015). *Complicated grief treatment.* Columbia Center for Complicated Grief, Columbia University. https://complicatedgrief.columbia.edu/professionals/manual-tools

Shipherd, J., Berke, D., & Livingston, N. (2019). Trauma recovery in the transgender and gender diverse (TGD) community: Extensions of the minority stress model for treatment planning. *Cognitive and Behavioral Practice, 26,* 629–646.

Shipherd, J. C., Maguen, S., Skidmore, W. C., & Abramovitz, S. M. (2011). Potentially traumatic events in a transgender sample: Frequency and associated symptoms. *Traumatology, 17,* 56–67.

Sibrava, N. J., Bjornsson, A. S., Pérez Benítez, A. C. I., Moitra, E., Weisberg, R. B., & Keller, M. B. (2019). Posttraumatic stress disorder in African American and Latino adults: Clinical course and the role of racial and ethnic discrimination. *American Psychologist, 74,* 101–116.

Spinazzola, J., Hodgdon, H., Liang, L., Ford, J. D., Layne, C. M., Pynoos, R., . . . Kisiel, C. (2014). Unseen wounds: The contribution of psychological maltreatment to child and adolescent mental health and risk outcomes. *Psychological Trauma: Theory, Research, Practice, and Policy, 6,* S18–S28.

Sripada, R. K., Rauch, S. A. M., Tuerk, P. W., Smith, E., Defever, A. M., Mayer, R. A., . . . Venners, M. (2013). Mild traumatic brain injury and treatment response in prolonged exposure for PTSD. *Journal of Traumatic Stress, 26,* 369–375.

Steil, R., & Ehlers, A. (2000). Dysfunctional meaning of posttraumatic intrusions in chronic PTSD. *Journal of Consulting and Clinical Psychology, 38,* 537–558.

Storebø, O. J., Stoffers-Winterling, J. M., Völlm, B. A., Kongerslev, M. T., Mattivi, J. T., Jørgensen, M. S., . . . Simonsen, E. (2020). Psychological therapies for people with borderline personality disorder. *Cochrane Database of Systematic Reviews, 5,* CD012955.

Sue, D. W., Capodilupo, C. M., Torino, G. C., Bucceri, J. M., Holder, A. M. B., Nadal, K. L., & Esquilin, M. (2007). Racial microaggressions in everyday life: Implications for clinical practice. *American Psychologist, 62,* 271–286.

Swan, S., Keen, N., Reynolds, N., & Onwumere, J. (2017). Psychological interventions for post-traumatic stress symptoms in psychosis: A systematic review of outcomes. *Frontiers in Psychology, 8,* 341.

Swenson, C. R. (2016). *DBT principles in action: Acceptance, change, and dialectics.* New York: Guilford Press.

Szymanski, D. M., & Balsam, K. F. (2011). Insidious trauma: Examining the relationship between heterosexism and lesbians' PTSD symptoms. *Traumatology, 17,* 4–13.

Tarrier, N., Sommerfield, C., Pilgrim, H., & Faragher, B. (2000). Factors associated with outcome of cognitive-behavioural treatment of chronic post-traumatic stress disorder. *Behaviour Research and Therapy, 38,* 191–202.

Tolin, D. F., & Foa, E. B. (2006). Sex differences in trauma and posttraumatic stress disorder: A quantitative review of 25 years of research. *Psychological Bulletin, 132,* 959–992.

Ullman, S. E. (2007). Relationship to perpetrator, disclosure, social reactions, and PTSD symptoms in child sexual abuse survivors. *Journal of Child Sexual Abuse, 16,* 19–36.

U.S. Census Bureau. (2019). *Quick facts: United States.* www.census.gov/quickfacts/fact/table/US/PST045219

Valera, R. J., Sawyer, R. G., & Schiraldi, G. R. (2001). Perceived health needs of inner-city street prostitutes: A preliminary study. *American Journal of Health Behavior, 25,* 50–59.

van den Berg, D. P. G., van der Vleugel, B. M., Staring, A. B. P., de Bont, P. A. J., & de Jongh, A. (2013). EMDR in psychosis: Guidelines for conceptualization and treatment. *Journal of EMDR Practice and Research, 7,* 208–224.

van Minnen, A., & Foa, E. B. (2006). The effect of imaginal exposure length on outcome of treatment for PTSD. *Journal of Traumatic Stress, 19,* 427–438.

van Minnen, A., Harned, M. S., Zoellner, L., & Mills, K. (2012). Examining potential contraindications for prolonged exposure therapy for PTSD. *European Journal of Psychotraumatology, 3,* 18805.

Weathers, F. W., Litz, B. T., Keane, T. M., Palmieri, P. A., Marx, B. P., & Schnurr, P. P. (2013). *The PTSD Checklist for DSM-5 (PCL-5).* National Center for PTSD. https://www.ptsd.va.gov/professional/assessment/documents/PCL5_Standard_form.PDF

Williams, M. T., Malcoun, E., Sawyer, B., Davis, D. M., Bahojb-Nouri, L. V., & Leavell Bruce, S. (2014). Cultural adaptations of prolonged exposure therapy for treatment and prevention of posttraumatic stress disorder in African Americans. *Behavioral Sciences— Special Issue: PTSD and Treatment Considerations, 4,* 102–124.

Wilson, L. (2018). The prevalence of military sexual trauma: A meta-analysis. *Trauma, Violence, and Abuse, 19,* 584–597.

Wisco, B. E., Marx, B. P., Wolf, E. J., Miller, M. W., Southwick, S. M., & Pietrzak, R. H. (2014). Posttraumatic stress disorder in the US veteran population: Results from the National Health and Resilience in Veterans Study. *Journal of Clinical Psychiatry, 75,* 1338–1346.

Wolf, G. K., Kretzmer, T., Crawford, E., Thors, C., Wagner, H. R., Strom, T. Q., . . . Vanderploeg, R. D. (2015). Prolonged exposure therapy with veterans and active duty personnel diagnosed with PTSD and traumatic brain injury. *Journal of Traumatic Stress, 28,* 339–347.

World Health Organization. (2018). *International classification of diseases for mortality and morbidity statistics* (11th revision). https://icd.who.int/browse11/l-m/en

Zanarini, M. C., Hörz, S., Frankenburg, F. R., Weingeroff, J., Reich, D. B., & Fitzmaurice, G. (2011). The 10-year course of PTSD in borderline patients and axis II comparison subjects. *Acta Psychiatric Scandinavica, 124,* 349–356.

Zang, Y., Su, Y., McLean, C. P., & Foa, E. B. (2019). Predictors for excellent versus partial response to prolonged exposure therapy: Who needs additional sessions? *Journal of Traumatic Stress, 32,* 577–585.

Zoellner, L. A., Roy-Byrne, P. P., Mavissakalian, M., & Feeny, N. C. (2019). Doubly randomized preference trial of prolonged exposure versus sertraline for treatment of PTSD. *American Journal of Psychiatry, 176,* 287–296.

Index

Note. Page numbers followed by *f* or *t* indicate a figure or a table.

Identity, 266*t*
If–then relationships, 39–42
Ignoring treatment type of invalidating
    behavior
  overview, 24*t*
  treating racial and ethnic minorities,
      342*t*
  treating sexual and gender minorities
      and, 350*t*
  See also Traumatic invalidation
Imaginal exposure
  anger and, 289
  anxiety regarding, 172–173
  avoidance during, 213–215, 214*t*
  case examples illustrating, 175–178,
      181–183, 189–191, 190*f*, 211–213,
      215, 225–227, 226*f*, 231–233
  case formulation and, 102, 104
  child sexual abuse and, 306–307
  conducting during Session 3, 183–191,
      190*f*
  continuing to practice following the end
      of treatment, 236–238
  corrective information and, 260–261
  emotional activation and, 254, 258–259
  fear and, 281
  during the final session, 230–233
  instructions on how to do, 179–183
  during the intermediate sessions
      (sessions 4+), 208–220, 214*t*, 217*f*
  joint and family sessions and, 167–169
  ordering of target traumas for, 124–125
  orienting to DBT PE protocol in
      pretreatment and, 36*t*
  planning for, 135
  progression of, 216–220, 217*f*
  rationale for, 174–179, 175*t*
  selecting treatment targets and, 117–118
  sexual assault and rape and, 324
  theoretical influences of DBT and, 8
  Trauma Interview and, 115, 124–129
  trauma narratives and, 125–129
  traumatic invalidation and, 318–319
  treating racial and ethnic minorities
      and, 344
  See also Exposure techniques; Post-
      Exposure DBT Skills Plan; Trauma
      narrative; Trauma
      processing
Imminent threat, 18, 19*t*
Impairment
  client readiness and, 78–79
  determining appropriateness for
      integrated DBT + DBT PE
      treatment and, 27
  pretreatment preparation for integrating
      DBT PE into DBT and, 34
  selecting treatment targets and, 118,
      119–120
  See also Disability
Implementation, 15–16, 102, 104
Improvement, lack of, 235
In vivo exposure
  case examples illustrating, 144–146,
      155–159, 162, 234–235
  case formulation and, 102, 104
  constructing a hierarchy for, 147–162,
      150*t*, 152*t*

continuing to practice following the end
    of treatment, 236–238
disgust and, 299
emotional activation and, 254, 258–259
Exposure Recording Form and, 161–162
fear and, 281
following session 3, 205
following sessions 4+ (intermediate
    sessions), 228
instructions on how to do, 160
joint and family sessions and, 165,
    167–169
orienting to DBT PE protocol in
    pretreatment and, 36*t*
rationale for, 143–146, 144*t*
rerating the exposure hierarchy and
    reviewing progress during the
    final session, 233–235
reviewing in session 3, 173–174, 174*t*
selecting tasks for, 150–155, 150*t*, 152*t*
selecting tasks for homework and,
    159–160
shame and, 296
theoretical influences of DBT and, 8
traumatic invalidation and, 318, 319
treating males and, 335–336
treating racial and ethnic minorities
    and, 345–346
treating sexual and gender minorities
    and, 352–353, 355
types of *in vivo* tasks, 147–150
See also Exposure techniques;
    Homework assignments
Incompleteness (stage 4 of disorder), 19*t*,
    20. *See also* Stages of disorder
    model
Independence, detached, 138–139
Individual therapy, 91–93
Informal exposure, 57–59, 237–238. *See
    also* Exposure techniques
Information processing, 261–265
Informed consent, 95–96
Inhibited grieving, 300. *See also* Sadness
Inhibitory learning theory
  mechanism hypotheses on the case
      formulation and, 98
  theoretical influences of DBT and, 8
Institutional contexts, 23–24, 24*t*
Integrated DBT + DBT PE treatment
  determining appropriateness for, 21–28,
      22*f*, 24*t*
  final stage of treatment and, 359–363
  overview, 363
  pretreatment preparation for, 33–42,
      36*t*
  structuring treatment, 90–95
  See also DBT Prolonged Exposure
      (DBT PE) protocol; Dialectical
      behavior therapy (DBT)
Intellectual disability, 264–265
Intensity of emotions. *See* Emotion
    regulation; Emotional intensity;
    Emotions
Intermediate sessions. *See* Session
    structure
Internalized racism, 346–347
International Classification of Diseases
    (ICD-11), 22

Interpersonal effectiveness skills training,
    57, 58*t*. *See also* Skills training
Interpersonal functioning
  determining appropriateness for
      integrated DBT + DBT PE
      treatment and, 27
  joint and family sessions and, 166
Interpretation
  anger and, 290*t*
  disgust and, 297*t*
  fear and, 281*t*
  mechanism hypotheses on the case
      formulation and, 99, 99*f*
  sadness and, 302*t*
  shame and, 293*t*
  See also Beliefs
Intimacy, 194*t*
Intimate partner relationships
  intimate partner violence and, 325–328
  sexual assault and rape and, 320
  traumatic invalidation and, 23–24,
      24*t*, 316
  See also Relationships
Invalidating environments
  explaining to clients, 34
  finding validating environments, 320
  mechanism hypotheses on the case
      formulation and, 99*f*, 101
  pervasive emotion dysregulation and,
      24–25
  theoretical influences of DBT, 7
  See also Environmental factors;
      Traumatic invalidation
Invalidation. *See* Traumatic invalidation
Irreverent communication, 199. *See also*
    Communication
Isolation, 316, 319

Joint sessions
  case examples illustrating, 169–170
  guidelines for, 163–165
  information processing problems and,
      265
  ongoing joint sessions, 171
  orientation session, 166–170
  overview, 163, 171
  preparing for, 165–166
  psychotic disorders and, 271
  structuring treatment, 94–95
Joy, 221*t*
Judgment
  child sexual abuse and, 308, 309–311
  trauma processing and, 194*t*
  treating sexual and gender minorities
      and, 355
  validation and, 196–197
Justice
  child sexual abuse and, 311
  problems with changing problematic
      beliefs and, 266*t*
  treating racial and ethnic minorities
      and, 347
Justified emotions
  anger as, 288–292
  disgust as, 298, 299–300
  fear as, 281
  guilt as, 282, 286–287
  overview, 221, 221*t*